S0-BZZ-861

Ex-Library: Friends of
Lake County Public Library

# HEARING INSTRUMENT TECHNOLOGY
## for the Hearing Healthcare Professional

# HEARING INSTRUMENT TECHNOLOGY

## for the Hearing Healthcare Professional

## *Third Edition*

**Andi Vonlanthen**

Phonak AG
Stäfa, Switzerland


**Horst Arndt, Ph.D.**

Unitron Hearing Ltd.
Kitchener, ON, Canada

**THOMSON**

**DELMAR LEARNING**

Australia Canada Mexico Singapore Spain United Kingdom United States

LAKE COUNTY PUBLIC LIBRARY

3 3113 02495 0000

**THOMSON**

**DELMAR LEARNING**

**Hearing Instrument Technology: for the Hearing Healthcare Professional, Third Edition**
by Andi Vonlanthen and Horst Arndt, Ph.D.

**Vice President,
Health Care Business Unit:**
William Brottmiller

**Editorial Director:**
Matthew Kane

**Acquisitions Editor:**
Kalen Conerly

**Product Manager:**
Molly Belmont

**Marketing Director:**
Jennifer McAvey

**Marketing Coordinator:**
Christopher Manion

**Production Editor:**
Anne Sherman

COPYRIGHT © 2007 by Thomson Delmar Learning, a part of The Thomson Corporation. Thomson, the Star logo, and Delmar Learning are trademarks used herein under license.

Printed in the United States of America

2 3 4 5 6 7 XXX 08 07 06

For more information, contact Thomson Delmar Learning,
5 Maxwell Drive, Clifton Park, NY 12065-2919

Or you can visit our Internet site at
http://www.delmarlearning.com

ALL RIGHTS RESERVED. No part of this work covered by the copyright hereon may be reproduced or used in any form or by any means—graphic, electronic, or mechanical, including photocopying, recording, taping, Web distribution or information storage and retrieval systems—without the written permission of the publisher.

For permission to use material from this text or product, contact us by

Tel (800) 730-2214
Fax (800) 730-2215
www.thomsonrights.com

Library of Congress Cataloging-in-Publication Data
Vonlanthen, A. (Andi), 1961–
  Hearing instrument technology for the hearing healthcare professional
  / Andi Vonlanthen, Horst Arndt.
— 3rd ed.
    p. ; cm.
  Includes bibliographical references and index.
    ISBN 1-4180-1491-5
    1. Hearing aids. 2. Cochlear implants. I. Arndt, Horst, 1940– .
II. Title.
    [DNLM: 1. Hearing Aids. 2. Cochlear Implants. WV 274 V947h 2007]
RF300.V66 2007
617.8'9—dc22

2006005624

## Notice to the Reader

Publisher does not warrant or guarantee any of the products described herein or perform any independent analysis in connection with any of the product information contained herein. Publisher does not assume, and expressly disclaims, any obligation to obtain and include information other than that provided to it by the manufacturer.

The reader is expressly warned to consider and adopt all safety precautions that might be indicated by the activities described herein and to avoid all potential hazards. By following the instructions contained herein, the reader willingly assumes all risks in connection with such instructions.

The publisher makes no representations or warranties of any kind, including but not limited to, the warranties of fitness for particular purpose or merchantability, nor are any such representations implied with respect to the material set forth herein, and the publisher takes no responsibility with respect to such material. The publisher shall not be liable for any special, consequential, or exemplary damages resulting, in whole or part, from the reader's use of, or reliance upon, this material.

# Contents

## 3 DIGITALLY PROGRAMMABLE HEARING INSTRUMENTS 53

# Preface to the Third Edition

This book was written primarily for educational purposes as part of a course of studies for hearing health care professionals. The book also serves as a good introduction to the hearing instrument designer.

The second edition was published in 2000, but hearing instrument technology has changed and advanced very rapidly since that time. In particular, the very rapid increase in the application of digital technology during the last five years, to the point where the operation of hearing instruments is almost totally dependent on digital signal processing, is the main reason for introducing this third edition. It provides new information about digital hardware and digital processes in hearing instruments. Since software and data transmission are fundamental to the operation of all signal processors, these topics are discussed in some detail in several new chapters.

## ORGANIZATION

The authors have attempted to introduce these new concepts in an easy-to-understand way by providing technical details only where necessary in order to illustrate a particular concept, process, or operation. Formulas and mathematical calculations are therefore kept to a minimum. Since digital data and data transfer are so important to the operation of a digital processor, some effort is made to explain the binary numbering system. Some very basic concepts in binary mathematics and data formats are presented.

Several chapters of the second edition have been merged together while a number of chapters are new to the third edition. For example, much of the content about hearing instrument types that appeared in Chapter 2 of the second edition has been merged with the material of Chapter 1 to produce a new Chapter 1 called "Historical Overview." Chapter 2 in the third edition deals with hearing instrument components and covers the material of the chapter on hearing instrument transducers as well as new material that has emerged since the publication of the second edition. New material has been added to almost every chapter, with the exception of Chapter 4, "Hearing Instrument Functions" in the second edition and "Signal Processing Strategies" in the third edition.

# NEW TO THIS EDITION

It is generally true that almost every chapter of the second edition has been enhanced with content pertaining to the transition from analog to digital technology. The chapter on the digital hearing instruments is expanded to include description of several signal processing algorithms for noise reduction, directional processing, and feedback cancellation. The chapter on hearing instrument measurements and standards is updated to include the most recent revisions of the applicable product standards, as well as discussions of new standards that deal with the measurement of cell phone emissions and hearing instrument immunity to cell phone interference. A summary of applicable standards is also added to this chapter.

Four entirely new chapters are added in the third edition. A chapter on digital mechanics describes the influence of computer technology and the application stereolithography and laser sintering on the hearing instrument shell-making process. The interference between hearing instrument and cell phones is acknowledged as a significant issue for the hearing-impaired cell phone user in a chapter of its own. Data concepts and data transmission techniques are fundamental elements of all digital signal processors and these are described in a new chapter in the third edition.

The importance of implanted devices is growing and a chapter is added to the book to describe various classes of implanted devices. However, a thorough treatment of this topic is well beyond the principal scope of this book and the reader is reminded that this chapter is only a brief overview of the topic.

The reader is reminded that the digital technology used in hearing instruments is similar to the digital technology used in products such as MP3 players and digital cameras in which software enhancements and adding memory capacity lead to regular performance improvements. It is to be expected that new and improved hearing instrument models will be introduced at a much more rapid pace than in the past.

Finally, the authors wished to improve on the educational nature of this book by adding a number of review questions at the end of each chapter and a set of answers at the end of the book.

# ACKNOWLEDGMENTS

Many people made technical contributions and provided guidance to all three editions of this book. We wish to thank Sonja Krienbühl, Andrea Gnädinger, Allison Cygan, Catherine Jennings Melia, Laura Voll, Herbie Bächler, Michael Boretzki, Helmut Ermann, Res Gerber, Volker Kühnel, Chas Kuratko, Stefan Launer and Tobias Zürcher for contributions to the first and second editions. The third edition benefited immensely from contributions from Henry Luo on the topic of digital technology and from Hans Hessel on the topic digital mechanics. Finally we wish to thank Michael Jones for his tireless efforts and support throughout the production of the second and the third editions.

Andi Vonlanthen
Horst Arndt

# CHAPTER 1

# Historical Overview

## INTRODUCTION

Hearing instruments are sound amplifiers. Their function is to amplify sound to a level such that a hearing-impaired person can both detect and, most importantly, make effective use of the acoustic signal (Veit, 1978).

Amplification is certainly the primary function of hearing instruments, but different degrees and etiologies of hearing impairment and associated problems of frequency and temporal discrimination place varying demands on hearing instrument design. Despite enormous progress in hearing instrument technology during the last few years, hearing instruments still only partially compensate for hearing loss and do not correct it completely. The current state of hearing instrument technology will be comprehensively described in this book.

## EVOLUTION OF AMPLIFICATION

Advances in hearing instrument technology can be divided into five somewhat overlapping phases. The intervals shown in Figure 1–1 give a general indication of the duration of each phase.

The first phase was an acoustic (mechanical) phase in which acoustic amplification was achieved by means of acoustic resonances in different types of resonators and ear trumpets. The first hearing instrument was a hand cupped behind the ear. (Unfortunately, this is still the most common means of assisting hearing during the early stages of hearing loss.) Figure 1–2 illustrates how a hand cupped behind the ear changes the acoustics of the signal. There is a resonance with an amplitude of approximately 10 dB between 1 and 2 kHz. At higher frequencies, there is actually an attenuation of the signal. (Note: The diagram represents an insertion gain measurement. The reader is referred to the section in Chapter 9 on in situ measurements and insertion gain.)

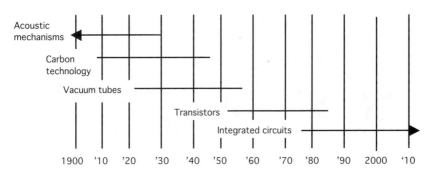

**Figure 1–1.** The five phases of hearing instrument technology development. *(Courtesy of Phonak AG.)*

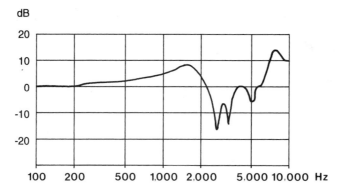

**Figure 1–2.** The insertion gain produced by a hand behind the ear. *(Courtesy of Phonak AG.)*

At the beginning of the nineteenth century, various kinds and shapes of ear trumpets (Figure 1–3) were produced. A significant amount of amplification could be achieved using an ear trumpet (Figure 1–4).

It was clear that a stereophonic arrangement (Figure 1–5) would be optimal.

The second phase in the development of hearing instrument technology took place in the early part of the twentieth century. In this phase, some elements of telephone technology were used in developing hearing instruments. For example, the use of a carbon microphone provided electrical amplification in addition to the amplification provided by mechanical and acoustical resonances inherent in the construction of electroacoustic transducers. The problems with carbon hearing instruments were twofold: first, the large distortion produced through the resonances of the microphone and the receiver and, second, excessive noise from the microphone.

Figure 1–6 shows the gain response of a carbon hearing instrument from 1922 and Figure 1–7 shows its components. The large round component is the carbon microphone while the smaller round component is the ear piece. The small rectangular component contains a volume control and the large rectangular can houses the batteries.

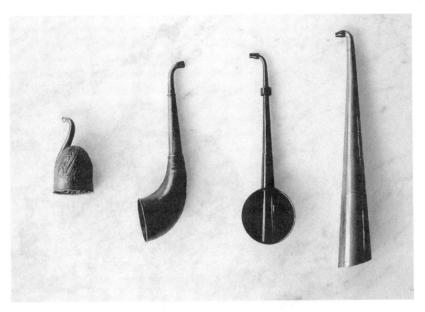

**Figure 1–3.** Various types of ear trumpets. *(Courtesy of Phonak AG.)*

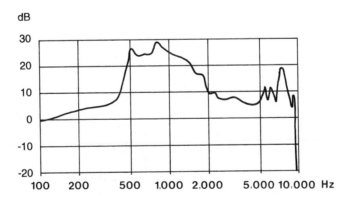

**Figure 1–4.** The insertion gain of an ear trumpet. *(Courtesy of Phonak AG.)*

In the third phase, vacuum tubes were utilized in the construction of hearing instruments (Figures 1–8 and 1–9). This made a much greater acoustical amplification possible than with carbon hearing instruments.

The invention of the transistor in the late 1940s led hearing instrument technology into the fourth phase. Vacuum tubes were replaced by much smaller transistors (Figure 1–9). This made it possible to produce hearing instruments that could be worn on the head.

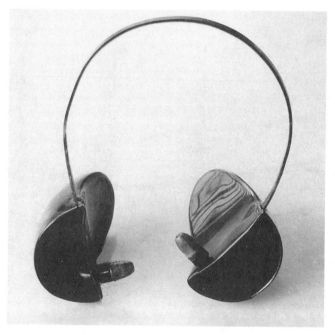

**Figure 1–5.** Ear trumpets for a stereophonic fitting (1930). *(Courtesy of Phonak AG.)*

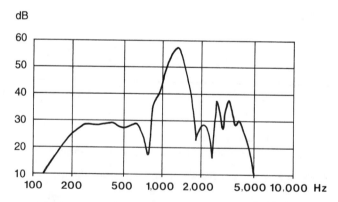

**Figure 1–6.** The frequency response of a carbon hearing instrument. *(Courtesy of Phonak AG.)*

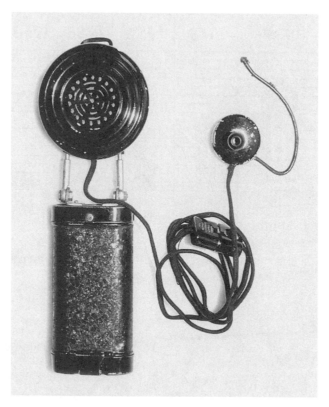

**Figure 1–7.** A carbon hearing instrument. *(Courtesy of Phonak AG.)*

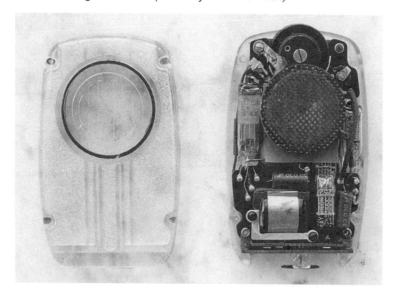

**Figure 1–8.** A body hearing instrument with three vacuum tubes (1939). *(Courtesy of Phonak AG.)*

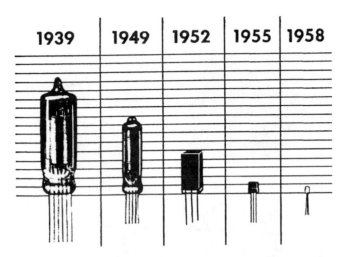

**Figure 1–9.** The size reduction from vacuum tubes to the transistor (approximate scale: 1:1) (Berger, 1984).

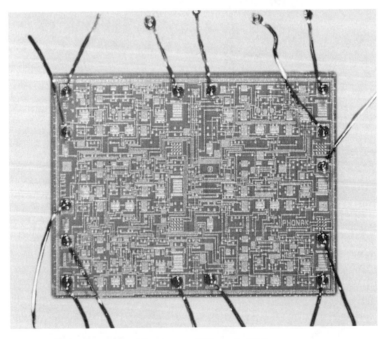

**Figure 1–10.** An integrated circuit (IC). *(Courtesy of Phonak AG.)*

Today, the fifth phase of technical development is well advanced and the integrated circuit (IC), often containing 100,000 or more transistors (see Figure 1–10), is the fundamental building block for electronic amplifiers. During the mid-1990s, digital technology replaced many of the analog functions in the hearing instrument amplifier. This important technical advance enabled hearing instruments to go beyond traditional frequency-dependent amplification. Many advanced features like noise reduction, feedback cancellation, directional processing, and adaptation to varying sound environments are made possible with digital technology. The application of digital signal processing is leading to intelligent, adaptive hearing instrument performance. Today, three out of every four hearing instruments sold are fully digital hearing instruments. Totally analog instruments could eventually disappear.

# HEARING INSTRUMENT TYPES

Various types of trumpets and horns, carbon and vacuum technologies allowed primarily tabletop and body instruments to be produced. The advent of the transistor, however, stimulated rapid progress in device miniaturization. In a relatively short time, body aids became smaller, only to be eventually displaced by behind-the-ear (BTE) instruments and eyeglass devices. The popular in-the-ear (ITE) instruments were developed during the late 1970s. Even this latter category has experienced advances in miniaturization from the original full concha instruments to in-the-canal (ITC) and eventually completely-in-the-canal (CIC) instruments. These developments evolved in parallel with semi-implanted and fully implanted devices.

## BODY HEARING INSTRUMENTS

The body hearing instrument is the oldest form of construction for an electronic hearing instrument. The microphone and the amplifier circuit, together with all the user and fitter controls, are in a housing which is normally carried on the body or in a pocket. The receiver is inserted in the ear and connected to the main unit by a cord (see Figures 1–11 and 1–12).

Although the market share of the body unit is steadily becoming smaller, its use is, in certain cases, advantageous compared to other types of hearing instruments.

**Advantages of body units:**

▼ A body hearing instrument offers the greatest possible acoustic amplification due to the maximal distance between the receiver and the microphone.
▼ Body hearing instruments have large user controls which make them easy to operate for those with poor manual dexterity.
▼ Body hearing instruments offer the greatest maximum output sound pressure level due to the large receiver.
▼ Body hearing instruments are cost-effective as they use large batteries.
▼ In the case of bone conduction receivers, the body hearing instrument offers the advantage of there being no mechanical feedback.

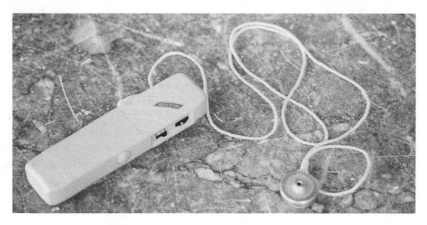

**Figure 1–11.** Body hearing instrument. *(Courtesy of Phonak AG.)*

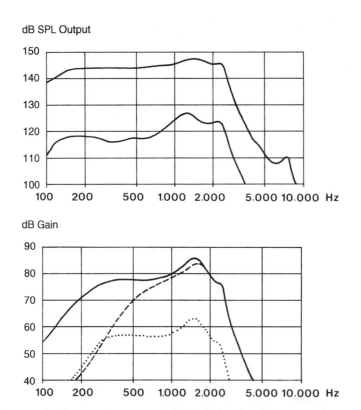

**Figure 1–12.** Output and gain response curves of a body hearing instrument (ear simulator measurement). The two curves in the top graph are the maximum and the minimum output levels the instrument can produce. Any output level between these extremes can be selected using a continuous output control trimmer. In the lower graph, the solid line represents the maximum gain (amplification) of the instrument and the dotted curve represents the minimum gain the instrument is designed to produce. Any value of gain between these extremes is selected with a continuous gain control trimmer. The dashed curve in the lower graph shows the effect of a low-tone control trimmer on the frequency range of the instrument. *(Courtesy of Phonak AG.)*

In addition to being cosmetically unappealing, the body hearing instrument has the following significant disadvantages:

- Its cumbersome size, as well as the one or two cords connecting the instrument to the receiver, make it awkward to wear.
- The microphone is not on the head, precluding directional and stereophonic hearing.
- Clothing rubbing against the microphone results in amplified noise.
- The button receiver does not produce a wideband frequency response (see Figure 1–12).

## EYEGLASS HEARING INSTRUMENTS

The first eyeglass hearing instruments were produced in the early 1950s.

In the eyeglass hearing instrument, all of the components are built into the temple bars of the eyeglass frame (see Figure 1–13).

The inlet for the microphone is located either at the hinge or behind the ear. The further forward the microphone inlet is located, the less is the danger of feedback. However, the directional hearing of the wearer suffers with a forward placement of the microphone.

The receivers are at the nonhinged ends of the temple bars and are joined to the earmold by plastic tubing.

**Advantages of eyeglass hearing instruments:**

- They can be configured with bone conduction receivers.
- Eyeglass hearing instruments are preferred for CROS applications since the wires can be mounted in the temple bars of the frame.
- In the case of an open ear fitting, it is possible to mount the microphone right at the front (near the hinge) so as to have as large a distance as possible between the microphone and the receiver, resulting in less feedback.

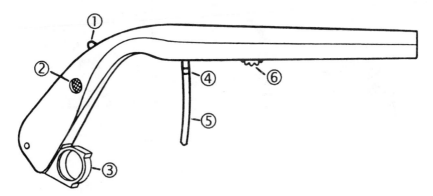

**Figure 1–13.** Eyeglass hearing instrument: (1) on/off switch, (2) microphone inlet, (3) battery compartment, (4) sound outlet, (5) sound tube to earmold, and (6) volume control wheel.

**Disadvantages of eyeglass hearing instruments:**

▼ Creating an interdependency between hearing and seeing is undesirable. With eyeglass hearing instruments the person cannot hear when he or she removes his or her eyeglasses. Likewise, the wearer must do without his eyeglasses if the hearing instrument needs repair. In the case of loss, the person loses both hearing instrument and optical correction.
▼ Conventional eyeglass hearing instruments are very heavy and seldom considered cosmetically acceptable.

Today, hearing instruments built into eyeglasses are rarely fitted. Instead a behind-the-ear instrument can be mounted on the temple bar of the glasses by means of an adaptor. This is often an attractive solution, especially in the case of an open ear fitting. The result is both elegant and inconspicuous since there is only a small length of tubing from the temple bar of the glasses to the ear canal and no earmold. Statistics show that a BTE instrument is preferred for open ear fittings. Figure 1–14 shows the ideal in elegance and discretion for a hearing instrument with a spectacles adaptor.

## BEHIND-THE-EAR (BTE) HEARING INSTRUMENTS

Today the behind-the-ear hearing instrument is still the most frequently used hearing instrument in Europe and is commonly used in North America. The receiver, microphone, and amplifier are built into a housing which is worn behind the ear. Sound is carried via soft plastic tubing to the ear canal.

Over the last thirty years, several different types of behind-the-ear hearing instruments have been developed. In the first generation of behind-the-ear hearing instruments, great care was taken to place the microphone and receiver as far from each other as possible. The reason

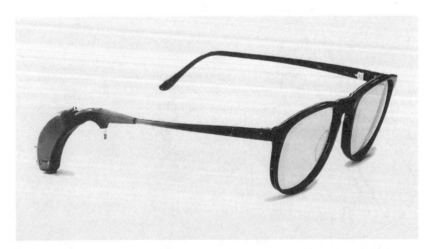

**Figure 1–14.** A behind-the-ear hearing instrument attached to eyeglasses using an eyeglass adaptor. *(Courtesy of Phonak AG.)*

for this was mechanical and acoustic feedback. Behind-the-ear hearing instruments were also constructed with external receivers (these were built into the earmold to obtain a better acoustic transmission), but the electrical connection between the receiver and amplifier failed to meet the mechanical demands. Figure 1–15 shows how the components are typically arranged in today's behind-the-ear hearing instrument.

The gain and output responses of a typical BTE hearing instrument are shown as a function of frequency in Figure 1–16. The top graph shows a series of curves that illustrate the effect of the tone control on the amplification in the low frequencies. The bottom graph shows a series of curves that illustrate how the maximum power output (MPO) is reduced by rotating the MPO control.

**Advantages of a behind-the-ear hearing instrument:**

▼ Open ear fittings are possible.
▼ Directional microphones can be utilized.

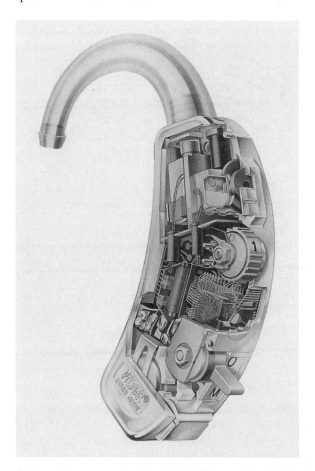

**Figure 1–15.** A view of internal components of a behind-the-ear hearing instrument. *(Courtesy of Phonak AG.)*

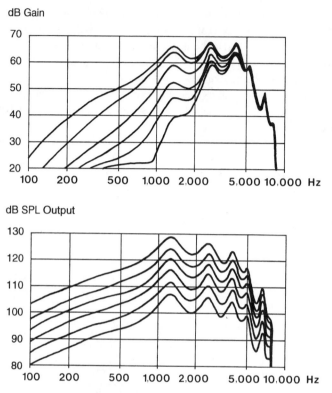

**Figure 1–16.** The gain and output frequency response curves of a behind-the-ear hearing instrument measured in a 2-cc coupler. The top graph shows the adjustment range of the tone control and the bottom graph shows the adjustment range of the output control. *(Courtesy of Phonak AG.)*

▼ A BTE represents a good compromise between the more powerful but large and unwieldy body hearing unit and the smaller but less powerful in-the-ear unit.
▼ BTE instruments are inconspicuous.
▼ The BTE hearing instrument has a housing which is roomy enough to accommodate new technological developments.
▼ Possibility of including acoustic transducers that produce a broadband frequency response (see Figure 1–16).

**Disadvantages of a behind-the-ear hearing instrument:**

▼ Resonance of the soft plastic tubing negatively affects natural sound quality.
▼ The microphone is not in the ear.

## IN-THE-EAR (ITE) HEARING INSTRUMENTS

In the case of in-the-ear hearing instruments, the components are all built into a housing which fits into the concha or ear canal.

Today, there are two types of in-the-ear units which differ in their construction:

1. The custom ITE hearing instrument
2. (Semi) modular instruments

In the case of the custom ITE (see Figure 1–17), a shell is first produced from an impression of the user's ear and the components (the microphone, receiver, amplifier, volume control, and potentiometers) are assembled onto a faceplate. The faceplate is an injection-molded plastic plate, slightly contoured for a pleasing appearance and with a tooled opening to accommodate the battery holder and molded-in battery contacts. The receiver is attached to the amplifier with sufficiently long wires so that it can be positioned as deep as possible into the canal portion of the shell. This faceplate assembly is then glued to the shell so that the microphone opening and the user controls are conveniently located in the concha. In programmable instruments, a programming socket replaces the potentiometers.

Modular ITE instruments (see Figure 1–18) are built into a standard housing which is then attached to a custom earmold. In a semimodular unit, the receiver is installed in the custom earmold.

A custom ITE is advantageous in that it makes optimal use of the entire space occupied by the shell. A custom ITE is the smallest form of hearing instrument.

The gain and output frequency responses of a typical ITE instrument are shown in Figure 1–19. The top graph shows the maximum gain and the ranges over which the low-tone and high-tone responses can be adjusted. The lower graph shows the maximum output as well as the minimum output when the MPO control is activated.

The advantage of a modular unit is that it is manufactured to more exact specifications, resulting in better-quality control (fewer rejects).

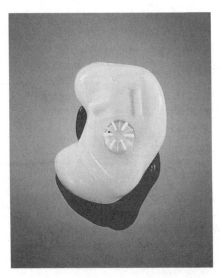

**Figure 1–17.** Custom in-the-ear hearing instrument. *(Courtesy of Phonak AG.)*

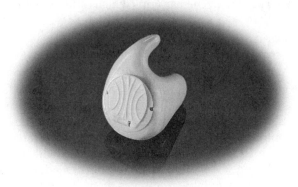

**Figure 1–18.** Modular in-the-ear hearing instrument. *(Courtesy of Phonak AG.)*

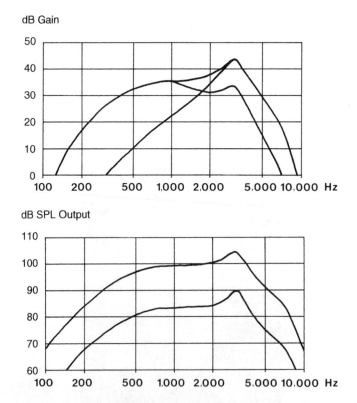

**Figure 1–19.** Gain and output frequency response graphs of an in-the-ear hearing instrument measured in a 2-cc coupler. The effects of low-tone and high-tone controls are shown in the top graph. The effect of a maximum output control is shown in the lower graph. *(Courtesy of Phonak AG.)*

Advantages and disadvantages of in-the-ear hearing instruments (custom-built or modular):

▼ Acoustically, ITE instruments are superior to other types. The microphone is situated within the ear, thereby taking advantage of the pinna's function. The receiver is located as near the tympanic membrane as possible, resulting in enhancement of high-frequency information due to the small cavity enclosed by the instrument (see Figure 1–19).
▼ ITE instruments are inconspicuous.
▼ ITE instruments are generally comfortable to wear.

▼ Acoustic feedback is more likely to be a problem, especially with the high levels of amplification required in the case of more severe hearing losses.
▼ The small size of ITE instruments sometimes necessitates compromises in construction at the cost of sound quality.
▼ ITE instruments are less durable than other types.
▼ ITE hearing instruments can frequently malfunction because of the intrusion of debris (earwax and moisture).
▼ The small batteries necessitate frequent battery changes.
▼ ITE instruments are frequently tight-fitting due to space limitations. This results in reduced wearer comfort due to occlusion.

## COMPLETELY-IN-THE-CANAL (CIC) HEARING INSTRUMENTS

In 1993 completely-in-the-canal (CIC) hearing aids (see Figure 1–20) were introduced to the market. In 1994 and 1995 they grew quickly in popularity and have leveled off to about 10–15% of hearing instrument sales in the European and North American markets. A properly fitted CIC fits deeply in the ear canal with the canal tip terminating in the bony part of the external

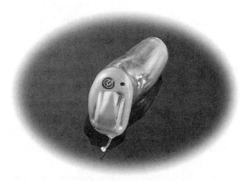

**Figure 1–20.** Completely-in-the-canal hearing instrument. Note the removal string at the bottom of the faceplate. *(Courtesy of Phonak AG.)*

auditory canal. It has a faceplate which is situated just inside the opening of the ear canal. Both the canal tip and faceplate placement are critical in achieving success with this model.

Without a doubt, the initial appeal of CICs is cosmetic. Often called the "contact lens for the ear," CICs have made hearing instruments a reality for many individuals with mild to moderate hearing loss who would not tolerate a more conspicuous hearing aid. Even with its cosmetic appeal, the CICs offer some unique benefits that should not be overlooked (Kochkin, 1994; Kochkin, 1995).

## Reduced Occlusion Effect

The occlusion effect is the perception of enhanced low frequencies of one's own voice when speaking. Hearing aid wearers who experience occlusion often complain of feeling like they "are talking in a barrel" or that their voice sounds "hollow."

Occlusion is caused by the enhancement of low-frequency vibrations of a person's voice when the ear canal is blocked. Inside the in-the-ear and behind-the-ear instruments a large vent is used to reduce the occlusion effect. Because of the size constraint of the CIC, a large vent is often not possible. However, it is sometimes possible to produce a vent by carving a trench on the outside of the shell. In this case, the shell must be sufficiently thick in the region of the vent so that an adequate amount of material can be carved away. If the ear canal is large, a CIC instrument may be able to accommodate a large enough vent to reduce the occlusion effect. However, this is often not the case. The best way to combat occlusion in a CIC fitting is to seal the canal tip deep into the bony portion of the canal.

A small vent is used to relieve pressure, but it has little effect on frequency response or occlusion effect.

## Gain, Output, and Frequency Response

CIC fittings require less gain and output from the hearing aid to achieve the same insertion gain benefit, especially in the high frequencies. There are two reasons for this: the deep placement of the microphone and the deep placement of the receiver.

The microphone location has long been known to affect the output and frequency response. As the microphone is placed deeper into the ear (such as in an ITC versus ITE), the hearing instrument produces more gain and more high-frequency response.

Placing the receiver deeper into the ear canal will also increase the gain and output in the ear. The residual volume of air between the canal end of the hearing instrument and the eardrum is smaller for deep canal fittings than with conventional fittings. Theoretically, halving the residual volume of air should result in a doubling of sound pressure for an increase of 6 dB SPL. However, the increase in gain will be greater for high frequencies than for low frequencies (Brüel & Kjaer, 1981). The higher compliance of the middle ear for low frequencies results in a larger effective volume in the ear canal for low frequencies, and a smaller effective volume for high frequencies. The end result is more output at high frequencies than at low frequencies (see Figure 1–21).

**Advantages and disadvantages of completely-in-the-canal (CIC) instruments:**

▼ Acoustically, CIC instruments come as close as possible to natural hearing because of their placement. The microphone is situated within the ear, thereby taking advantage

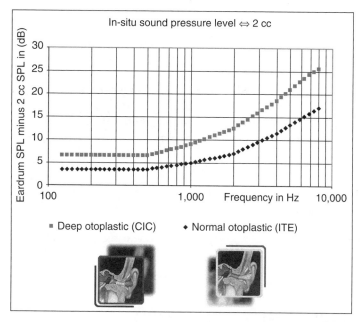

**Figure 1–21.** The influence of the effective residual volume between the hearing instrument and the eardrum on the in situ response. *(Courtesy of Phonak AG.)*

of the pinna's and the canal's functions. The receiver is located as near the eardrum as possible.

▼ Cosmetic appeal.
▼ Reduced occlusion effect.
▼ Directionality; the deep placement of the microphone can take advantage of the natural function of the outer ear.

▼ Acoustic feedback can be a problem, especially with the small distance between microphone and receiver. (See the section in Chapter 8 on feedback.)
▼ Handling of such small devices can be difficult for those with poor dexterity.
▼ Microphones and receivers are more susceptible to damage from ear wax.
▼ The small size of the CIC instrument does not generally allow control elements like volume controls and trimmers to be included. (This limitation has, to some degree, been overcome in digital instruments where multiple programs can be selected with a small push button switch. Different loudness and responses can be incorporated into these programs.)
▼ No space available to use directional microphones.
▼ The small microphone used in CICs has a higher equivalent input noise level.
▼ CICs use very small batteries (10A and 5A) which are difficult to handle and necessitate frequent battery changes.

## IMPLANTED HEARING INSTRUMENTS

A newly introduced style of hearing aid is the implanted device. These devices are surgically implanted into the skull.

**Hearing implants have some advantages over conventional hearing instruments:**

▼ Implants do not use sound to transmit the signal; therefore, there is no acoustic feedback.
▼ No earmold is needed, so there is no occlusion effect.

It is necessary to divide the group of implants into two types:

1. Implants that have no negative effect on the ear (no destruction of the ear).
2. Implants with an additional destruction of the ear.

Group 1 consists of systems like bone-anchored hearing aid (BAHA) and middle-ear implants; group 2 consists of cochlear implants (CI). These devices are discussed in greater detail in Chapter 15.

## HEARING INSTRUMENT STATISTICS

It is interesting to study the distribution of the types of hearing instruments used today.
The trend is towards increasingly smaller units, that is, to in-the-ear units.
There are two main reasons for the success of the in-the-ear units:

1. The rapid development of electronic and acoustic transducers over the last fifteen years has made it possible to produce higher fidelity ITE instruments than ever before.
2. An inconspicuous hearing instrument is often more appealing to the wearer.

Table 1–1 summarizes percentages of BTE, ITE (which include full-shell, half-shell, and canal instruments), and CIC hearing instruments sold in the two major markets in the world: North America and Europe. Approximately two million hearing instruments are sold annually in each of these markets.

The percentage of BTE instruments sold in North America has grown by about 5% over the last five years, possibly due to the high penetration of digital technology in this market and the availability of attractive and small BTE instruments. The situation has remained relatively constant in Europe for the last five years.

**Table 1–1.** Proportion of hearing instruments sold in North America and Europe.

| Region | BTE | ITE | CIC |
|--------|-----|-----|-----|
| NA | 26% | 59% | 15% |
| Europe | 65% | 31% | 4% |

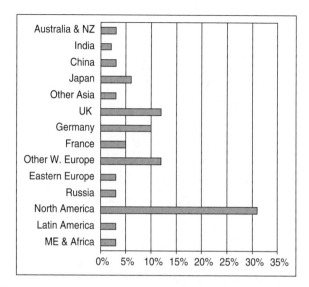

**Figure 1–22.** Annual hearing instrument consumption in selected countries expressed as a percentage of total annual world consumption. For example, about 12% of all hearing instruments produced in the world every year are distributed in the United Kingdom (U.K.), while 31% of the world's production is consumed annually in North America. *(Courtesy of Unitron Hearing Ltd.)*

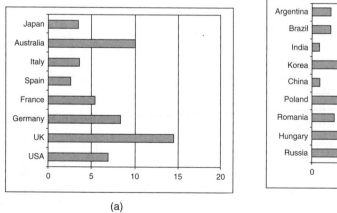

(a)

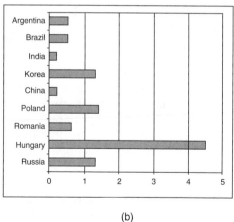

(b)

**Figure 1–23.** Hearing instrument ownership per 1,000 capita in selected countries in (a) developed markets and (b) emerging markets. For example, nearly fifteen people in every 1,000 people in the United Kingdom (U.K.) own hearing instruments while about seven people in every 1,000 own hearing instruments in the USA. On the other hand, just over one person per 1,000 owns a hearing instrument in Poland and Korea. *(Courtesy of Unitron Hearing Ltd.)*

In addition to the hearing instruments sold in North America and Europe, an additional three million hearing instruments are sold in the rest of the world. Figure 1–22 shows the percentages sold in those countries as well.

The per-capita consumption of hearing instruments varies widely in different countries as is shown in Figure 1–23 for a number of selected countries.

## SUMMARY

1. Hearing instrument performance and appearance have changed significantly as a result of technology improvements intended primarily for advancing communications and entertainment equipment.
2. Hearing instrument manufacturers have, as a rule, quickly adopted any new technology that could contribute to size reduction of hearing instruments and improve their ability to provide effective amplification for people with a hearing loss.
3. The invention of the transistor initiated a successful period of hearing instrument miniaturization which continues to this day by the ever-greater capabilities of integrated circuits.
4. The development of the in-the-ear type of device made hearing instruments less visible.
5. The most popular types of hearing instruments are ITE, CIC, and BTE.
6. Europe and North America are the two largest markets for hearing instruments.

## REVIEW QUESTIONS

1. What physical phenomena provided amplification in horns and ear trumpets?
2. What invention led to dramatic reduction in the size of hearing instruments?
3. Which hearing instrument type is most popular in North America?
4. What is the smallest type of hearing instrument?
5. Which statements are correct when comparing ITEs with BTEs?
   - **A.** ITEs have a greater tendency to feedback            A ☐
   - **B.** ITEs have reduced localization                       B ☐
   - **C.** BTEs have more resonances in the acoustic tubing     C ☐
   - **D.** BTEs require less effort to acoustically modify the shell/earmold   D ☐

# CHAPTER 2

# Hearing Instrument Components

## INTRODUCTION

While a hearing instrument contains many components, its electroacoustic transducers, the microphone and receiver, are extremely important components in any hearing instrument. Every hearing instrument contains a microphone to pick up the acoustic signal and to convert it into an electrical signal. The hearing instrument amplifier then modifies this signal according to the hearing loss requirements and feeds the amplified signal to the receiver. The receiver converts the amplified electrical signal again into a sound signal appropriate for the hearing-impaired user.

A wide variety of electroacoustic transducers is available and the different types may be characterized primarily in terms of:

- ▼ Technology
- ▼ Size
- ▼ Quality
- ▼ Price

The correct choice of electroacoustic transducers is important for an optimal acoustic fitting. The different types of transducers that are used in hearing instruments are discussed in the following paragraphs.

## BASIC COMPONENTS OF A HEARING INSTRUMENT

Hearing instruments are available in several different styles: behind-the-ear, in-the-ear, eyeglass, or body hearing instruments. All hearing instruments are intended to amplify sound and therefore the essential components used in their assembly are fundamentally the same. Hearing instrument style does, however, imply major differences in component packaging and appearance of the instrument.

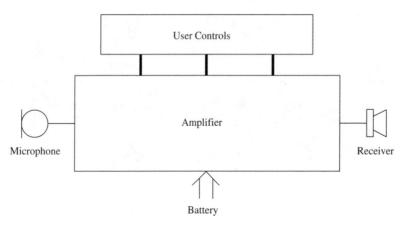

**Figure 2–1.** Block diagram of a basic hearing instrument. *(Courtesy of Phonak AG.)*

A hearing instrument consists of the following basic components, usually connected as shown in Figure 2–1.

| Component | Function |
|---|---|
| Microphone | Converts input acoustic signals into electrical signals. |
| Amplifier | Amplifies the electrical signal. |
| Battery | Supplies power to the hearing instrument. |
| User controls | Influences the output, amplification, and frequency response, etc., of the hearing instrument; can be adjusted by the user of the hearing instrument, or by the hearing health care professional. |
| Receiver | Converts the processed electrical signal back into an acoustic signal. |

The behind-the-ear (BTE) hearing instrument is examined in detail here in order to facilitate a better understanding of its construction. Figure 2–2 illustrates several fundamental concepts in BTE hearing instrument technology and assembly. Hearing instrument transducers, control elements, telecoils, and amplifiers are discussed in this chapter. However, detailed discussion of acoustic modifications and accessories other than the telecoil occurs in Chapters 6 and 7.

BTE hearing instrument shell design strives to achieve the smallest possible size and the best cosmetic appearance within the constraints imposed by the components intended to be used in the instrument. The receiver, microphone, and battery are generally the most important components in determining the size of BTE housings. Large receivers can deliver higher acoustic outputs than smaller receivers, but they also need a larger battery to produce high maximum output levels and a useful battery life. Power instruments intended for use with severe to profound hearing losses are therefore usually larger than instruments in-

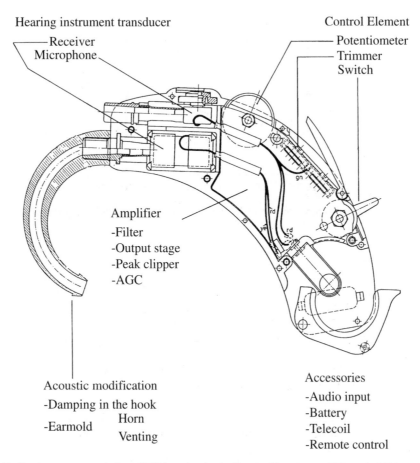

Hearing instrument transducer
—Receiver
Microphone

Control Element
— Potentiometer
— Trimmer
Switch

Amplifier
-Filter
-Output stage
-Peak clipper
-AGC

Acoustic modification
-Damping in the hook
Horn
-Earmold
Venting

Accessories
-Audio input
-Battery
-Telecoil
-Remote control

**Figure 2–2.** Basic components in a BTE hearing instrument. *(Courtesy of Phonak AG.)*

tended for mild to moderate hearing losses. Besides the large receiver and battery, power instruments also need space to accommodate sufficient isolation between the microphone and receiver to avoid feedback. This also takes up space and needs to be provided for in the shell design. Microphones play a less critical role. A microphone of a particular size will perform well in all types of hearing instruments. However, the shell design needs to accommodate requirements for directional properties provided with either a single microphone cartridge with two sound inlets or two omnidirectional microphones and additional signal processing in the amplifier. These options need to be considered in the shell design and sufficient space needs to be provided for these features. Regardless of the requirements, particularly good results can be achieved with a careful choice of transducers and careful component placement.

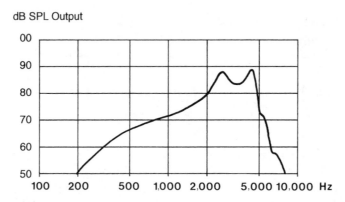

**Figure 2–3.** Typical frequency response of a Swisscom Tritel telephone (1990). *(Courtesy of Phonak AG.)*

## THE MICROPHONE

### *A Historical Perspective*

Following World War II, a number of research projects were undertaken with the purpose of determining a communications frequency band that would allow optimal understanding of speech under various conditions. These studies showed that, under favorable conditions, a frequency band of 300 Hz to 3,000 Hz was most suitable for people with normal hearing.

Under worse conditions where loudness, noise, and distortion interfered with listening tasks, this band (300 Hz to 3,000 Hz) still gave the best speech understanding (i.e., better than a narrower or broader frequency band). This research had a strong influence on the entire field of telecommunications. Today, telephones still have a frequency band of around 400 Hz to 5,000 Hz (see Figure 2–3).

The optimal frequency band for speech understanding with a hearing instrument has also been the focus of much post–World War II research. In these studies, speech comprehensibility tests with and without background noise were given to hearing-impaired subjects. Results indicated that a frequency band that was either flat or increasing at 6 dB/octave between 300 Hz and 4,000 Hz (the frequency band is sharply cut above and below this range) was best for speech understanding for nearly all the hearing-impaired subjects.

At that time, the electroacoustic transducer that provided approximately this frequency pass band was the electromagnetic microphone (Figure 2–4).

In the mid-1960s it became clear that the electromagnetic microphone could not meet the increasingly greater demands for better hearing instrument performance. Most importantly, a broader and flatter frequency response was desired (so that one could fully enjoy the music of the Beatles). More and more people with slight hearing impairments were being diagnosed and fitted with hearing instruments. For them, enjoyment of music and natural sounds as well as recognition of voices were important.

In the late 1960s, technical developments produced a microphone with a broader and flatter frequency response for application in hearing instruments. This was the piezoelectric ceramic microphone.

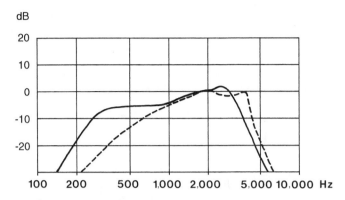

**Figure 2–4.** Comparison of the frequency responses of an electromagnetic microphone (dashed curve) and the ideal frequency response for speech understanding (solid curve). Both curves are normalized to 0 dB at 2,000 Hz. *(Courtesy of Phonak AG.)*

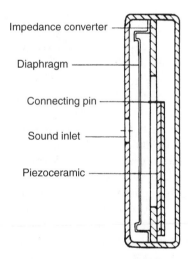

**Figure 2–5.** Construction of a ceramic microphone. *(Courtesy of Knowles Electronics.)*

Figure 2–5 shows the construction of a ceramic microphone. It contains a flexible element made out of two strips of a piezoceramic bonded together. Sound pressure variations move the diaphragm. These movements are then mechanically transmitted to the piezoceramic via the connecting pin. When this piezoceramic moves in phase with the sound, an alternating voltage is produced (again in phase with the sound). This element is extremely sensitive to electrostatic interference because of its exceptionally high impedance. Therefore, an electrical impedance converter (amplifier) is necessary and is positioned directly adjacent to the element in the microphone housing. This element converts the electrical impedance so that there is a relatively low-resistance output at the external microphone terminals.

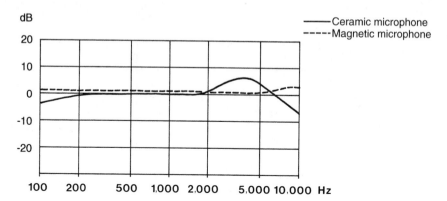

**Figure 2–6.** Frequency responses of a ceramic and a magnetic microphone normalized at 1,000 Hz (Killion & Carlson, 1969). *(Courtesy of Audio Engineering Society.)*

The power required for the microphone is drawn from the hearing instrument into which the microphone is built. Such an impedance converter contains a field effect transistor. Figure 2–6 shows the frequency responses of a ceramic and a magnetic microphone.

The ceramic microphone has, in fact, a broader frequency response than the magnetic microphone (of the same size). Yet, despite its superiority to the magnetic microphone, the ceramic microphone has become obsolete in hearing instrument production due to a very basic shortcoming.

The main problem with the ceramic microphone was its high sensitivity to vibrations at low frequencies (e.g., mechanical feedback, friction noise). This led the microphone manufacturers to look for other, low vibration systems and, at the beginning of the 1970s, it became possible to produce an even better microphone suitable for use in hearing instruments.

This was the electret condenser microphone. The electret condenser microphone works according to the electrostatic transducer principle. Condenser microphones consist of a thin metal diaphragm and a rigid metal backplate making up the electrodes of an air dielectric capacitor. A dc voltage (polarization voltage) is applied across the two electrodes. The effect of sound pressure on the diaphragm is a variation of capacitance in accordance with the sound pressure variations. This variation in capacitance is, in turn, transformed into voltage variations. An ac voltage appears over a high ohmic resistor (being part of the polarization circuit) and represents an analog of the sound picked up.

The dc voltage required for normal condenser microphones is not needed for electret microphones, which possess a permanent electrical field and are comparable to permanent magnets. The charged electret film provides the necessary polarization voltage.

The electret element is manufactured from high-insulation plastics such as Teflon™, in which a permanent electrostatic charge has been set up through special processes.

The electret condenser microphone has as high a resistance as the ceramic microphone. Therefore, the electret microphone also requires an impedance converter (field effect transistor; see Figure 2–7), which is built into the microphone capsule. It is because of this impedance converter that a current supply is required for the electret condenser microphone.

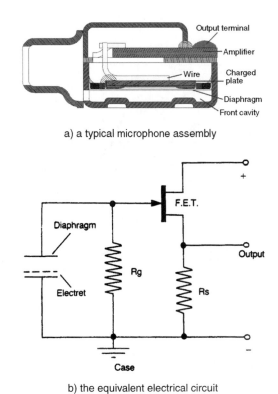

a) a typical microphone assembly

b) the equivalent electrical circuit

**Figure 2–7.** a) Cross-sectional view of an electret condenser microphone and b) equivalent electrical circuit of an electret microphone with a preamplifier (from Knowles Electronics Datasheet: Miniature Microphones and Miniature Receivers). *(Courtesy of Knowles Electronics.)*

As noted above, the piezoceramic microphone was extremely sensitive to mechanical vibrations. It is generally true that the heavier the diaphragm, the more sensitive it is to vibrations. As the thin, metal film diaphragm is extremely light in the case of an electret condenser microphone, it is much less sensitive to vibrations than ceramic and electromagnetic microphones (see Figure 2–8).

Figure 2–9 shows the frequency response of an electret condenser microphone. It is also possible to maintain an extended linear frequency response (100 Hz to 15 kHz). While this is advantageous in producing a high-frequency fidelity hearing instrument, such a broad response can lead to excessive sensitivity to and interference from ultrasonic sources, unless appropriate filtering is provided in the amplifier. A microphone with a resonance of 4 kHz is frequently used in hearing instrument applications.

This resonance can be reduced in frequency to around 2.5 to 3 kHz by using a sound tube to the microphone (extension of the microphone in the hearing instrument housing). The intent of such an acoustic modification is to compensate for the loss in acoustical amplification due to the natural resonance of the ear canal when it is occluded with closed earmolds.

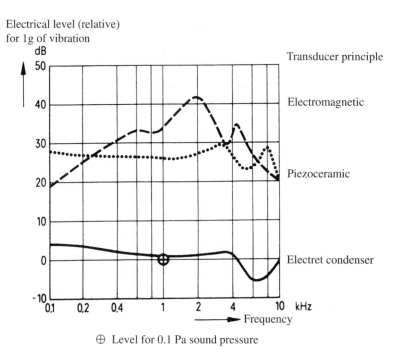

**Figure 2–8.** Vibration sensitivity of different microphones (Killion & Carlson, 1973). *(Courtesy of Audio Engineering Society.)*

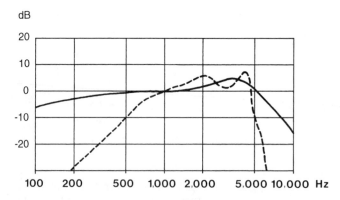

**Figure 2–9.** Frequency responses of electret condenser microphones: The dashed curve is a broadband response and the solid curve is a typical response for hearing instrument applications. *(Courtesy of Phonak AG.)*

## The Omnidirectional Microphone (Pressure Sensor)

The omnidirectional microphone is a pressure sensor because its diaphram moves in response to sound pressure level fluctuations at the diaphram. When the pressure sensor is located in a sound field, the diaphragm movement depends only on sound pressure variations regardless

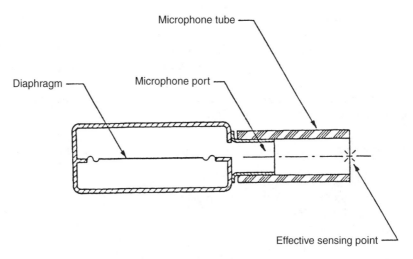

**Figure 2–10.** Cross-sectional view of an omnidirectional microphone. *(Courtesy of Knowles Electronics.)*

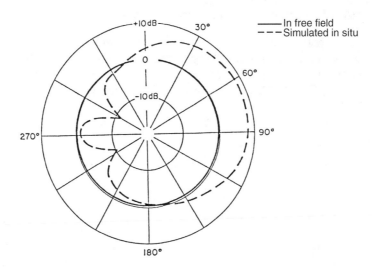

**Figure 2–11.** Polar response of an omnidirectional microphone in free field and simulated in situ (KEMAR) (from Knowles Electronics Technical Bulletin, TB21). *(Courtesy of Knowles Electronics.)*

of which direction the sound is coming from. A pressure sensor is, in fact, a microphone with a spherical pickup characteristic.

Figure 2–10 shows a longitudinal section of an omnidirectional microphone. The omnidirectional microphone has one sound inlet and the sound is directed at one side of the diaphragm.

A polar plot is often used to show the directional characteristic of a microphone. Such a plot is produced by moving the sound source in a circle around the microphone, and plotting the microphone's output relative to that at 0° incidence. Figure 2–11 shows the polar response for an omnidirectional microphone measured in the horizontal plane around the microphone. The solid circular line represents the directional characteristic in a free field. Since there are no reflections in a free field environment, the omnidirectional microphone has a circular characteristic, which means that sound emanating from all directions is picked up with equal strength.

The dashed curve in Figure 2–11 represents the KEMAR (Knowles Electronics Manikin for Acoustic Research) response for the omnidirectional microphone and clearly demonstrates the influence of the head (head shadow, reflections).

### Advantages and disadvantages of the omnidirectional microphone:

▾ Small
▾ Full sonority, good low-frequency transmission
▾ Good vibrational damping
▾ Low noise

▾ Spherical characteristic is problematic in background noise

## *The Directional Microphone (Pressure Gradient Sensor)*

Directional microphones have two sound ports that direct sound to the front side and also to the rear side of the diaphragm. By careful dimensioning of the sound paths, different directional characteristics can be produced. The directional microphone reacts better to sound emanating from a certain direction. Figure 2–12 shows a section of a directional microphone. The two sound inlets lead to a small cavity that is divided into two chambers by the diaphragm. This diaphragm reacts only to the difference in air pressure between the two sides and converts this difference

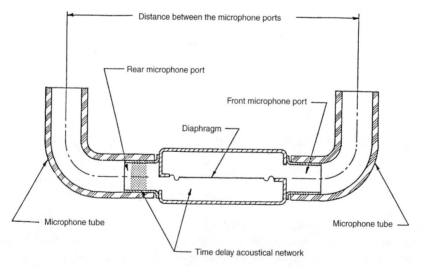

**Figure 2–12.** Cross-sectional view of a directional microphone (from Knowles Electronics Technical Bulletin, TB21). *(Courtesy of Knowles Electronics.)*

into an electrical output signal. When the air pressure in both chambers is of equal level and phase, there is no net effect of pressure on the diaphragm and thus, no electrical output signal.

To prevent sound originating behind the microphone from reaching the diaphragm first, a time delay element (fine filter, mesh) is built into the rear sound inlet. This time delay is designed to equal the time required for the sound wave to pass from the rear sound inlet opening to the front sound inlet opening. In this way the sound originating from the rear produces a pressure fluctuation at both sides of the diaphragm simultaneously. Thus, the pressure on both sides of the diaphragm will be equal and there will be no movement of the diaphragm (i.e., no electrical signal).

A directional microphone tested in free field typically shows a cardioid polar pattern, as illustrated by the solid curve in Figure 2–13. However, the directional characteristic of the microphone is quite different when the head shadow effect is taken into account (dashed curve).

The effective polar sensitivity of the directional microphone depends on how it is built into the hearing instrument. This is influenced by a number of factors, including arrangement of the microphone inlets and distance from one another, the dimensions of the delay tube and the time delay element, and the shape of the hearing instrument housing. The directional characteristics are primarily influenced by the properties of the acoustic delay filter and the distance from the front to the rear port.

The calculation of the spatial directivity pattern for a microphone is extremely complex. To be completely accurate, the directivity of a microphone is a three-dimensional quantity normally defined in a polar coordinate system where $\theta$ degrees defines azimuth and $\Phi$ is the angle of elevation. For simplicity, it is common to describe the directional response of a hearing instrument in a two-dimensional plane at zero elevation ($\Phi = 0°$). In that case the directional sensitivity is described by Eq. (1) shown below:

$$D(\theta, \omega) = (\beta + \cos\theta) \cdot k \cdot \Delta d \qquad \text{Eq. (1)}$$

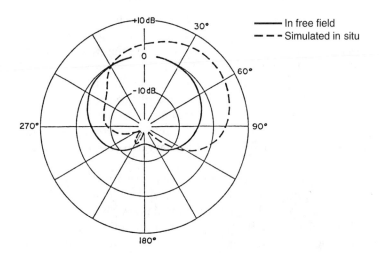

**Figure 2–13.** Polar response of a directional microphone in free field and simulated in situ (KEMAR) (from Knowles Electronics Technical Bulletin, TB21). *(Courtesy of Knowles Electronics.)*

$$\text{where } \beta = \frac{c \cdot \tau}{\Delta d}$$

▼ $\beta$ is the ratio of the internal to the external delay
▼ $c$ is the speed of sound in air, 344 m/s
▼ $\tau$ is the acoustic time delay of the filter
▼ $\Delta d$ is the distance from the front to the rear port
▼ $\omega$ is the frequency of the signal (several of the parameters in Eq. [1] are frequency dependent)
▼ $k$ is a constant

It was noted above that directionality is a three-dimensional quantity and its measurement is complicated and time-consuming. In comparison to a three-dimensional directivity measurement, the measurement of the two-dimensional spatial response (at 0° elevation) given in Eq. (1) is relatively simple and involves measuring microphone sensitivity at a number of angles in a plane at a number of different frequencies. The measurement is performed in a horizontal plane by rotating the sound source in this plane in 15° increments around a circle with the microphone located at its center. The output of the microphone in response to a constant input is measured at each point. Figure 2–13 shows examples of directivity patterns for a directional microphone alone and the directional microphone placed at ear level on KEMAR. The microphone shown in Figure 2–13 has been designed to produce a cardioid response in free field. Both measurements are performed in a reflection-free environment, such as an anechoic chamber. An azimuth of 0° is the position directly in front of the test microphone, while 180° azimuth indicates a position directly behind the microphone.

## Free Field Characteristics of Different Types of Microphones

The polar sensitivity pattern of a microphone depends on the ratio of the internal to external time delay, $\beta$. Different idealized free field characteristics are shown in Figure 2–14. Specific directivity properties can therefore be achieved by selecting the two design variables $\tau$ and $\Delta d$.

A single number, the directivity index (DI), is used to express the improvement in signal to noise ratio provided by a particular directional response. This quantity is very useful for comparison purposes. Additional information on the derivation of $DI$ is given in Chapter 9.

The distance from the front to the rear port determines the external delay. Therefore, it is possible for the same directional microphone to exhibit different polar pickup characteristics. Figure 2–15 shows the difference in directionality that can result from changes in the port spacing parameter.

It will be shown in Chapter 9 (measurement of hearing instruments with directional microphones), that the directional microphone has a frequency response with greater amplitude in the high frequencies than does the omnidirectional microphone.

The distance from the front to the rear port strongly influences this effect. Changing the microphone port spacing will change the response curve and therefore the signal to noise ratio of the microphone. The smaller the distance, the higher the frequency roll-off and therefore the lower the sensitivity.

| Characteristic | Omnidirectional | Bidirectional | Cardioid | Hypercardioid | Super Cardioid |
|---|---|---|---|---|---|
| Polar Response Pattern | 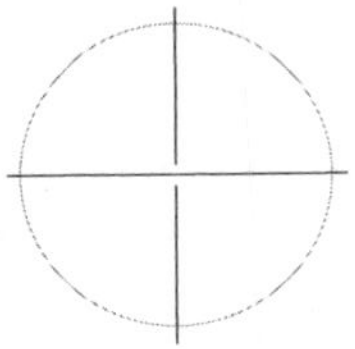 | 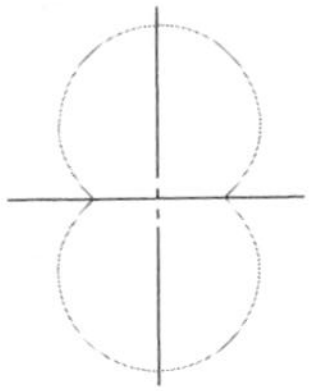 | 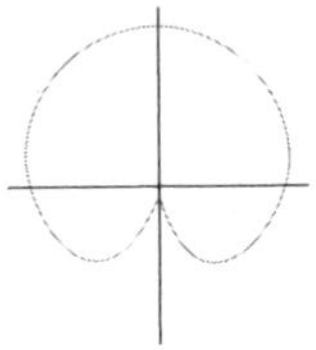 | 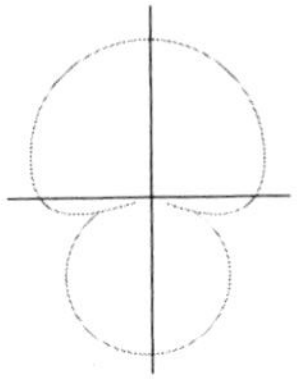 | 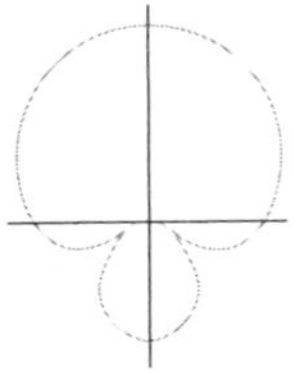 |
| D (θ) | 1 | COS θ | ½ (1 + COS θ) | ¼ (1 + 3 COS θ) | $\frac{1}{(1+\sqrt{3})}$ (1+ √3 COS θ) |
| β | ∞ | 0 | 1 | 0.333 | 0.577 |
| Front to Back Response Ratio | 0 dB | 0 dB | ∞ | 6.0 dB | 11.4 dB |
| Directivity Index | 0 dB | 4.8 dB | 4.8 dB | 6.0 dB | 5.7 dB |

**Figure 2–14.** Free field directional characteristics of different types of microphones (from Knowles Electronics Technical Bulletin, TB21). *(Courtesy of Knowles Electronics.)*

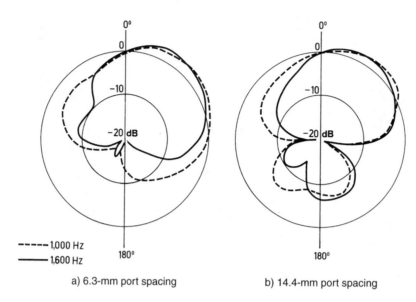

a) 6.3-mm port spacing          b) 14.4-mm port spacing

**Figure 2–15.** Polar plots for a directional microphone with a 24.9-μs delay in the rear port and a port spacing of a) 6.3 mm and b) 14.4 mm on a BTE hearing instrument on KEMAR (Madaffari, 1983). *(Courtesy of Knowles Electronics.)*

Figure 2–16 shows the difference in sensitivity of a directional microphone. The reduction in sensitivity gives the same amount of reduction in signal to noise, because of amplifying the microphone loss with the amplifier.

## Making an Omnidirectional Microphone Out of a Directional Microphone

If the rear inlet in a directional microphone is closed, the microphone exhibits the spherical characteristic and flat frequency response shown in Figure 2–17.

In certain hearing instruments, the hearing health care professional can close the rear microphone inlet by means of a mechanical slide, thereby effectively making it a hearing instrument without a directional microphone. (*Tip:* When possible, fit the hearing instrument with the directional microphone operative [slide open]; the hearing-impaired wearer will likely be pleased with the effect.)

Closing of the rear inlet is only possible, however, for hearing instruments with an amplification of less than 60 dB (2-cc coupler); at greater levels of amplification internal feedback (whistling) results from closing the rear inlet.

Another reason that few powerful hearing instruments utilize a directional microphone is that directional microphones are more sensitive to vibration than omnidirectional microphones. That is, the vibration damping of a directional microphone in a hearing instrument requires considerably more space than an omnidirectional microphone. In general, hearing instruments with directional or multiple microphones are becoming popular,

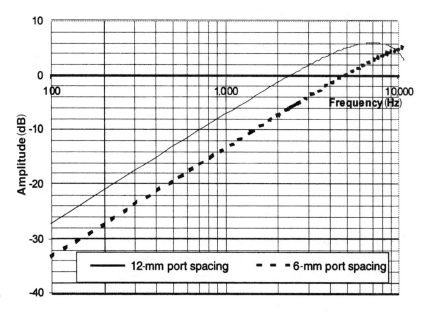

**Figure 2–16.** Frequency response of microphones with different port spacing. *(Courtesy of Phonak AG.)*

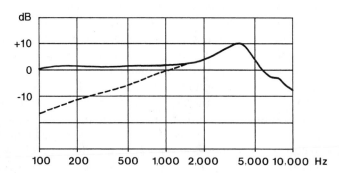

**Figure 2–17.** Relative frequency responses of a directional microphone with open and closed rear sound inlets. *(Courtesy of Phonak AG.)*

and are being more frequently prescribed and fitted because of the advantages they offer in noisy surroundings.

The main reasons are:

1. Many hearing instrument manufacturers offer units with directional microphones as a standard feature or as an option.
2. The hearing health care professional is now more aware of the enormous advantages of directional microphones.

**Advantages and disadvantages of directional microphones:**

▼ As yet, the most effective method for improving speech understanding in noisy environments (Hawkins and Yacullo, 1984; Soede, 1990)

▼ Poorer vibration damping than omnidirectional microphones
▼ Directional effect is not desirable in all listening situations (e.g., music)

## Multimicrophone Technology

Multimicrophone technology has been available in hearing instruments since 1993. The development goal was to allow a combination of two microphone characteristics in the same hearing instrument. Today, many manufacturers offer products with multiple microphone instruments.

While directional microphones have advantages for listening in noise, they can also have disadvantages in certain situations. The reduction of low-frequency amplification can negatively influence subjective judgments of sound quality, especially during conversation in quiet and when listening to music. An additional disadvantage is seen in situations where it may be undesirable to attenuate signals from the sides and the rear, particularly in traffic and for the detection of warning sounds.

To allow optimal listening conditions in both quiet and noise, a modern communications system must offer a choice of both directional and omnidirectional microphones. The introduction of the multimicrophone technology has made this possible. The directional microphone effect is achieved electronically by processing the outputs from two individual microphones. The hearing instrument user can easily switch from an omnidirectional to directional mode by pressing a key on the remote control or by using a manual switch on the hearing instrument.

The conventional directional microphone as illustrated in Figure 2–12 basically measures the pressure difference between two cavities. Pressure differences occur due to an external signal delay between the two sound ports and an internal signal delay produced by an acoustical filter built into one port. The same effect is achieved with increased efficiency by utilizing two separate omnidirectional microphones and finely tuning their combined electrical output signals via an electronic network. The parameters $\tau$ and $\Delta d$ are responsible for optimizing the directivity patterns. Provided the two microphones are perfectly matched for sensitivity and phase, every directional characteristic can be achieved with this multimicrophone technology.

The multimicrophone approach yields a number of advantages. If two independent microphones can be used to form the directional characteristics, there is a significant degree of additional freedom for design optimization. The internal propagation delay $\tau$ can be realized either by acoustic means or with an electronic delay line, or a combination of both. Furthermore, the frequency responses of the two microphones can be shaped differently. This additional design freedom does have one production-related drawback. Since the goal is to achieve reliable directional properties in each individual hearing instrument, it is necessary to precisely calibrate the two microphones by means of electronic tuning in every single hearing instrument. However, the advent of digital hearing instruments allows this matching to be accomplished inside the hearing instrument amplifier.

Many possibilities are available, especially in a digital platform.

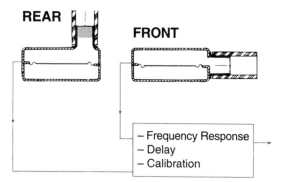

**Figure 2–18.** Cross-sectional view of a directional array using two omnidirectional microphones, one mounted to the front and the other mounted facing to the rear of a BTE hearing instrument. The electrical outputs of the microphones are combined and the directional characteristic is controlled with electronic circuitry. *(Courtesy of Phonak AG.)*

## *Second-Order Directional Microphone*

The advantage of a directional microphone is that it reduces signals from other directions and enhances signals from the front. The quality of a directional microphone is expressed by the directivity index (DI). With a single directional microphone a maximum DI of 6.0 dB can be achieved. A single directional microphone is also called a first-order directional microphone. The naming comes from the high pass characteristic of the frequency response, a high pass characteristic with a slope of 6 dB/octave. To achieve a directional microphone with a higher suppression of the surrounding noise, the DI has to increase. This is not possible with the first-order or single directional microphone (shown in Figure 2–19).

The operation of a multimicrophone system was described earlier in this chapter. The system shown in Figure 2–18 employs two omnidirectional microphones to achieve a first-order directional characteristic.

Using two directional microphones, delaying the input from one, mixing the signals together, and taking the signal difference of the two directional microphones results in a second-order directional microphone with a DI of about 8.8 dB.

The big advantage of the second-order directional microphone is that it achieves maximum noise suppression not only from the back (180°), but also from the side (90°), as shown in Figure 2–20.

**Disadvantages of second-order directional microphones are:**

▼ With every second-order system, the frequency response has a steeper high pass filter characteristic with a slope of 12 dB/octave.
▼ Second-order microphones are much more sensitive to microphone matching. Imperfect matching causes a drastic reduction of the DI.
▼ Two directional microphones require a lot of space.

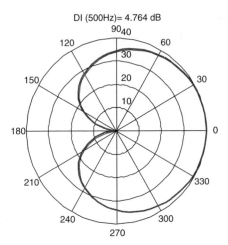

**Figure 2–19.** Cardioid polar response of a first-order directional microphone. *(Courtesy of Phonak AG.)*

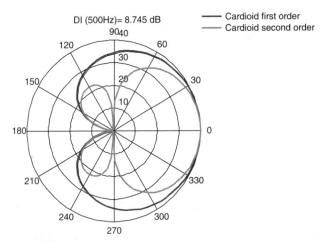

**Figure 2–20.** Polar responses of a first-order and a second-order directional microphone. *(Courtesy of Phonak AG.)*

Second-order directional microphones are designed for use in very noisy environments. Because of the size, the best application of the second-order directional microphone is a handheld system (handheld microphone or FM transmitter with microphone).

Increased miniaturization will make it possible to build second-order systems into headworn hearing instruments.

## Special Microphones

At the beginning of this chapter, two types of microphones that differ in their directional characteristics were discussed. In this section, another microphone that differs in its ampli-

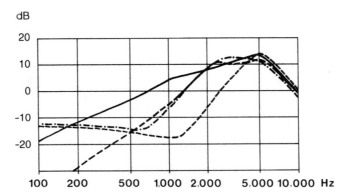

**Figure 2–21.** Frequency responses of microphones with different low-frequency slopes. *(Courtesy of Phonak AG.)*

tude response will be touched on: the slope microphone. This microphone is an omnidirectional microphone.

The amplitude response of the slope microphone differs primarily in the low-frequency range. Compare the flat frequency response of an omnidirectional microphone as shown in Figure 2–9 with the four different slope microphone frequency responses in Figure 2–21. One can clearly see the drop in sensitivity in the lower frequencies.

Slope microphones were used principally in small in-the-ear units. Slope microphones allow the elimination of a sophisticated filter circuit from the hearing instrument. The main disadvantage of slope microphones is their relatively poor signal-to-noise ratio at low frequencies. The advent of digital amplifiers with very capable filters has made the use of these microphones impractical.

## *Summary*

The electret condenser microphones used in hearing instruments today are of superior quality. They exhibit a (desirable) flat frequency response to well above 10 kHz and an equivalent input noise of 22 dB SPL (A-weighted). (This A-filter approximates the sensitivity of human hearing, i.e., low- [f<500 Hz] and high- [f>5000 Hz] frequency components are less emphasized than frequencies in the intermediate band in which the human ear is most sensitive.)

The 22 dB SPL equivalent input noise is almost always the dominant noise source in the hearing instrument and it is interesting to consider this in relation to ambient noise. Consider the following table (Figure 2–22) in which natural ambient noises are compared.

It can be seen that the microphone noise (22 dB SPL) is far below the level of most natural ambient noises and thus cannot be detected in their presence.

The maximum current consumption of an electret condenser microphone in a hearing instrument is 50 μA (typically 30 μA). This means (how often this is misunderstood) that the microphone current consumption in relation to that of the hearing instrument as a whole is negligible.

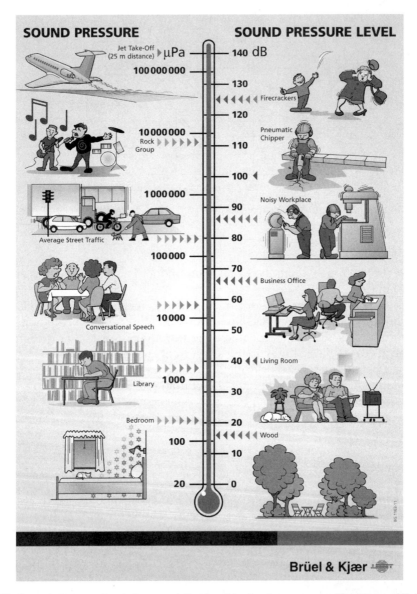

**Figure 2–22.** Sound pressure levels for a variety of ambient noise sources. *(Courtesy of Brüel & Kjær.)*

**Future considerations:**

Various research institutes are working on the next generation of microphones → the silicon microphone.

It will be produced in a manner similar to that for an integrated circuit.

The advantages of a silicon microphone are "simple" mechanical production and tighter sensitivity tolerances.

The disadvantage is that as yet there is still too much noise.

The target of a new silicon microphone, a much smaller microphone with the same performance as an electret microphone, has yet to be achieved.

## HEARING INSTRUMENT RECEIVERS

### Design Principles

The function of the hearing instrument receiver is to convert an amplified electrical signal into an acoustic signal. The hearing instrument's receiver must be highly efficient and capable of producing very high output SPLs.

The hearing instrument receiver works in accordance with the electromagnetic principle. A current flowing through a coil causes it to behave like a magnet. That is, it forms a magnetic North and South pole depending on the direction of the current. An alternating current flowing through the coil causes a shift in polarity of the coil corresponding to the alternating current and thus, a continual change in the direction of the magnetic field lines. An alternating magnetic field is the result.

Figure 2–23 shows a section of a hearing instrument receiver and its principal parts.

The armature of the receiver is a thin, magnetically permeable metal reed with a coil of fine wire around it. When the receiver is not in operation, the armature rests between the two yokes of the magnetic system. When current flows through the coil, a North or South pole is produced at the free-moving end of the armature according to the direction of the current. The armature is thus alternately attracted to or repelled from the permanent magnets.

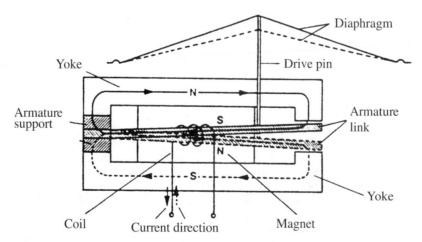

**Figure 2–23.** Cross-sectional view of an electromagnetic receiver for hearing instruments. *(Courtesy of Knowles Electronics.)*

In other words, an alternating current flowing through the coil results in deflections of the armature to either side of the air gap in the yoke corresponding to the change of direction of the current. The armature acts on the diaphragm via the drive pin causing the development of sound pressure variations in the adjacent volume of air.

Various resonances are present in an electromagnetic sound transducer:

*Electrical resonance:* Coil and own capacitance

*Mechanical resonance:* Diaphragm size and material

*Acoustic resonance:* Receiver volume, tube length and diameter, residual ear cavity

These resonances and several external factors together shape the frequency response. Particularly in the case of behind-the-ear units, the angle of the hearing instrument and the sound bore in the earmold affect the acoustic resonances. Lengthening of the receiver tube or reduction of its diameter causes the resonances of the receiver frequency curve to be displaced towards the lower frequencies and vice versa. (See Chapter 6.)

## The Class A Receiver

Earlier in this chapter the basic properties of an electromagnetic receiver were described. In the three following sections, electromagnetic receivers will be considered together with a given amplifier (output stage). The name of the receiver is determined by the type of output amplifier employed. Thus Class A receivers are connected to Class A output amplifiers.

The Class A receiver has two terminals (see Figure 2–24). A dc operating current flows through the receiver and produces a dc magnetic field. The reed of the receiver is positioned

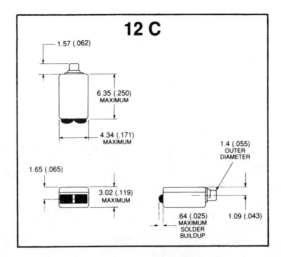
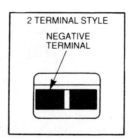

**Figure 2–24.** Class A receiver (from Knowles Electronics Datasheet: Miniature Microphones and Miniature Receivers). *(Courtesy of Knowles Electronics.)*

in the middle of the air gap by this dc field. As soon as the operating current is modulated by the amplified signal the reed swings freely in the air gap.

*Important:* It is for this reason that the Class A receiver must be correctly polarized (i.e., the receiver wires must not be reversed).

→ **Note:** As shown in Figures 2–25 and 2–26, the operating point of the hearing instrument receiver is close to the battery voltage. The amplifier cannot cause a deflection above the battery voltage (UB), but the high inductivity of the receiver (= coil) enables energy to be stored in the coil. This energy is released when the supply voltage is exceeded to produce a maximum alternating voltage of about 2.2 V across the receiver.

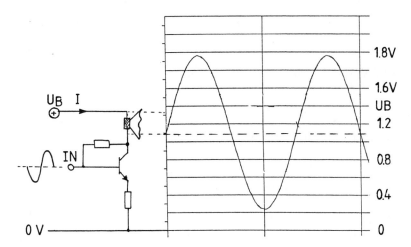

**Figure 2–25.** Circuit diagram and operation of a Class A receiver and amplifier. *(Courtesy of Knowles Electronics.)*

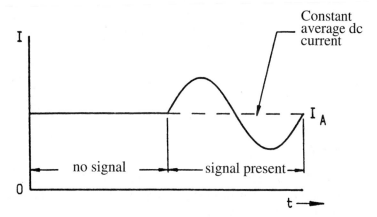

**Figure 2–26.** Current consumption of a Class A receiver. *(Courtesy of Knowles Electronics.)*

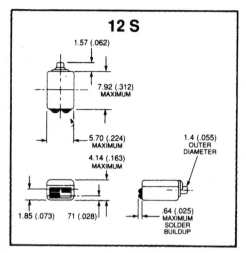
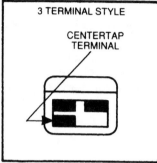

**Figure 2–27.** Class B (push-pull) receiver (from Knowles Electronics Datasheet: Miniature Microphones and Miniature Receivers). *(Courtesy of Knowles Electronics.)*

**Advantages and disadvantages of Class A receivers:**

▼ As long as the receiver does not exceed its limits, there is little distortion
▼ Better than previous receiver solutions

▼ Class A receivers require a fixed operating current which is relatively high

## The Class B Receiver (Push-Pull Receiver)

In contrast to the Class A receiver, the push-pull receiver shown in Figure 2–27 has three terminals.

The push-pull receiver has a coil with a center tap. This center tap is connected to the supply voltage UB which results, in fact, in two Class A receivers. Both halves of the receiver now receive equal signals, but out of phase by 180° (see Figure 2–28).

As the receiver again inverts the two signals through its winding with the center tap, the resultant effect (deflection of the diaphragm) is an addition of the two signals as seen in Figure 2–29.

The result is a maximum amplitude which is about twice that of a Class A receiver's output.

### Current consumption

A further advantage of Class B receivers over Class A receivers is that the Class B amplifier consumes current dependent on the control signal. That is, the smaller the electrical signal at the receiver, the smaller the current consumption.

If no signal is present, then only a very small quiescent current flows (see Figure 2–30).

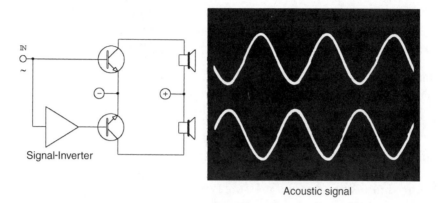

Acoustic signal

**Figure 2–28.** Circuit diagram and operation of a Class B (push-pull) receiver and amplifier indication equivalence to two Class A receivers. *(Courtesy of Phonak AG.)*

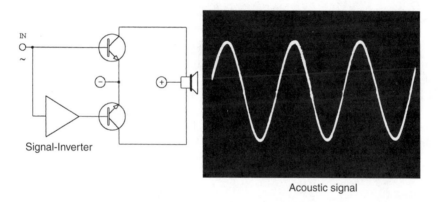

Acoustic signal

**Figure 2–29.** Circuit diagram and operation of a Class B (push-pull) receiver. *(Courtesy of Phonak AG.)*

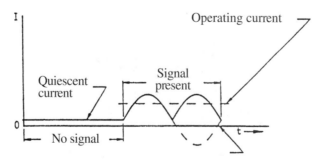

**Figure 2–30.** Current consumption of a push-pull amplifier and receiver (Ditthardt, 1990). *(Courtesy of Knowles Electronics.)*

As the reed (armature) of the receiver is only deflected by the signal from the central position (only a small quiescent current is flowing), the push-pull receiver has no definite polarity; that is, the two signal inputs of the push-pull receiver can be reversed.

→ **Note:** The reversal of the receiver terminals inverts the acoustic output signal (acoustic signal and magnetic field are phase displaced by 180°). This can cause acoustic problems when the induction coil is in operation, especially in the case of powerful behind-the-ear units (feedback!).

**Advantages and disadvantages of push-pull receivers:**

▾ Higher maximum output sound pressure is possible (6 dB higher than with Class A)
▾ Negligible quiescent current and high current consumption only when necessary

▾ The method of operation of the Class B amplifier results in crossover distortions when the signal passes through zero. The distortion varies inversely with the quiescent current.

## The Class D Receiver

A Class D receiver shown in Figure 2–31 is an electromagnetic receiver with an integrated Class D amplifier; that is, the output amplifier, in this case a Class D amplifier, is built into the housing of the receiver.

The Class D receiver has three terminals which are:

1. battery positive (current supply for the Class D amplifier)
2. battery negative
3. input signal

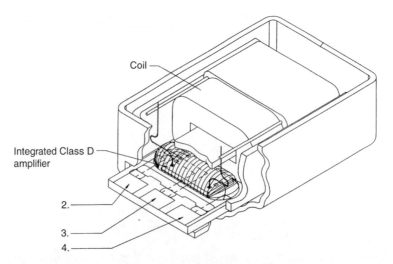

**Figure 2–31.** Sectional view of a Class D receiver (Ditthardt, 1990). *(Courtesy of Knowles Electronics.)*

## Operation of the Class D receiver

The Class D amplifier (also called a switching amplifier) converts the analog input signal into a digital signal. More precisely, a pulse-width modulated signal (PWM) is produced from the analog signal by means of a square wave generator and a comparator. The sampling frequency is at about 100 kHz (see Figure 2–32).

The pulse-width modulated square wave signal controls a power switch that alternately charges the coil of the receiver with a positive and negative supply voltage.

As the receiver coil cannot transfer the high sampling frequency (100 kHz), an analog signal is again produced from the pulse-width modulated square wave signal (see Figure 2–33).

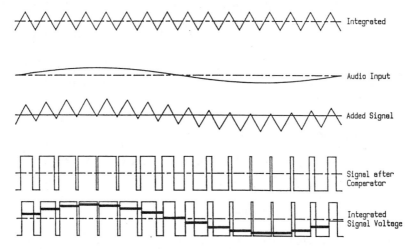

**Figure 2–32.** Electrical signal at various points in a Class D amplifier of a Knowles Class D receiver. *(Courtesy of Knowles Electronics.)*

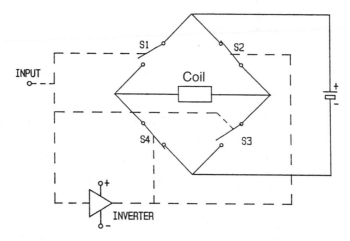

**Figure 2–33.** Schematic circuit diagram for a Class D receiver. *(Courtesy of Knowles Electronics.)*

## Current consumption

The main advantage of the Class D receiver is its low current consumption. Although the quiescent current is more or less equivalent to that of the Class B receiver, the operating current of the Class D receiver is 20 to 40% lower.

>   **Advantages and disadvantages of a Class D receiver:**

> ▼ Current consumption
> ▼ Small size (by integration of the output stage into the receiver housing)

> ▼ Good acoustic properties as long as the receiver is not operated at its performance limits (maximum sound pressure)
> ▼ High cost (particularly for in-the-ear units where the receiver is often invaded by debris and needs to be replaced)
> ▼ If the Class D receiver is operated at its performance limit then additional disturbing frequencies can occur due to the sampling of 100 kHz (subharmonics of the 100 kHz signal appear at the output).

## The Zero Bias Receiver

The zero bias receiver is a two-terminal receiver similar to the Class A receiver but with the armature centered in the air gap between the magnetic pole pieces.

## Zero Bias Direct Drive Amplifiers

Today, almost all digital hearing instrument integrated circuits (ICs) contain end amplifiers, or output amplifiers, to drive a zero bias receiver. This practice combines the advantages of the reduced current consumption of a Class D–type amplifier and the two terminals of the zero bias receiver. This advance almost completely eliminated the need for Class D receivers leading to a simpler manufacturing process and lower service costs. It is less costly to replace a zero bias receiver than a Class D receiver when the receiver fails.

## The Dual Receiver

The "dual receiver" is a special receiver that is sometimes used in hearing instruments. The dual receiver is made out of two standard receivers (Class A ED receiver). The two receivers are glued "back to back," and the two outlets lead into one port (see Figure 2–34).

The advantage of dual receivers is a doubling of the output and a significant reduction of mechanical vibration. Because of the back-to-back design, it is possible to cancel some of the vibration of the receiver.

Velocity and force measurements were made using laser interferometry to compare the vibration output of ED-1932 and EJ-3026 (essentially a dual ED-1932). The EJ typically exhibits at least 12–15 dB less vibration normal to the diaphragm at the same voltage drive level. When the vibration is referred to the acoustic output instead of the drive voltage, the EJ produces 18–21 dB less vibration normal to the diaphragm.

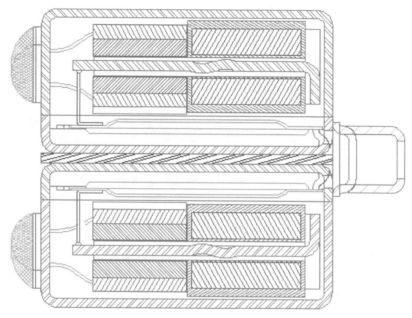

**Figure 2–34.** Dual receiver. *(Courtesy of Knowles Electronics.)*

The acoustic output from the two receivers is added in phase so that the maximum acoustic output is doubled. But nothing comes for free—the battery drain is four times higher than for a single ED receiver. It is common practice to increase the coil impedance to provide sensitivity equal to a "standard" ED. But it is also possible to get 6 dB increased maximum output if the impedance is low enough to avoid electrical clipping.

Because of the higher price of the dual receiver it is hardly used.

## CONTROL ELEMENTS

Control elements traditionally found in analog hearing instruments are a function switch, volume control, and several trimmer potentiometers (see Figure 2–35). More modern programmable and totally digital hearing instruments often contain a program select button, or switch, to select programs associated with microphone and telecoil inputs and other specialized programs such as directional processing or noise reduction. Although digital instruments now offer automatic loudness adjustment features, the volume control is still preferred by many hearing instrument users to enable rapid changes in loudness in response to sudden noises in the environment. Trimmers are the analog controls that the hearing health care professional sets in to best compensate for the individual hearing loss during fitting. These are no longer required in programmable instruments as adjustments are carried out electronically and eventually stored in the memory of the hearing instrument. However, digital instruments with trimmers are now being developed for emerging markets where computers are not widely available in dispensing offices.

VC    Trimmers   Switch

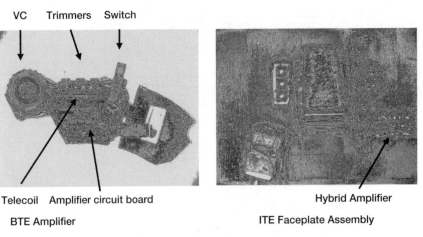

Telecoil   Amplifier circuit board           Hybrid Amplifier

BTE Amplifier                    ITE Faceplate Assembly

**Figure 2–35.** Typical BTE and ITE amplifier assemblies. *(Courtesy of Unitron Hearing Ltd.)*

## AMPLIFIER

The amplifier (see Figure 2–35) contains most of the electronics in the hearing instrument and consists of various circuit elements. The amplifier is fed the signal from the microphone, amplifies it according to the settings, and sends the appropriately amplified signal on to the receiver. Recent technological developments have made it possible to replace the traditional analog amplifier with a digital signal processor consisting of analog-to-digital converters, signal processors, filter banks, and other digital functional blocks. These components are contained in an integrated circuit which is usually packaged in a hybrid package. The hybrid contains additional components such as capacitors required for power supply regulation, filtering, and decoupling.

## TELECOIL

The telecoil (see Figure 2–35) is a series of windings on a magnetically permeable core that is used to sense magnetic fields in the vicinity of the hearing instrument. Such magnetic fields exist in telephones and in loop systems and provide an alternate input to a hearing instrument amplifier. The advantage of picking up the magnetic field from a telephone earpiece and using it as the input signal during a telephone conversation is that the hearing aid avoids amplifying the ambient acoustic signal in the environment and thereby produces a less noisy telephone signal. Unfortunately, such a magnetic field is not available from all telephone sets.

Loop systems are designed to work specifically with hearing aids and are installed in many public places such as schools, places of worship, theaters, and concert halls. These spaces have a wire loop installed in the periphery of the space. An amplified microphone signal drives a current through the loop and a magnetic field is established inside the loop. This magnetic field is sensed by the telecoil in the hearing instrument.

In the past telecoils were passive, namely a number of turns of fine wire on a magnetic core. They can now be provided with an integrated amplifier in a single, small package. This type of telecoil uses a shorter coil with fewer turns of wire, and is therefore less sensitive. The loss in sensitivity is made up by the gain of the integrated amplifier. The amplified telecoil is particularly useful in the construction of a small instrument.

An important goal in hearing instrument design is equalization of microphone and telecoil sensitivities. This ensures that the loudness of the amplified signal does not change significantly when the instrument is switched from an acoustic to a magnetic input mode to accommodate loop system or telephone use.

Switching between the microphone and telecoil modes can be tedious and at times difficult for people with limited dexterity. Many hearing instruments now feature an automatic telecoil referred to by a variety of names like "Easy Phone," "Easy Coil," "Touchless Telecoil," etc. This feature relies on activating a reed switch in the hearing instrument input circuit with a static magnetic field. This static magnetic field is sometimes present in the vicinity of the telephone handset. Unfortunately, this field is usually quite weak or may not be present at all. Reliable operation is assured by attaching a permanent magnet to the handset. When the handset is placed near the ear, the magnetic field activates the reed switch and the associated amplifier circuit turns off the microphone signal and turns on the telecoil signal. When the magnetic field is removed from near the ear at the end of the telephone conversation, the reed switch opens and the microphone input mode becomes active again.

Loop systems produce only a magnetic field that oscillates in harmony with the transmitted speech signal. No static magnetic field is present and the so-called automatic telecoils do not function with loop systems. It is therefore necessary to manually switch on the telecoil input mode when a loop system is to be used and also when the telephone does not produce a sufficiently strong static magnetic field. Automatic telecoils will become available for these cases as well when circuits are developed to detect the presence of alternating magnetic fields in the vicinity of the hearing instrument.

## SUMMARY

1. Performance and size of components continue to be the important drivers for advancement in hearing instrument performance and size.
2. Performance and size are both important.
3. The microphone and receiver have a critical influence on the performance and size of hearing instruments.
4. If components are large the instrument will also be large and lack cosmetic appeal for the user.
5. The never-ending challenge is to ensure that performance parameters like bandwidth, distortion, current consumption, and maximum output of the component are not adversely affected by the ongoing miniaturization process.
6. A small instrument that does not deliver adequate performance for the user is of little value.

## REVIEW QUESTIONS

1. **A.** Draw a longitudinal section of a directional microphone.
   **B.** How can the directional characteristics of the microphone be influenced?
2. What occurs when the port spacing of a directional microphone is divided by two?
3. What are the advantages and disadvantages of a Class D receiver in an ITE?
4. What are the features of a directional microphone?
   **A.** Frequency response with high-frequency emphasis　　　　　A ☐
   **B.** Reduced sensitivity to mechanical vibration　　　　　　　B ☐
   **C.** Polar response independent of the head shadow effect　　　C ☐
   **D.** It is a pressure gradient sensor　　　　　　　　　　　　D ☐
5. What happens if the connections of the two wires between the amplifier and the Class A receiver are reversed?
   **A.** No effect　　　　　　　　　　　　　　　　　　　　　　A ☐
   **B.** There will be more distortion　　　　　　　　　　　　　B ☐
   **C.** There will be a higher current consumption　　　　　　　C ☐
   **D.** The receiver will be destroyed　　　　　　　　　　　　　D ☐
6. Which is correct?
   **A.** Class A receivers have equal quiescent and working current　　A ☐
   **B.** Class A receivers have unequal quiescent and working current　B ☐
   **C.** Class B receivers have a current consumption depending on the sound pressure level being produced　　　　　　　　　　　　C ☐
   **D.** The quiescent current of a Class A receiver is smaller than a Class B receiver　　　　　　　　　　　　　　　　　　　　　D ☐
7. The microphone equivalent input noise:
   **A.** Is independent of the size of the microphone　　　　　　　A ☐
   **B.** Is less the smaller the microphone　　　　　　　　　　　B ☐
   **C.** Is less the bigger the microphone　　　　　　　　　　　　C ☐
   **D.** The microphone doesn't have an equivalent input noise　　　D ☐
8. An increase of the port spacing of a directional microphone creates:
   **A.** An improved directional polar pattern　　　　　　　　　　A ☐
   **B.** A reduction of the sensitivity at low frequency　　　　　　B ☐
   **C.** An improved high-frequency response　　　　　　　　　　C ☐
   **D.** An improved signal-to-noise ratio of the microphone　　　　D ☐
9. A reduction of the inlet (port) opening of a microphone due to debris creates:
   **A.** A sensitivity loss at low frequencies　　　　　　　　　　A ☐
   **B.** A sensitivity loss at all frequencies　　　　　　　　　　　B ☐
   **C.** A sensitivity loss at high frequencies　　　　　　　　　　C ☐
   **D.** No change in the response curve of the microphone　　　　D ☐

# CHAPTER 3

# Digitally Programmable Hearing Instruments

## INTRODUCTION

Hearing instrument technology has changed greatly over the past few years. Component and device miniaturization is an ongoing activity and progress is continually being made to produce ever-incrementally smaller instruments with better cosmetic appearance and improved fit. Hearing instrument design also benefits from major technology developments that create new classes of instruments.

Digitally programmable hearing instruments are a new class of instruments. This development offers the possibility for better matching the instrument to the audiological need of the user.

## WHAT IS A DIGITALLY PROGRAMMABLE HEARING INSTRUMENT?

A digitally programmable hearing instrument is an instrument without traditional trimmer potentiometers. Instead, the hearing instrument is equipped with the means to be electrically connected to a personal computer (PC) or a manufacturer's proprietary programming device via a cable connection for the purpose of adjusting its operating parameters. The hearing health care professional adjusts the parameters of the hearing instrument in this way and receives visual confirmation of the changes from the PC.

A distinguishing feature of the digitally programmable instrument is that it is designed to be part of a system (see Figure 3–1). The system consists of the hearing instrument, a cable, a programming interface, and a software-based fitting module that is installed on a PC for the purpose of manipulating the operational parameters of the hearing instrument. The full system is required to adjust the hearing instrument. Once this step is completed, the hearing instrument is disconnected and its operation is like a traditional non-programmable instrument.

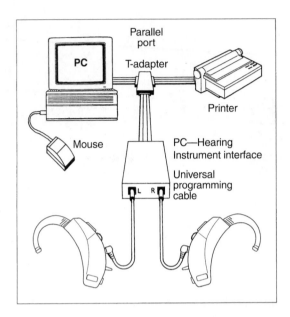

**Figure 3–1.** Digitally programmable system components including hearing instruments, personal computer system, programming interface, and cables. *(Courtesy of Phonak AG.)*

The introduction of the digitally programmable hearing instrument was a major advance in hearing instrument technology. On the one hand, there was no previous development that offered more possibilities for better audiological fitting flexibility and accuracy than the programmable hearing instrument. And on the other hand, the introduction of the PC in the selection and fitting process made a wide range of support tools available to the health care professional. This chapter presents a discussion of this new generation of instruments.

Prior to the introduction of digitally programmable hearing instruments, such a high degree of flexibility was unknown. The following are just a few of the parameters that can be changed by a mere press of a button: overall amplification, low-frequency amplification, high-frequency amplification, maximum output sound pressure, output limiting system (PC or AGC [Automatic Gain Control]), AGC kneepoint, and compression ratio.

*Important:* Several parameters can be changed and compared simultaneously. The possibility for switching rapidly between various settings allows the hearing instrument wearer to judge which setting best facilitates understanding of speech in noise or which sounds best in quiet surroundings.

Subsequent to fitting the hearing instrument, the various parameters (amplification, filter coefficients, etc.) are stored digitally in the hearing instrument. This stored data will not be lost, even when the hearing instrument's battery is changed.

It is important to distinguish between a digitally programmable and a fully digital hearing instrument. In the case of a digitally programmable hearing instrument, only the settings are changed and stored digitally. The analog signal is processed using analog principles.

A fully digital hearing instrument utilizes digital signal processing in the signal path. This means that the analog signal is converted to a digital one and processed digitally.

*Important:* A digitally programmable hearing instrument is not a digital hearing instrument.

The hearing health care professional can, as a routine follow-up procedure, connect the hearing instrument to the programming device or the computer, read the stored data, and make any necessary alterations in the settings. A further advantage of some programmable hearing instruments is that various groups of settings can be stored as programs in the hearing instrument. This enables the wearer to select the most advantageous program with a push button or a remote control for any given listening environment. For example, the hearing instrument may have a program for quiet surroundings, and another for listening to music (with bass and treble boosting), as well as a program designed to optimize speech understanding under noisy listening conditions.

It is clear that a programmable system requires both hardware and software. Both components of digitally programmable systems are discussed next.

# HARDWARE

During the last few years, digitally programmable hearing instruments (analog and digital) have come to dominate the market. The hearing health care professional can use a special programming device, if it is available, or a personal computer for fitting these instruments.

## THE PROGRAMMABLE HEARING INSTRUMENT

The first programmable hearing instruments had a traditional analog signal path fabricated with BiPOLAR semiconductor processes (see Figure 3–2). The innovative part in a programmable hearing instrument is that the analog trimmer potentiometers were replaced by

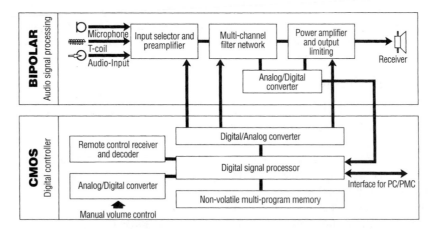

**Figure 3–2.** Block diagram of a digitally programmable hearing instrument. *(Courtesy of Phonak AG.)*

integrated electronic networks whose electrical resistance was determined by electronic data stored in a memory in the hearing instrument. A new component, a socket for connecting the programming cable, needs to be provided in the programmable instrument.

Trimmer potentiometers occupy physical space in a hearing instrument. Their numbers, and hence the number of adjustment possibilities, are limited in practice by the available space in the instrument.

There is practically no limitation on the number of programmable resistive networks that can be constructed on a complementary metal oxide semiconductor (CMOS) IC of an area occupied by a single trimmer potentiometer. Programmable hearing instruments therefore offer a significant increase in the number of programmable parameters and greater fitting flexibility.

## PROGRAMMING DEVICES

A second key element of a programmable system is the programming device.

### Dedicated Proprietary Programming Devices

At first glance, a programming device dedicated to a specific hearing aid manufacturer's hearing instrument would appear to be the best and certainly most straightforward solution. In the beginning, hearing health care professionals who had no experience with personal computers generally preferred programming devices offered by hearing instrument manufacturers because their operation was easily learned and mastered. The disadvantages of such an approach became clear quite quickly. Since each hearing instrument manufacturer needs to offer a dedicated programming device, it is necessary for the hearing health care professional to have three or four different devices on hand to be able to fit just a few of the instruments on the market. To avoid this, Siemens collaborated with other hearing instrument manufacturers (Hansaton, Philips, Phonak, Rexton) to produce a universal programming interface called PMC. The objective of PMC becoming an industry standard programming interface was not embraced because many manufacturers began exploiting the flexibility of the personal computers (PCs).

The PC rapidly became the industry standard as manufacturers developed fitting software to run on these machines to adjust digitally programmable instruments.

### The Personal Computer

The personal computer (PC) presents the most complete solution for hearing instrument adjustment. The following components are required for this:

- ▼ IBM-compatible PC (Requirements vary with manufacturer. It is not unusual that PCs three or four generations older than the current model are not supported by the most recent fitting software release.)
- ▼ Programming interface.
- ▼ Specific hearing instrument manufacturer adjustment software.

The PC has none of the disadvantages of the programming devices. The PC offers:

- ▾ Virtually limitless display possibilities.
- ▾ Adequate storage capacity.
- ▾ High computational capacity.
- ▾ The ability to be updated to the most current fitting software release.
- ▾ The ability to run fitting software from different manufacturers.

The PC provides the flexibility and capability to adjust digital hearing instruments today and in the future.

## PROGRAMMING INTERFACES

Programmable hearing instruments can differ enormously from one another, as does their corresponding PC software. In addition, it is necessary to utilize an interface specific to the manufacturer when programming a given hearing instrument. Obviously, it would involve considerable inconvenience and expense for the hearing health care professional to be able to fit programmable hearing instruments from different manufacturers. This has been the impetus behind standardization of hardware (interface) and software in the area of programmable hearing instrument fitting.

Hardware interface standardization led to the development of the HI-PRO programming interface. Software standardization (NOAH) is discussed in the "Software" section later in this chapter.

### HI-PRO

HI-PRO (see Figure 3–3) was a parallel development to NOAH to develop a standard hardware interface between the PC and a hearing instrument. The interface allows the hearing health care professional to adjust all programmable hearing instruments from various manufacturers with the same interface. The interface is automatically configured to the programming voltage levels and data structure requirements of the specific hearing instrument to be programmed. The PC and hearing instrument can therefore communicate with one another. Consequently, HI-PRO was developed as a means of saving the hearing health care professional the inconvenience and cost of acquiring and managing many proprietary interface devices. HI-PRO is an interface designed by Madsen Electronics for standardization around NOAH and includes the requirements of all hearing instrument manufacturers.

### NOAHlink

NOAHlink is a new programming interface designed to replace the HI-PRO interface for programming advanced hearing instruments of today and tomorrow. NOAHlink is compatible with NOAH 3 fitting modules and provides faster data communication between NOAH 3 and the hearing instrument.

NOAHlink is worn by the patient during programming (see Figure 3–4) and provides a wireless Bluetooth technology link to the PC. Short cables connect the interface to the hearing instrument(s).

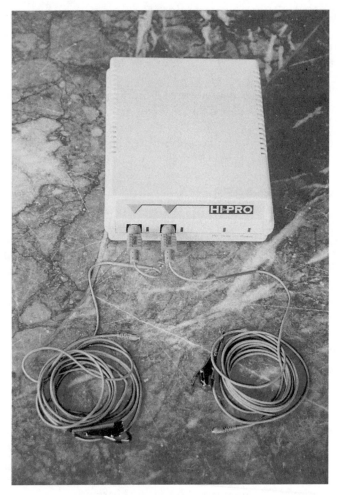

**Figure 3–3.** HI-PRO programming interface. *(Courtesy of GN ReSound as A/S.)*

The wireless Bluetooth connection allows programming at a distance of up to five meters for the computer and the patient is free to move about within that distance during programming. NOAHlink is operated on rechargeable batteries with an estimated life of fifteen hours.

## OTHER PROGRAMMING INTERFACES

Although the Hi-Pro programming interface is a standard configurable programming interface, it is not a particularly portable device. Smaller, more versatile interfaces were developed shortly after the introduction to make portable programming of hearing aids more convenient through the use of laptop computers or Personal Digital Assistants (PDAs). This was a particular need for audiologists and dispensers working in rural and home-care settings.

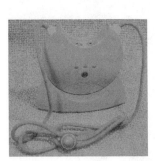 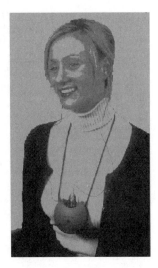

**Figure 3–4.** NOAHlink programming interface. *(Courtesy of HIMSA A/S.)*

### Microcard

The first such interface was the Microcard, developed by Microtech on a modified PCMCIA card. (PCMCIA stands for the Personal Computer Memory Card Interface Association.) This device slides into the PCMCIA slot of a laptop computer or a PDA. The Microcard requires a cable adaptor to use standard programming cables to interface the PCMCIA card to the hearing aid. The Microcard is hardwired and configured with firmware to make it a dedicated interface for a specific manufacturer's hearing instrument models. It is not generally configurable for more than one manufacturer.

### Microconnect

The Microconnect (see Figure 3–5) was an improved version of the Microcard. Standard DIN connectors were incorporated into the mechanical package, making it more rugged and compatible with standard hearing instrument programming cables. Furthermore, Microconnect featured optical isolation between the laptop power supply and the hearing instrument, ensuring patient safety in accordance with applicable requirements.

## SOFTWARE

The importance of software in the hearing instrument industry has grown immensely since the advent of digitally programmable and fully digital hearing instruments. Software has found a permanent place in two principal areas: PC-based software (fitting software, etc.) and digital signal processing firmware or algorithms.

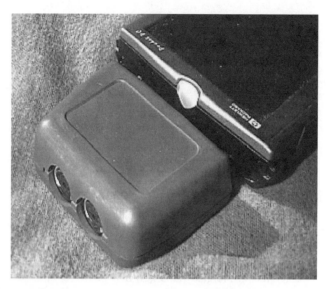

**Figure 3–5.** Microconnect programming interface fitted into the PCMCIA slot of a PDA. *(Courtesy of Micro-Tech Hearing Instruments.)*

## HEARING INSTRUMENT FIRMWARE AND ALGORITHMS

Digital hearing aids use two different types of software. In general terms, software is a sequence of instructions that determines the operation of a signal processor or a computer. The computer, often referred to as a microprocessor, consists of series logic devices such as "AND" and "OR" gates connected in specific ways in an integrated circuit (IC) to perform a variety of arithmetic functions. A DSP (digital signal processor) microprocessor is a type of microprocessor designed for rapid math calculations. It often has a pipeline and/or Harvard architecture. The logic gates can be connected permanently during IC fabrication to perform a specific function. In this case the sequence of logic events is referred to as firmware. Alternatively, the logic gates can be connected through electronic switches that can be opened or closed according to a sequence of instructions. This series of instructions constitutes an algorithm. Changing the algorithm changes the function of the processor.

When a system uses only firmware, it is referred to as a closed system. An algorithm-based system is referred to as an open system. The functionality of a closed system can be changed or modified only by physically changing the IC. Good IC design will contain most or all the connections between logic elements in one or two layers and only these layers need to be altered. On the other hand, in an open system, the functionality can be improved and other problems can often be corrected with an algorithm change.

A preferred hearing aid IC design strategy often uses a combination of open and closed function blocks. It is advantageous to use a closed firmware-controlled approach for repetitive and often-used functions. A filter bank that implements the well-known and standard Fast Fourier Transform calculation is more efficient when implemented with a dedicated hardwired block. On the other hand, it is more efficient to implement newly developed noise reduction and feedback cancellers in an algorithm on an open DSP processor. The latter case allows algorithms to be further refined and upgraded with changes to the algorithm.

Firmware is either hardwired during IC fabrication or stored in read-only memory (ROM) during fabrication. In this way firmware can be updated in the ROM section of an IC. Algorithms are stored in electrically erasable, programmable memory (EEPROM). This type of memory is usually a second silicon chip that makes up the digital chip set for a hearing aid application. The algorithm can therefore be erased and rewritten to EEPROM as required.

The capabilities of this type of software are discussed in more detail in Chapter 5, "Digital Hearing Instruments."

## PC-BASED SOFTWARE (FITTING SOFTWARE, ETC.)

Aside from advances in software-based fitting modules, rapid developments are occurring in software-based product delivery options such as order and repair forms, order tracking, and automated billing. These latter features form the backbone of a new software tool called e-TONA, an acronym for "electronic transmission of NOAH actions." The purpose of e-TONA is to assist users, manufacturers, and business partners in processing electronic communications associated with orders, returns, and repairs. These electronic communications are stored in a standardized format as actions in the NOAH database.

Clearly, it is not desirable or logical for every hearing instrument manufacturer to undertake these types of developments on their own. Instead, industry-sponsored development association was created to produce standard products for manufacturers and hearing health care professionals.

### HIMSA

HIMSA (Hearing Instrument Manufacturer Software Association) is a development association founded by the hearing instrument companies Danavox, Oticon, Phonak, and Widex in Denmark in 1993. The objective of HIMSA was to develop a software standard for hearing instrument adjustment (especially for programmable hearing instruments). This software was launched at the end of 1993 under the name NOAH.

### NOAH

NOAH is the software platform (in Windows) for the adjustment of programmable hearing instruments. It makes it possible for the hearing health care professional to control and manage his or her whole field of work on the PC with an easily operated program interface. NOAH enables optimal hearing instrument adjustment and programming, as well as efficient management of client data, audiometric data, and administrative affairs (see Figure 3–6).

The industry-standard NOAH software framework allows every manufacturer of hearing instruments, audiometers, office systems, etc., to develop proprietary modules (software packages). These are made available by the hearing instrument manufacturers as separate software modules and are specially geared to their products' possibilities. Many different fitting modules can be installed in NOAH and any one of these fitting modules can be started and run within the NOAH framework when a hearing instrument needs to be adjusted. Through the direct link between NOAH and an audiometer, the adjusted data can be checked directly "in situ." Practically all manufacturers of hearing instruments, audiological equipment, and office automation systems are compatible and work with the NOAH standard (see Figure 3–6).

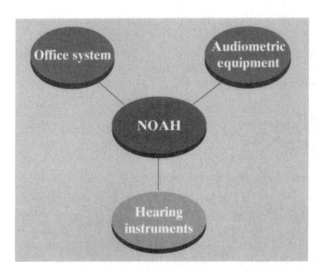

**Figure 3–6.** Interconnection possibilities with NOAH. *(Courtesy of Phonak AG.)*

NOAH, now in its third revision, offers Windows XP Professional and NOAHlink compatibility. In the future, NOAH 3 will offer the ability to order hearing instruments electronically (see the discussion on e-TONA) and to store standardized questionnaire data such as COSI and APHAB (refer to later in the chapter and to Chapter 11 for details) in the NOAH database.

## FITTING SOFTWARE

In 2001 approximately two of every four hearing instruments sold were programmable. By mid-2004, just over four of five instruments sold were programmable. It is clear that fitting software has become an indispensable tool for hearing instrument selection and fitting and is, therefore, an integral part of the product offering from every manufacturer.

Fitting software is the dispenser's and dispensing audiologist's principal tool. Intuitive operation, ease of use, professional appearance and comprehensive coverage of product lines are essential elements for the acceptance of a manufacturer's fitting software by the dispensing community.

New and updated fitting software must accompany every new product release from a manufacturer and there is no doubt that each manufacturer must support significant software development expertise to be able to release new fitting software for each new hearing aid model. Furthermore, each new fitting software release must keep pace with PC hardware and operating system developments as well as work in harmony with other manufacturers' fitting software products. HIMSA provides a certification service to ensure that no major compatibility problems exist.

As product life cycles become shorter, the number of new software products must keep pace with new product releases. Rapid-fitting software development makes use of the most modern architectures and development tools. In general, object-based architectures are now in common use. This means that each new model release is structured as a self-contained block of code. Data structures and input/output communications are designed in accordance with predetermined protocols. Standard operations such as target gain calculations and frequency response adjustments for a variety of fitting formulas, or a manufacturer's proprietary fitting formula, are shared object functions. These can be called up as required at any time in the hearing aid adjustment process, but always within the confines of the predetermined data and communications protocol.

Following these design rules allows new models to be easily added to the fitting software without affecting older models and without needing to undo previous features and options.

While digital hearing aids provide greater adjustment flexibility and improved functionality, these hearing aids also offer a greater number of adjustment parameters to the hearing instrument clinician. For example, consider a sixteen-band digital hearing instrument with basic wide dynamic range compression in each band. Each band then has a unique input/output characteristic defined by a linear gain section, a first threshold (T1) for the onset of compression, a second threshold (T2) for the onset of output limiting, and a fixed high-level output limiting ratio. T1 and T2 are defined by an input value and an output value from which the gain and compression ratio in each band can be derived. Even in this simple case, $16 \times 4 = 64$ parameters must be adjusted to best match the target gain predicted for a particular hearing loss. Increasing the number of thresholds, adding low-level expansion ratios, and other options such as noise cancellation, directional processing, and so on, in two or three different user-selected programs, makes the proper adjustment of a digital hearing aid a formidable task.

Therefore, there is an increasing reliance on automated fitting processes which can achieve an optimal match to the target gain based on the audiogram, preferred fitting formula, and lifestyle information. The objective is to achieve spontaneous acceptance by the hearing-impaired user when the hearing aid has undergone the initial adjustment of the fitting process. Subsequent fine-tuning can then be performed on several levels depending on the desires of the fitting professional: simple fine-tuning, automated fine-tuning and expert level fine-tuning (Hayes, 2004).

### Fitting Software Organization

The organizational flow of an ideal fitting software structure consists of the following elements:

- Patient profile: personal information and lifestyle information.
- Diagnostics: audiogram and in situ data (see Figure 3–7 for an example of a selection screen).
- Pre-calculation of targets: formula driven with correction factors for individual ear canal resonance and individual real-ear to coupler level differences.
- Fitting and fine-tuning (see Figure 3–8 for an example of a fitting screen).
- Outcome and verification: using speech discrimination, auditory scene verification (audio streaming), COSI, APHAB, etc.

## OTHER SOFTWARE FEATURES

Lifestyle information is now commonly used to achieve refined fitting targets. This type of information can be obtained from a number of different assessment scales. These scales are

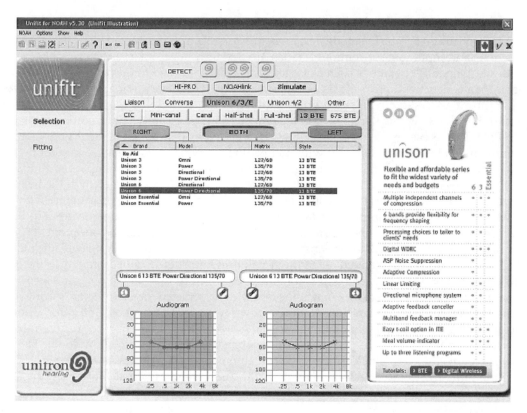

**Figure 3–7.** Example of a hearing instrument selection screen. The audiogram for the right and left ears are displayed and different models can be selected for each ear. *(Courtesy of Unitron Hearing Ltd.)*

derived from standardized questionnaires, also now available in electronic form and often included as a module in fitting software packages that attempt to measure the degrees of difficulty individuals have in everyday listening situations. Some of the more common assessment scales are:

APHAB (abbreviated profile of hearing aid benefit)

HHIE (hearing handicap inventory for the elderly)

COSI (customer-oriented scale of improvement)

They provide a subjective rating of the perceived disability or handicap (without and with a hearing aid) and of the efficacy of amplification. These questionnaires are discussed in more detail in Chapter 11.

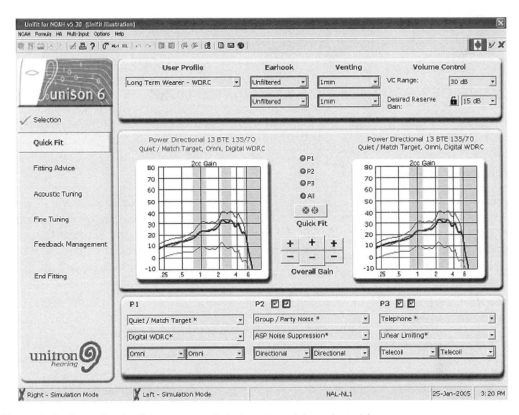

**Figure 3–8.** Example of a fitting screen. Gain targets and the selected frequency response curves are closely matched. Upper and lower adjustment limits for the instrument are also shown for both ears. *(Courtesy of Unitron Hearing Ltd.)*

## *e-TONA*

e-TONA is developed by HIMSA to assist users, manufacturers, and business partners in processing electronic communications such as orders, returns, and repairs. The electronic communication will be stored in standardized formats as actions in the NOAH database.

# ADVANTAGES AND DISADVANTAGES OF PROGRAMMABLE HEARING INSTRUMENTS

Although programmable hearing instruments open up a world of possibilities, the new technologies involved made them seem at first to be rather a mixed blessing. Drastic changes were required of both hearing instrument manufacturers as well as fitters to be able to successfully use the new technologies. The manufacturers had to struggle with the usual bugs inherent in new products, while the hearing health care professionals had to abandon tried and true fitting strategies. Although it has only been a few years since its commercial debut, the advantages of the programmable hearing instrument are already clearly apparent.

## ADVANTAGES FOR THE HEARING-IMPAIRED USER

The benefits of digitally programmable hearing instruments for the wearer are perhaps the most important.

### Instrument Complexity

- ▼ Digitally programmable hearing instruments have much more complex electronics. This means that overload of the instruments is better controlled, resulting in less distortion.
- ▼ There is greater filtering potential, enabling a better fitting for the individual hearing loss.
- ▼ Various sound pressure limiting systems are possible in one unit so that the user can select the one best suited for him.

### Remote Control

- ▼ With remote control, simpler operation of the hearing instrument is possible.
- ▼ It is only with remote control that some functions are possible (e.g., various hearing programs).
- ▼ Users with decreased manual dexterity can easily operate the hearing instrument.
- ▼ Binaural control is possible.

### User Programs

- ▼ A digitally programmable hearing instrument can have several programs, each of which can be set to amplify and filter the signal in different ways. The user can then select the program best suited for a particular situation (e.g., noise, music, party, etc.).

### Service

- ▼ Mechanical parts (e.g., trimmers) are replaced by electronic components in the digitally programmable hearing instrument. As a consequence, there is not so much wear and tear on the instrument, making it less prone to needing repair

## ADVANTAGES FOR THE HEARING HEALTH CARE PROFESSIONAL

### Fitting

- ▼ Simpler programming (no tiny trimmers to be manipulated).
- ▼ "Compare mode"; instrument settings differing by more than just one trimmer setting can be compared.
- ▼ Two instruments can be adjusted simultaneously.

## *Computer*

▼ A given setting including the effects of various acoustic parameters (venting, horn, damper, etc.) can be calculated.

▼ Storage of fitting data in the client database.

# INTERNET ACCESS

As in other phases of daily life and business, the Internet has a profound impact on the hearing health business. e-TONA is already providing Internet-based services for the dispenser by enabling electronic transactions for order entry, order tracking, and maintenance activities.

In addition, hearing assessment and hearing aid adjustment will also be enabled over the Internet.

## SUMMARY

1. Programmable hearing instruments represent a significant advance in hearing instrument capability.
2. The transition to digital technology in hearing instruments began by replacing the traditional controls such as resistive trimmer potentiometers with solid-state circuit elements.
3. The period of the digitally programmable instrument with analog signal processing was of a very short duration, somewhat less than ten years, but it represents the beginning of the transition from analog to totally digital instruments.
4. Digitally programmable hearing instruments have an analog signal path whose operational parameters are stored in digital form.
5. Digitally programmable hearing instruments are not digital instruments, but initially all digital hearing instruments were digitally programmable.
6. The number of available adjustment parameters in a programmable instrument exceeded the number of trimmer potentiometers that could be accommodated in the shell of a BTE instrument or on the faceplate of an ITE instrument. This type of instrument therefore offered more flexibility for use with a wide variety of hearing losses.
7. Digitally programmable hearing instruments offered the advantage of multiple programs optimized for several listening environments.
8. The programmable hearing instrument period mandated the use of PCs for hearing instrument selection and fitting into the hearing health care professional's office.
9. The fitting software modules which ran on the PC managed the complexities of hearing instrument selection, adjustment, and optimization.
10. In addition, the extensive use of PCs in dispensing offices enabled progress in office automation and record keeping.

## REVIEW QUESTIONS

1. Digital programmable hearing instruments:
   A. Are the first products with integrated circuits      A ☐
   B. Use a digital signal processing                       B ☐
   C. Have a built-in Class D receiver                      C ☐
   D. Use analog signal processing but digital storage of fitting parameters   D ☐
2. Describe the components of a programmable system.
3. Name three different programming interfaces.

# CHAPTER 4

# Signal-Processing Strategies

## INTRODUCTION

Modern hearing instrument amplifiers are required to perform two basic tasks. The first is signal amplification to best correct for a loss in hearing sensitivity and non-linear loudness growth. These functions have been applied extensively in analog hearing instruments but they are also the fundamental amplification functions in digital devices. The second task is to improve signal quality and to provide a clean amplified signal to the eardrum. This chapter is concerned with fundamental signal-processing strategies aimed at signal amplification. A variety of hearing instrument amplification functions will be thoroughly described in this chapter. Signal-processing strategies aimed at improving signal quality, which can be applied in conjunction with these basic amplification strategies, are discussed in Chapter 5.

## FILTER FUNCTIONS

Electrical filters are built into hearing instrument amplifiers to allow the frequency response of the instrument to be altered in order to best meet the requirements of a particular hearing loss. These filters were traditionally constructed using electronic components such as resistors and capacitors.

As hearing instrument amplifiers became more advanced, filter functions also became more flexible. The most basic filter function in a hearing instrument is a high-pass filter. Such a filter passes signals in the high-frequency band, generally referred to as the passband, and attenuates lower frequencies. Similarly, a low-pass filter has a passband in the low-frequency region and attenuates signals with frequencies above the passband. The transition from the passband to the frequency region where attenuation occurs, generally referred to as the stop band, is a gradual transition after which the attenuation increases with frequency.

Two additional filters have also found application in hearing instruments. These are the bandstop filter and the bandpass filter. The bandstop filter attenuates the signal over a narrow frequency band and passes signals outside that band. Such a filter can be used to suppress a feedback signal. The bandpass filter passes signal in a band between two frequencies and blocks higher and lower frequencies. Adjacent bandpass filters are used to produce hearing instruments with several independent frequency bands, or multiband instruments.

In order to be able to change the frequency response of the hearing instrument, a filter component, usually a resistor, is replaced with an adjustable resistor, or trimmer. For example, a simple high-pass filter using an adjustable resistor, $R$, and a fixed capacitor, $C$, has a transition frequency, or corner frequency $f_c = 1/(2\pi RC)$. The corner frequency $f_c$ is defined as the frequency where the signal level is reduced by 3 dB from the signal level in the passband. The hearing health care professional needs only a small screwdriver to alter the resistance value and thus best match the hearing instrument's frequency response to the slope in the hearing loss. Adjusting the low-pass and high-pass filters in this way allows the frequency range of the instrument to be controlled. A simple $RC$ filter is a first-order filter in that the attenuation outside the passband changes with frequency at a rate of 6 dB/octave. Higher-order filters require additional filter stages (i.e., more components), but analog instruments commonly contain second- and third-order filters with 12 dB/octave and 18 dB/octave slopes.

Modern digital hearing aids use signal processors to implement filter functions by means of mathematical operations on a digitized version of the signal passing through the hearing instrument. Every filter type described above can be implemented in a digital processor and the effect of the filter on the signal is the same for the analog and the digital case.

Additional details and terminology associated with hearing aid filters are presented in the following paragraphs.

## HIGH-PASS FILTER (LOW CUT)

A high-pass filter allows, as the name suggests, the higher frequencies to pass unattenuated through the filter.

By changing the resistance value, the corner frequencies are changed as shown in Figure 4–1. For simplicity, the transition from the passband to the attenuation band is shown as an abrupt one rather than a gradual one as described previously. The order of the filter indicates the slope of the filter curve.

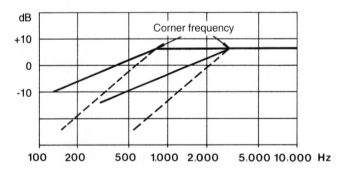

**Figure 4–1.** High-pass filter response, with adjustable corner frequencies and stop-band slopes. *(Courtesy of Phonak AG.)*

First order → slope = 6 dB/octave

Second order → slope = 12 dB/octave

First-order filters are usually passive filters. That is, the filter function is achieved with only one resistor and one capacitor (i.e., a simple *RC* circuit). Higher-order filters (second to fourth order) will often be active filters. These filters also have active components (amplifiers) in addition to the passive components (*R* and *C*).

The advantage of active filters over passive ones is that active filters can cover a greater frequency range and steep or slopes. Modern hearing instruments (particularly digitally programmable units) all have active filters, but digital hearing instruments rely on signal processors to implement filters. The advantage of digital processing is that any type of filter can be implemented using computational techniques. The filter parameters for different corner frequencies and slopes are contained in the algorithm and implemented computationally when required. This eliminated the need to add components or manually manipulate component values to achieve the required filter performance.

## LOW-PASS FILTER (HIGH CUT)

A low-pass filter allows low frequencies to pass unattenuated through the filter (see Figure 4–2). Since most hearing instruments are lacking in high-frequency gain (too narrow a receiver band), the low-pass filter is mostly used when there is a feedback problem.

However, a low-pass filter can also be of help during a new wearer's acclimatization to the hearing instrument. Since the hearing impaired with a high-frequency loss have not heard the high frequencies for years (or decades), most hearing instruments initially sound too shrill.

The low-pass filter can be used to reduce gain in the higher frequencies, which can make the hearing instrument easier for the new wearer to accept. The frequency response of the hearing instrument can be widened as the wearer becomes accustomed to again being able to hear high-frequency sounds.

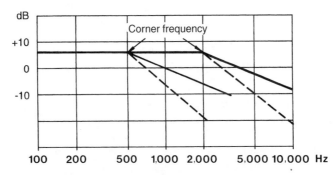

**Figure 4–2.** Low-pass filter response, with adjustable corner frequencies and stop-band slopes. *(Courtesy of Phonak AG.)*

Research has not demonstrated any immediate improvement in speech understanding subsequent to fitting with a hearing instrument with a wide-band frequency response. However, speech understanding scores have been shown to improve significantly after a couple of months of hearing instrument use.

# FILTERING STRATEGIES: ASP, BILL, AND TILL

## BACKGROUND

A common hearing instrument user complaint is that the amplified signal is too noisy. It is, therefore, not surprising that filters are often employed in an attempt to improve the signal-to-noise ratio (SNR) in a hearing instrument. Two fundamentally different approaches are used in noise suppression techniques for hearing instruments: adaptive electronic filtering and directional microphones or beamforming. The most important difference between these two approaches is their position within the signal processing chain. The directional microphone acts on the signal before it enters the hearing instrument's signal-processing path, while the adaptive filter is placed within the signal-processing path. Since the signal entering the hearing instrument contains both the signal of interest and the background noise, it is very difficult for traditional nonadaptive filters to separate these two signals. Identifying and suppressing particular frequency regions of a noise will suppress the same frequency region of the signal of interest and to the same degree. As a result, the SNR can't be improved. Directional microphones, on the other hand, improve the SNR before the combined signal and noise enters the rest of the signal-processing pathway.

## ADAPTIVE ELECTRONIC FILTERING

The term automatic signal processing (ASP) has become synonymous with more recent hearing instruments with level-dependent automatic filtering. Hearing instruments with automatic gain control (AGC) circuits, which were first introduced about fifty years ago, must also be categorized as automatic signal-processing devices. ASP is thus too general a term which does not describe sufficiently the actual properties of the applied signal-processing scheme. Killion et al. (1990) categorized current systems according to their mode of operation. Two initial categories and terms are important to note in this context:

**FFR (Fixed Frequency Response):** This refers to devices with linear filtering.

**LDFR (Level-Dependent Frequency Response):** This refers to devices with nonlinear filtering.

Within the LDFR category, they further defined three subcategories. The most important differentiating criteria is the filtering process that takes place at low-input levels.

**BILL (Bass Increase at Low Level):** This scheme is characterized by a relatively flat frequency response at low-input levels with increasing high-frequency emphasis as the input level increases (see Figure 4–3).

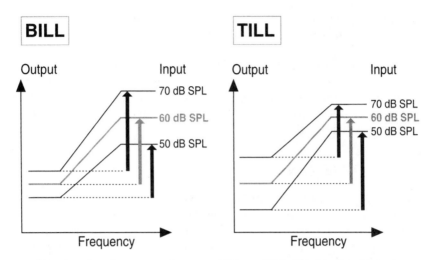

**Figure 4–3.** Level-dependent frequency response BILL vs. TILL: The idealized input/output responses are plotted as a function of frequency for different input levels. As a reference, the 60 dB SPL input response is identical for both processing schemes. Notice that BILL is flatter at low levels than TILL, which is flatter at high levels. *(Courtesy of Phonak AG.)*

**TILL (Treble Increase at Low Level):** High-frequency emphasis occurs at low-input levels with the response becoming flatter at higher input levels (see Figure 4–3).

**PILL (Programmable Increase at Low Level):** The behavior of the frequency response at low- and high-input levels can be programmed.

Thus a PILL can be programmed to act as a BILL, TILL, or even an FFR.

## REFERENCE TO PSYCHOACOUSTICS

Even though the BILL and TILL strategies are conceptually very different from each other, both are plausible approaches considering fundamental psychoacoustics. BILL was developed to counter the upward spread of masking effects associated with a sensorineural hearing loss. There is little evidence, however, to support a solution that offers a constant increase in filter steepness or increase in high-frequency amplification at high-input levels.

The goal behind the development of the TILL strategy was to restore the loudness growth function. In the presence of normal hearing, the equal loudness contours become flatter with increasing input level. TILL instruments attempt to reproduce this phenomenon with the hearing instrument in order to provide pleasant, natural-sounding amplification. On the surface, these two concepts seem to be pulling in entirely different directions. In reality, however, a BILL and a TILL hearing instrument fitted with a vented mold/shell and exposed to moderate input levels will provide similar insertion gain values. Significant differences exist only for low-level input signals. The input/output characteristics of BILL and TILL systems, measured with a composite noise instead of pure tones, show practically the same nonlinear compression characteristics (Fabry, 1991).

The BILL system has been studied thoroughly by a large number of authors. Fabry and Van Tassel (1990) calculated the theoretical effectiveness of a BILL instrument based on the Articulation Index, and verified their results in an evaluative study. They found that an improvement of speech discrimination in speechlike noise could neither be theoretically predicted nor measured in practice.

## INDIVIDUAL IMPROVEMENT

Despite the fact that, on average, no improvement was measured with adaptive filter systems, we must not conclude that these methods are useless for all individuals. First of all, it is important to remember that hearing loss cannot be quantified and classified based on pure-tone threshold data alone. Second, the listening requirements of different users vary significantly. It is also important to analyze several issues that can strongly influence the average results of such studies.

# BASIC SIGNAL-PROCESSING STRATEGIES

## THE AUTOMATIC GAIN CONTROL (AGC) CIRCUIT

AGC circuits alter the amplification as soon as a certain signal level (kneepoint) is reached. As long as these levels are not attained, the AGC functions as a linear amplifier.

If the kneepoint is reached and exceeded the AGC begins to reduce its amplification. → It enters the compression range (see Figure 4–4).

The compression ratio can be predetermined by the hearing instrument designer or it can be made programmable. A compression ratio of 2:1 means that the input signal must be increased by two parts in order to increase the output signal by one part (dB scale).

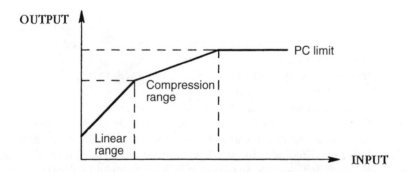

**Figure 4–4.** Input/output function of an AGC amplifier. *(Courtesy of Phonak AG.)*

If the AGC has a very high compression ratio (10:1 or more) then it can be utilized as a limiter.

The dynamic behavior of the compression amplifier is characterized by predetermined time constants for the onset (or attack) of compression and the release from compression. The compression ratio can be determined from the input/output relationship in the steady-state condition (as measured by the standard methods described in Chapter 9). Dynamic AGC activation (e.g., during speech) reduces the compression ratio when attack and release times are too long.

Unlike the peak clipper, the AGC circuit needs time to react. The time it takes the AGC to decrease the gain to the limiting level is called the *attack time*. Once the AGC is in operation and the input SPL is no longer high enough to require limiting, the time it takes for the hearing instrument to resume normal gain function is called the *release time* (see Chapter 9). Attack and release times are not set arbitrarily but are dependent on which functions the AGC possesses—that is, what type of hearing-impairment is to be fitted.

AGC circuits are divided into two types which are designed for different applications: AGCi and AGCo.

## Low-Level Expansion (LLE)

Low-level expansion is a relatively new feature in AGC amplifier circuits. Expansion is the complementary process to compression. While a compression circuit reduces gain as the input level is increased, an expansion circuit increases gain as the input level is increased. Expansion is used specifically in the low-level input region of the I/O curve in order to reduce low-level environmental signals and microphone noise.

The I/O curve of Figure 4–4 shows that a linear amplification region transitions to a compression region when a specific input level (say 60 dB SPL) is exceeded. On the other hand, when LLE is active, reduction of the input level below a preset level (e.g., 40 dB SPL) will cause the linear region to transition to the expansion region of the I/O curve and the I/O relationship becomes steeper than in the linear section. Thus, very low-level input signals receive very little amplification. Hearing instruments with LLE are perceived as very quiet instruments in quiet surroundings.

LLE is extensively used in digital amplifiers along with AGCi and AGCo as well as Wide Dynamic Range Compression (WDRC). It is common to mix these strategies in one amplifier, beginning with LLE for very low inputs, linear amplification for low inputs, AGCi for moderate inputs, and AGCo for loud inputs and output limiting. Peak clipping can also be used to limit the maximum output SPL.

## The Automatic Gain Control Input (AGCi) Circuit

An AGCi is defined as one where the AGC circuit is located before the volume control potentiometer (VC), so that the AGC circuit is activated by the input SPL (see Figure 4–5). The operation of an AGCi circuit is clearly illustrated by its input/output function (Figure 4–6).

In an AGCi circuit, the input SPL required to activate the circuit remains constant even with a reduction in gain via the volume control. Since the AGCi usually has a compression ratio of only 2:1 or 3:1, the maximum output sound pressure must be limited by either a PC or an AGCo with a high compression ratio.

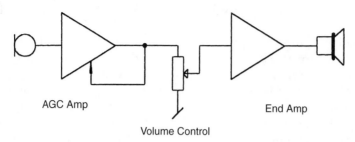

**Figure 4–5.** Schematic block diagram of an AGCi amplifier. The volume control is located after the AGC amplifier block and affects the maximum output of the amplifier. *(Courtesy of Phonak AG.)*

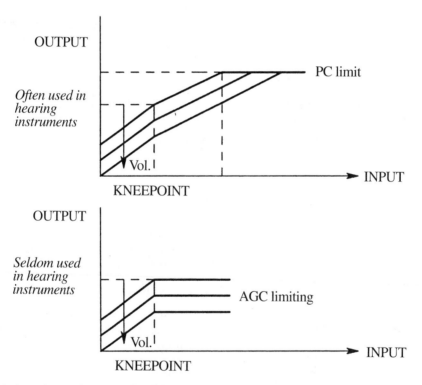

**Figure 4–6.** Input/output functions of AGCi amplifiers. *(Courtesy of Phonak AG.)*

The AGCi (e.g., compression ratio 2:1) is often used in cases where recruitment is a major problem for the wearer. In order to preserve good speech understanding, fast attack and release times are crucial. This means that syllabic compression must be provided which again indicates fast attack and release times. When AGCi is used as a syllabic compressor, attack time should be less than 5 ms and release time less than 30 ms.

The disadvantages of the AGCi utilized in this manner are harmonic distortions at low frequencies and, because of the controlling effects, high noise levels in the hearing instrument (pumping). The AGCi is seldom used today for output limiting since gain reduction via the volume control also reduces the output SPL by the same value.

## Wide Dynamic Range Compression (WDRC)

A special version of the AGCi is the WDRC. Almost all people with cochlear hearing loss have a reduced dynamic range (loudness recruitment). This probably results largely from the loss of a frequency-selective, fast-acting compression mechanism which operates in the normal cochlea. This compression reflects the operation of an active mechanism which depends on the integrity of the outer hair cells. A loss of the outer hair cells therefore has a direct impact on the cochlear mechanics by degrading the active process. This results in an increased threshold for soft sounds and a normal perception of loud sounds. The loudness growth function of such a person is steeper than that of a normal hearing person (see Chapter 12). WDRC compression amplifiers were designed especially for this group of people.

The WDRC is a syllable compressor with fast-attack (<5 ms) and fast-release (<50 ms) times. The input/output function is described in Figure 4–6 (the often-used type). The target of a WDRC circuit is to restore normal loudness perception. Low-level input signals are amplified more than high-level input signals to provide audibility and ensure a comfortable volume level at all times. To achieve this, the kneepoint of the WDRC has to be low (< 60 dB SPL) and the compression ratio should be between 1.5:1 to 3:1 (depending on the hearing loss).

WDRC circuits are designed to allow speech in quiet to be understood over a wide range of sound levels without discomfort and without any need to adjust the volume control on the hearing aid.

The level of the output signal of the hearing instrument is controlled in accordance with the compression factor or compression ratio. For a linear instrument, a 10-dB change in input (e.g., from 50 dB SPL to 60 dB SPL) will produce a 10-dB change in the output. A WDRC instrument with a kneepoint at 50 dB SPL and a compression ratio of 2:1 will produce a 5-dB change at the output for the same input range.

WDRC circuits are beneficial for those patients where loudness tolerance is an issue, but it can also produce the following disadvantages:

- ▼ The increase in gain for soft sounds can increase the ambient noise level in quiet, resulting in a complaint of "circuit noise."
- ▼ The increase in gain for soft sounds can increase the potential for feedback, especially when combined with large vents.

## The Automatic Gain Control Output (AGCo)

In an AGCo instrument the AGC circuit is positioned after the volume control (see Figure 4–7).

A characteristic of an AGCo circuit is that the kneepoint of the AGCo moves to the right (greater input SPL) when amplification is reduced with the volume control. The result is a large range of linear amplification as is evident in Figure 4–8.

Today, the AGCo is largely used for output limiting (compression ratio > 10:1) which has the advantage of little distortion even at maximum output sound pressure levels. In other words, in a hearing instrument with an AGCo as output limiter, there is never more than 10% distortion under any operating condition.

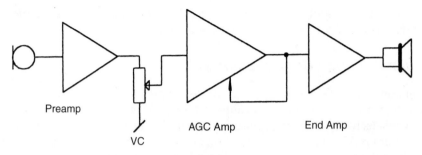

**Figure 4–7.** Schematic block diagram of an AGCo amplifier. The volume control is located before the AGC amplifier block and does not affect the maximum control of the amplifier. *(Courtesy of Phonak AG.)*

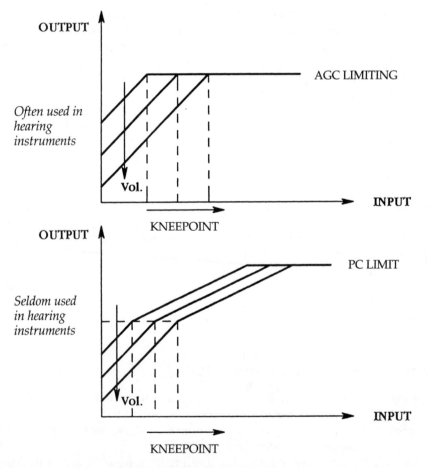

**Figure 4–8.** Input output functions of AGCo amplifiers. *(Courtesy of Phonak AG.)*

When used for this kind of output limiting, the AGCo should have an attack time of < 10 ms, and a release time of about 200 ms. However, this combination of attack and release times leads to the so-called "pumping effect," which occurs when the background noise level increases during speech pauses as the compression is released. To prevent this, an adaptive release time is used which can range from 50 ms to 1.5 s depending on how long the AGC circuit is activated.

An AGCo with a compression ratio as low as 2:1 or 3:1 is now seldom used.

More complex solutions can be found in systems where more than one AGC network is used, or different AGC systems are used in different filter bands. These are called multiBand or multichannel compression, and they are routinely implemented in digital hearing instruments.

## OUTPUT LIMITING

Output limiting plays an important role in a fitting. It prevents the maximum output sound pressure from exceeding the discomfort level of the wearer. There are a number of different ways of limiting the maximum output sound pressure. The decision as to which method of output limiting is most appropriate in a given case must be made by the hearing health care professional together with the hearing-impaired individual.

There is no single type of limiter that is optimal for every kind of hearing loss.

### Peak Clipping and Soft Peak Clipping

In the block diagram (Figure 4–9) is a simple presentation of output limiting by means of peak clipping (PC). In this context PC is a commonly used abbreviation for peak clipping. It should not be confused with the abbreviation PC when it denotes a personal computer.

A peak clipper, as its name suggests, "clips" the peaks of the signal that exceed a certain voltage (see Figure 4–10).

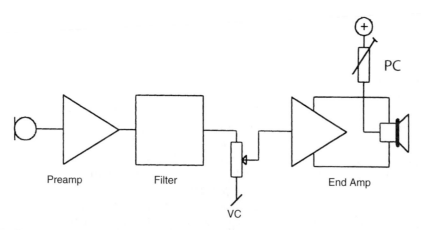

**Figure 4–9.** Block diagram of a peak clipping (PC) limiter in a Class B amplifier. *(Courtesy of Phonak AG.)*

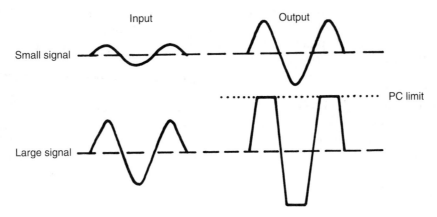

**Figure 4–10.** Operation of a PC on small and large signals. *(Courtesy of Phonak AG.)*

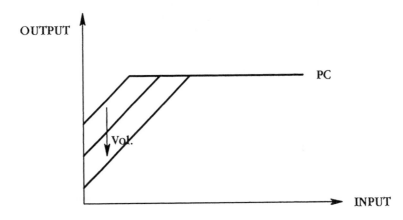

**Figure 4–11.** Input/output function with PC output limiting. *(Courtesy of Phonak AG.)*

Limiting of the output sound pressure by peak clipping leads to a large amount of distortion.

Since the peak clipper works very quickly, there is virtually no delay in the effect. PC is suitable for the hearing-impaired wearer with a limited dynamic range (requiring a great deal of gain, but having a relatively low uncomfortable loudness level).

The operation of a PC is shown in the input/output function (as shown in Figure 4–11).

The maximum sound pressure never exceeds the limit set by the PC. The PC limit is not changed by reducing gain with the volume control.

The PC limit is not changed when the overall hearing instrument gain is reduced with the volume control. As the gain is reduced by a given amount, the input sound pressure level must be increased by the same amount before peak clipping occurs and the hearing instrument goes into saturation. The result is that the kneepoint on the input/output graph moves to the right (greater input level).

**Advantages and disadvantages of a PC:**

▼ Peak clipping is the means of output limitation allowing the greatest possible amplification. (There is no gain reduction when limiting is reached.)
▼ Acts instantaneously.

▼ Results in a great deal of distortion.

## SOFT PEAK CLIPPING

The expression "soft peak clipping" is not defined. Probably every hearing instrument manufacturer has a different definition.

The expression "soft peak clipper" usually refers to a system with a peak clipper and a mechanism to reduce harmonic distortion. There are two common ways to achieve this goal: diode compression and slow acting compression.

## DIODE COMPRESSION

A peak clipper with diodes in the feedback of the output amplifier, as shown in Figure 4–12, reduces second harmonic distortion. Such a circuit could be called "diode compression" or "soft peak clipping." The diodes are connected in an "antiparallel" manner across the final stage. The diodes limit the signal to a maximum of one diode voltage (300 mV for Schottky diodes).

Diode compression is often used with Class A output amplifiers. It replaces the practice of using a resistor in series with the receiver. Using a resistor results in asymmetrical peak clipping with a great deal of second harmonic distortion, and poor speech understanding. Diode compression produces symmetrical peak clipping with much reduced amounts of second harmonic distortion.

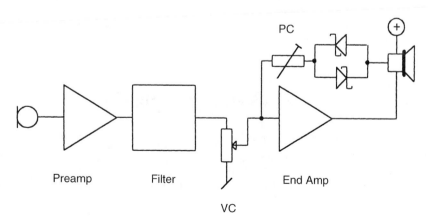

**Figure 4–12.** Block diagram for a diode compression limiting amplifier. *(Courtesy of Phonak AG.)*

## SLOW-ACTING COMPRESSION

The combination of an automatic volume control (AVC) and a peak clipper (PC) will also reduce harmonic distortion. The AVC has a slow attack and a slow release time. For fast signals, the AVC has no influence on the signal, and so maximum gain is added for speech signals. In a noisy environment, all signals become louder and the high input activates the AVC in a soft peak clipping system. This AVC reduces the gain of the hearing instrument to a level of output that is limited to 6 dB below clipping. Enough headroom exists again for higher speech signals. With a simple PC, all signals (noise floor and speech signal) would go into saturation and produce a lot of harmonic distortions.

The "soft PC" reduces the harmonic distortion, especially in noisy environments, and gives the user a more comfortable and better sound quality.

## SUMMARY

1. The strategies described in this chapter have been used for many years in analog instruments.
2. These signal-processing strategies are still of fundamental importance in digital hearing instruments. They are not implemented as circuits constructed from discrete components, but in the form of numerical calculations in a microprocessor controlled by an algorithm.
3. Different types of amplification strategies were developed in order to meet the individual requirements of different hearing loss configurations.
4. The audiogram alone, while a good indicator, will not always predict the best signal-processing strategy for a specific hearing loss.
5. Different signal-processing strategies are incorporated in some analog instruments and in many digital instruments.
6. Multiple processing strategies allow the user to select the best strategy for a specific acoustic environment.
7. Nonlinear processing strategies are designed to best meet the properties of nonlinear loudness growth sensation.

## REVIEW QUESTIONS

1. In an AGC instrument, the VC can be located either before or after the AGC. This produces either an AGCo or an AGCi.
   A. What is the difference for the end user?
   B. Describe the different functionality that occurs during a volume change.

2. An AGCi instrument has a compression ratio of 3:1 and a threshold of 55 dB SPL. The instrument has a gain of 40 dB in the linear part of the input/output (I/O) curve. There is a PC at 110 dB SPL for the MPO control.
   A. Make a drawing of the I/O curve.
   B. The gain is reduced by 10 dB with the VC. Draw the new I/O curve.
   C. Draw the I/O curve when the PC is reduced by 10 dB.

3. What is (are) the advantage(s) of a diode compression limiter?
   A. The large fitting range                                    A ☐
   B. The soft transition from linear to limiting                B ☐
   C. The reduction of the second harmonic distortion            C ☐
   D. The reduction of the third harmonic distortion             D ☐

4. What kind of limiting system has a relation between maximum MPO and the VC setting?
   A. ASP                                                        A ☐
   B. AGCi                                                       B ☐
   C. PC                                                         C ☐
   D. AGCo                                                       D ☐

5. Which relation of compression/limiting system and I/O curve is correct?
   A. X,1                                                        A ☐
   B. Y,2                                                        B ☐
   C. Z,2                                                        C ☐
   D. Y,3                                                        D ☐

6. A frequency response curve has a second-order, high-pass filter with a corner frequency at 800 Hz and a first-order, low-pass filter with a corner frequency at 5,000 Hz.
   A. Draw the frequency response curve.
   B. Draw the frequency response curve after the high-pass corner frequency is moved one octave higher.

7. List all the output limiting systems you know. What are their features?

# CHAPTER 5

# Digital Hearing Instruments

## INTRODUCTION

Digital signal-processing technology has found applications in almost every industry and the hearing aid industry is no exception (Murray and Hanson, 1992). Advances in IC technology have overcome the physical limitations of small size, low current consumption, and low operating voltage requirements and made possible powerful digital-signal processor (DSP) platforms for hearing instrument application. Now DSP-based hearing instruments can employ many well-known digital signal- processing techniques initially developed for communication, speech processing, radar, and sonar systems. More sophisticated digital platforms and more advanced digital signal-processing technologies will continue to be developed and implemented in order to advance hearing instrument performance. This chapter addresses DSP technologies and applications that relate to digital hearing instruments today and their ongoing development in the future. Three aspects of DSP are of interest: the digital signal-processor or the hardware that runs the digital signal-processing algorithm, the digital signal- processing algorithms that are at the core of digital processing applications in hearing instruments, and the future development of intelligent digital hearing instruments.

## DIGITAL SIGNAL-PROCESSING TECHNOLOGIES FOR HEARING INSTRUMENTS

Digital signal-processing technology has experienced a rapid evolution over the past three decades. Over this period, DSP technology has evolved from its origins in Fast Fourier Transforms (FFTs), analog-to-digital (A/D) and digital-to-analog (D/A) conversions, and general digital filter design to a wide range of applications in many areas such as: 1) speech encoding and decoding for telecommunications, 2) array signal processing for radar and sonar; 3) spectral analysis, 4) multimedia processing, 5) as well as appliances used in daily life and home entertainment. Many real-time applications require real-time processing of continuous flow data but general-purpose processors often limit the efficient implementation of digital signal-processing technologies in these applications. Special-purpose signal processors needed to be designed for the complex and computationally demanding digital signal processing of continuous flow data.

The hearing instrument industry fell behind other industries in applying digital technology because these special-purpose processors could not meet the small size requirement nor operate at the power levels available from hearing instrument batteries. During the last decade, however, practical low-voltage, low-power silicon technology became available. Now, advanced digital signal-processing technologies originally implemented in different fields have found powerful applications in hearing instruments.

## DSP HARDWARE FOR HEARING INSTRUMENTS

In a typical DSP-based hearing aid system, a preamplifier circuit and an analog-to-digital (A/D) converter acquire the analog signal from a microphone and convert it into a digital format. After applying the required correction for a specific hearing loss, a digital-to-analog (D/A) converter and post-amplifier convert the processed digital signal back into analog form to drive the loudspeaker that delivers the processed acoustic signal to the patient. Usually, these conditioning circuits, A/D and D/A, are integrated with the DSP and memory chips and are often packaged as a ceramic substrate-based hybrid amplifier. It is also possible to integrate the A/D and the conditioning circuit into the microphone (i.e., digital microphone) and to integrate the D/A and signal adjustment circuit into the receiver (i.e., digital receiver). A typical DSP-based hearing aid system with two microphone inputs is shown in Figure 5–1.

It is now possible to use DSP amplifiers in hearing instruments because of continued progress in feature size reduction for integrated circuits (ICs). Feature size is the smallest dimension that can be produced during the IC manufacturing process. The small feature size, which allows more semiconductor devices to be integrated into a given area of the IC, has led to a sufficiently high device density on a silicon chip no more than 2 or 3 mm on each side. It is also fortunate that devices with a smaller feature size require less current to operate. The evolution from a 5 μm (μm = micrometer = one millionth of a meter) feature size to a 0.13 μm feature size not only increases device density, and therefore increases computational power,

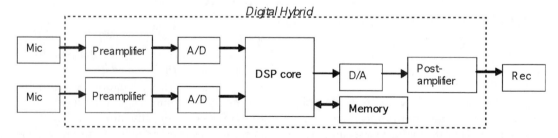

**Figure 5–1.** Block diagram for a typical DSP-based digital hearing instrument. *(Courtesy of Unitron Hearing Ltd.)*

but also reduces the current consumption in a given area of silicon chip. These factors have made digital ICs in hearing instruments practical.

For hearing instruments, the requirements of a DSP digital hybrid amplifier are:

1. Its physical size must be small enough to fit into the hearing aid housing, usually less than 20 mm² footprint and less than 3 mm thick.
2. The working voltage of the DSP has to be very low (1.0 ~ 1.3V) so that a hearing aid battery can drive the DSP system.
3. The current consumption of the DSP hybrid amplifier has to be very low (usually less than 1.0 mA) so that a standard battery can drive a hearing aid for 100 hours or more.

The first digital hearing aids were based on low-power application specific integrated circuit (ASIC) DSP cores. ASIC DSPs first made it possible to apply digital signal-processing technologies in hearing instruments, but they had limited flexibility. Long lead times are required to develop the digital hardware and, once the design is done, it is difficult to modify its functionality. However, since the design is optimized for a specific application, the DSP could be very efficient in performing dedicated signal-processing tasks such as converting signals from the time domain to the frequency domain using fast fourier transforms (FFTs), the inverse operation from the frequency to the time domain (iFFTs), and the application of gain and finite impulse response (FIR) filtering. Although these ASIC systems have a hardwired, or fixed, functionality, they do allow parametric changes via a programming interface so that parameters such as gain, frequency response and compression characteristics of the device can be optimized to best suit an individual's hearing loss. In essence, digital hearing instruments (with the exception of digital hearing instruments with trimmer controls) are also digitally programmable hearing instruments, although the opposite is not true.

The first commercially successful digital hearing instruments were introduced in 1996. At that time, the microprocessor was dedicated to a fixed instruction set, hardwired into the microprocessor and its memory. These electronic circuits in these devices were primarily of the ASIC type. Their operation could, however, be programmed by setting specific parameters in the chip as was the case for analog programmable hearing instruments.

More recently, software controlled, or quasi-open platform DSP systems with low-voltage and low-power consumption have been developed. These can run various digital signal-processing strategies, implemented in the form of algorithms. Additional technological advances now make it possible to overwrite old algorithms with new algorithms to improve or totally change the performance of the hearing instrument.

The time required for technology development and algorithm upgrades can be significantly shorter with the use of the open platform DSP system compared with ASIC-style fixed function hardware (Niellsen, 1998). However, completely open platform DSPs are usually designed for general-purpose digital signal processing. These are very flexible but not necessarily efficient enough, in terms of power consumption, processing power, and speed, for application in hearing instruments.

Digital signal processing for hearing aids usually requires computationally intensive operations such as time-to-frequency transformations, frequency-to-time transformations, and various types of filtering. These operations consume a large portion of the available DSP resource when they are performed exclusively by the DSP core.

The new generation of DSP for hearing instruments integrates an open platform programmable DSP core with dedicated ASIC DSP blocks. These dedicated blocks handle the repetitive computations of specific signal-processing tasks in the most efficient way. In this way, it is possible to meet the computational requirements within the power consumption constraints imposed by the hearing instrument environment. In addition, the advantage of open platform programmable DSP designs, namely the flexibility for design and algorithm upgrades, is maintained.

## DSP ALGORITHMS FOR HEARING INSTRUMENTS

Digital signal-processing technologies such as adaptive filtering, noise reduction, echo cancellation, and array signal processing (beamforming technology) have been widely used in digital hearing instruments as in other industry applications. In hearing instruments, digital signal processing for signal enhancement and hearing loss compensation can be implemented in the time domain, the frequency domain, or both. Therefore, time-to-frequency ($T{\rightarrow}F$) and frequency-to-time ($F{\rightarrow}T$) transforms such as fast fourier transforms or filter banks are usually required to convert the signal between the time domain and the frequency domain (see Figure 5–2).

Many adaptive processes can be integrated into hearing instruments to compensate for the detrimental influence of the acoustic environment in which the instrument has to operate, thereby maximizing the performance and benefit of digital hearing instruments for the hearing-impaired individual (Edwards et al., 1998). Major signal-processing algorithms such as noise reduction, adaptive hearing compensation, beamforming, and feedback cancelling are discussed in the following sections.

## SIGNAL PROCESSING FOR THE IMPAIRED EAR

Any fitting formula can predict target gains the hearing instrument should deliver at a number of frequencies for a specific hearing loss. Unfortunately, two individuals with identical audiograms may not perform equally well with the same gain prescription.

The problems associated with hearing loss are far more complex than the simple elevated hearing thresholds depicted in standard audiograms. Compensating for elevated hearing

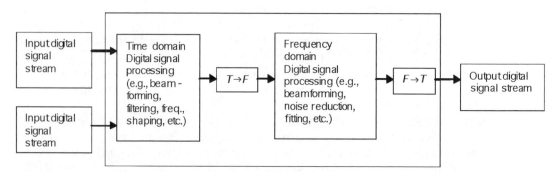

**Figure 5–2.** Digital signal processing in a DSP-based hearing instrument. *(Courtesy of Unitron Hearing Ltd.)*

thresholds is essential to restore audibility, but amplification alone is not enough to optimally compensate for a loss in speech understanding.

Therefore, hearing instruments must be even more sophisticated if they are to help the user take full advantage of residual hearing. They need to provide an undistorted and noise-free amplified signal to the impaired ear in order to minimize masking of important speech components. Hearing instrument users often complain that they hear well in quiet but not in noisy surroundings. The first-order effect in a noisy environment is that speech consonants, which are less intense than most vowel sounds, are masked by noise and are therefore not heard.

An important objective of any hearing instrument is to suppress the noise component and to amplify the desired component of a noisy signal. In most cases, the desired signal is speech and in some cases it is music. Digital hearing instruments offer new capabilities in this area with digital signal processing.

The increase in signal-processing complexity necessary to achieve such improvements can be realized in digital hearing instruments with appropriate hardware and software. This chapter explores a number of signal-processing features which are often combined with the traditional amplification strategies described in Chapter 4.

Damage to hearing can occur in any one of several areas of the ear. Damage to the outer and middle ear often causes a conductive loss which means that the signal strength reaching the middle ear is reduced. This type of loss is usually treated effectively with amplification of the types discussed in Chapter 4.

Damage to the inner ear, usually referred to as a sensorineural loss, can also cause attenuation of signal strength but various types of signal distortion can also be present. The inner ear contains rows of inner and outer hair cells which play an essential role in converting mechanical vibrations into electrical information (see Chapter 12, "Audiology and Psychoacoustics"). Damage to inner and outer hair cells usually causes a loss in sensitivity (which causes signal attenuation), a loss of dynamic range, and frequency selectivity (Moore, 2000). Hearing aids do not deal uniformly well with this type of loss.

The potential for correcting this wide variety of complex deficiencies in an impaired ear has improved significantly with the introduction of digital signal processing in hearing instruments, but much remains to be done in diagnosing as well as in correcting these deficiencies.

Sensitivity loss correction has traditionally been the main area of concern for analog instruments. These instruments provide frequency-specific amplification to reconstruct a preferred loudness level as required by commonly used fitting formulas such as the 1/2 gain rule, NAL, POGO, DSL, etc. (See Chapter 11 for definitions and detailed descriptions of these fitting formulas.)

Nonlinear amplification is quite effectively applied to remedy abnormal growth of loudness. Level-dependent compression, as described in Chapter 4, is a commonly used amplification strategy. A variety of input-output curves has been possible in analog instruments for some time, and these are also applied in digital instruments to achieve audibility for quiet sounds without undue discomfort for loud sounds (Baechler et al., 1997). Digital instruments can employ multiband amplification more effectively than analog instruments, and this is routinely done as required for the particular hearing loss. Proper choices must be made for the time constants of the dynamic compression as these do affect the overall sound quality of the amplified signal.

Binaural loss is usually corrected with hearing instruments fitted to both ears, which can be effective. But an optimal binaural hearing correction requires communication between the processors on either ear in order to achieve effective spatial hearing and localization. Noise reduction is an important element in this type of processing.

Central processor damage is difficult to diagnose and extremely difficult to correct with a hearing instrument. Noise reduction algorithms, directional microphones, and adaptive sound scene adaptation can all contribute to a solution for this problem.

These factors and loss of frequency and temporal discrimination, sensitivity to noise, and abnormal growth of loudness sensation require tools and methods that have only recently become available to hearing instrument developers and health care professionals with the advent of digital technology for hearing instruments.

Hearing instruments can now be designed to deal with more of the elements of hearing loss than ever before. No longer does a designer have to add components to an amplifier to increase or change functionality. Instead, functionality is now determined by the computational capacity of the small computer or microprocessor that has become an important component in the digital hearing instrument. Functionality of these systems is determined not by manipulating electronic components but by manipulating the set of sequenced instructions in the algorithm that are performed by the microprocessor or digital signal processor.

## WHAT IS DIGITAL SIGNAL PROCESSING?

Digital signal processing (DSP) is about numbers. Digital signal processors are extremely powerful calculators. DSP is the mathematics, the algorithms, and the techniques used to manipulate signals after they have been converted into a digital format. Before the calculations can begin, the everyday analog acoustic events are converted into numerically coded representations of these events. This means that the infinite resolution of analog signals, that are continuous in amplitude and time, is converted to a discrete sequence of numbers. This process of sampling the analog signal magnitude at a point in time and converting it to a number is performed with an analog-to-digital converter (ADC). Figure 5–3 shows the process of analog-to-digital (A/D) conversion.

Figure 5–3(a) represents an analog signal, such as the electrical output signal produced by a microphone. Time is shown on the horizontal axis and amplitude on the vertical axis. It is clear that this analog signal is continuous in amplitude and in time. The ADC performs a series of voltage measurements at discrete time intervals to capture the rapidly changing rise and fall of the electric waveform, as shown in Figure 5–3(b).

At each of these points in time the amplitude is quantized, or converted, to the closest numerical value available in the digital representation. Curve (c) shows the typical discrete amplitude-discrete time digital signal. The equivalent (digital) numerical values for the original analog signal are shown along the x-axis of curve (c). The numerical values use a binary numbering system, the numerical system used in digital computers and digital signal processors.

The temporal aspect of resolution is referred to as the sample rate and is expressed as a frequency in Hertz (Hz). The sample rate denotes the number of samples taken during one second. The digitizer resolution for amplitude is characterized in terms of quantization steps. To store the information in digital format a fixed number of binary digits (bits) is used. The number of bits (i.e., the width of a word of data) used during digital processing determines the dynamic range and signal to noise ratio. Note that four bits of information are contained in each data word in Figure 5–3.

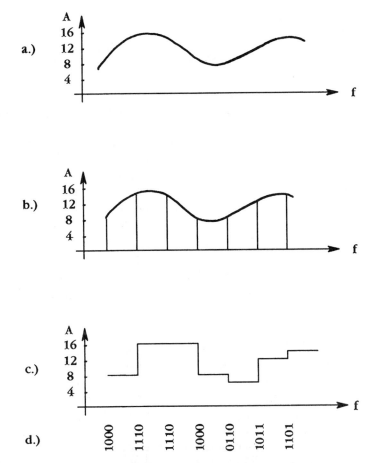

**a.)**

**b.)**

**c.)**

**d.)** 1000  1110  1110  1000  0110  1011  1101

**Figure 5–3.** Four stages of analog-to-digital conversion: a) an analog signal continuous in time and magnitude, b) analog signal sampled in time, c) signal converted to discrete levels of amplitude, and d) binary values of discrete amplitudes at the sampling intervals. *(Courtesy of Phonak AG.)*

Every decimal number that represents an analog quantity like a voltage or a current can be represented as a sequence of binary digits. The following decimal numbers can be represented with three binary bits.

| Decimal | 0 | 1 | 2 | 3 | 4 | 5 | 6 | 7 |
|---|---|---|---|---|---|---|---|---|
| Binary | 000 | 001 | 010 | 011 | 100 | 101 | 110 | 111 |

There are $2 \times 2 \times 2 = 2^3 = 8$ different values from 0 to 7. In other words, a three-bit analog-to-digital converter would assign one of eight binary values to an analog voltage. If the maximum analog amplitude is 1.0 V, the resolution of the converter is 1.0 V/8=0.125 V. For example, an analog signal amplitude of 0.125 V converts to a binary value of 001 and 0.250 V converts to a binary value of 010. On the other hand, 0.150 V converts to the closest binary value, namely 001, the same binary value that was assigned to 0.125 V. When this binary value, 001, is converted back to decimal, the result is 0.125, which is clearly different from the initial value of 0.150. The error of 0.025 appears as noise in the output.

On the other hand, a sixteen-bit ADC operating on the same 1.0-V signal would have a resolution of $2^{16}$ = 64,536 steps in amplitude, and will assign unique digital values to analog quantities that differ by as little as 0.0154 mV.

A small number of quantization levels results in insufficient smoothness compared to the analog signal. This lack of smoothness introduces noise that is called quantization noise.

In general, a one-bit increase of the data word width doubles the number of levels the ADC can discriminate, or for a given resolution, the ADC can convert a signal of twice the amplitude, or a signal increase of 6 dB. The total dynamic range of an ADC is therefore given by six times the number of bits. Some examples are given below.

| Data word width | 8 bit | 12 bit | 16 bit | 20 bit | 22 bit |
|---|---|---|---|---|---|
| Max. dynamic range | 48 dB | 72 dB | 96 dB | 120 dB | 132 dB |

Digital systems with complex mathematical operations can perform these operations using either fixed-point or floating-point arithmetic. The former usually uses positive or negative whole numbers like −3, −2, −1, 0, 1, 2, 3, . . . The problem with fixed-point arithmetic is that all numbers are represented with the same number of binary digits. If two big numbers of the same range are subtracted, the difference is a much smaller number. Further calculations with this small number have a smaller precision since the number of significant digits is reduced. These problems do not occur in numerical calculations that use floating-point numbers. Floating-point numbers use a scientific notation with a mantissa and an exponent to represent a numerical value. For example, the number 434,485,200 becomes $4.344852 \times 10^8$ in scientific notation. The mantissa is 4.344852 and the exponent is 8. In digital floating-point notation the exponent is not raised to the power of ten but to the power of two. While floating-point arithmetic produces more accurate results, floating-point DSPs are much more complex and consume more power than fixed-point DSPs.

The speed of the sample rate directly determines the frequency range of audio signal processing. This constraint is known as the Nyquist rule, or sampling theorem. To avoid a kind of digital noise called "aliasing errors," the sampling rate must be at least twice the intended frequency range. Aliasing is perceived as distortion in the analog output signal. Hence, to have a bandwidth of 10 kHz for the audio signals, the sampling rate has to be at least 20 kHz (20,000 samples per second) to avoid distortion due to aliasing. An analog antialias filter is usually placed before the A/D conversion process to ensure that the analog signal components above 10 kHz are attenuated.

Another way to overcome the limitation of the Nyquist rule is the use of a much higher sampling rate than would be suggested from the Nyquist rule. This procedure is called oversampling and has the advantage that the antialiasing filter requirement is much reduced or no

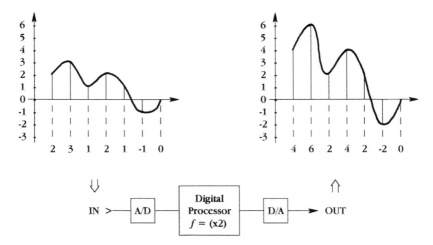

**Figure 5–4.** Conversion with signal processing. *(Courtesy of Phonak AG.)*

antialiasing filter may be needed at all. A modern design of such an A/D converter with over-sampling is called Sigma-Delta converter.

After reconversion of digital signals back to analog, a similar problem occurs that requires an anti-imaging filter or some other means to eliminate unwanted frequencies from the re-conversion process.

Transducer technology can be used to reduce extra components, such as a dedicated digital-to-analog converter (DAC). In this case, the digital amplifier contains a Class D output stage. The properties of the Class D output stage can be exploited since its operation is based on digital principles. The fast stream of switches can be modulated directly by the DSP to produce a pulse-width modulated (PWM) output signal (see Figure 2-32), or a digital-to-digital (D/D) conversion. The PWM signal is used to drive a zero bias receiver directly.

Figure 5–4 shows an example of the conversion of an analog signal into a digital one with additional signal processing. The numerical values are multiplied by a factor two and again converted into an analog signal.

The result of this multiplication in digital signal-processing produces an amplification of the input signal. In this way, complicated (nonlinear) signal changes are made possible by special computer algorithms. A further advantage is that the algorithms can be changed during signal processing. This means that the arithmetic functions adjust to the input or output signal (adaptive signal processing). Adaptive signal processing is used, for example, in feedback suppression in order to be able to react optimally under changing conditions (e.g., hand on the hearing instrument, chewing).

## WHY DIGITAL HEARING INSTRUMENTS?

Digital technology provides the hearing instrument designer a new set of tools to attempt to provide solutions to problems that have, to date, remained unsolved (Fabry, 1998). These tools are algorithms designed to run in real-time on the processor in the hearing instrument amplifier and can contribute, in addition to basic amplification, to providing clean signals free of noise, ensure listener comfort in all acoustic conditions, and provide effective localization and superior signal quality. In particular, digital technology enables the hearing instrument specialist to also begin to develop solutions for the nonlinear problems caused by damage to the inner ear, the auditory nerve, and the central processor in the cerebral cortex.

## TECHNOLOGY

The capabilities of analog technology are practically exhausted. Future potential lies in digital technology. As an example, in the next ten years, analog circuits could become about 20% smaller on the basis of possible technological improvements. In contrast, the degree of miniaturization possible with digital circuits is much greater.

## COMPLEXITY

Increasing computational power in the hearing instruments means greater flexibility and performance capabilities. Because digital technology enables more complex signal processing than analog technology, its advantages grow ever more apparent. While some improvements for simpler hearing instruments can be accomplished using analog technology (e.g., less power consumption), more complex instruments must be of digital construction. In fact, some solutions are simply not possible with analog technology (or only at enormous expense).

# DIGITAL HEARING INSTRUMENT FEATURES

Various sophisticated and innovative concepts can be realized by digital signal-processing techniques. The performance of hearing instruments will not be measured any longer by the number of AGC channels or the type of compression. We have to get used to the fact that these classical terms are not suited to describing new signal-processing concepts for the hearing impaired.

Basic psychoacoustical knowledge such as loudness perception or spectral masking can be described by mathematical equations and models. These models should be applied for controlling the gain of hearing instruments. Innovative control systems, such as inverse loudness models, will likely be implemented and provide optimal use of the residual area of audibility for the hearing impaired.

Physical or technical methods can suppress either environmental noises or annoying acoustical feedback whistling. The basic building blocks of these concepts are adaptive filters and control systems modifying the filter coefficients according to specific criteria such as: speech—present or not; or feedback whistling—yes or no.

Directional microphones or array processing can significantly enhance speech intelligibility in background noise. Today's solutions could go further if the size of the device were not an issue. We must still solve cosmetic issues to realize more efficient array processors.

# NOISE CANCELLERS

## *Noise Cancelling Using a Single Microphone*

Hearing instruments typically contain one single microphone. Even in the case of a dual microphone directional array, the microphones are so close together that using one of these microphones as a reference microphone in a noise reduction algorithm produces insignificant levels of noise reduction. The useful signals and the disturbing background noise are both present at the input of the whole system and a separation of these signals afterwards generally is very difficult.

A popular approach to reduce background noise is spectral subtraction. This technique estimates the noise spectrum N during speech pauses which is then subtracted from the spectrum of the noisy speech (S + N) as shown in Figure 5–5.

The subtraction is performed by a digital adaptive filter. This filter continuously adapts to the noise spectrum. Spectral subtraction assumes that the time intervals where the noise is constant are longer than those of speech. But the estimation of the noise spectrum is not perfect. The resulting processing artifacts are known as musical noise. Recent research efforts are concentrated on the reduction of this processing noise.

For narrowband noise such as car noise, it can give significant improvements in signal-to-noise ratio (SNR). Especially when low-frequency noise is suppressed, the speech intelligibility can be increased because of a reduced masking effect. If the spectrum of the speech signal and the noise are very similar, which naturally is the case for speechlike noise (party noise), the spectral subtraction only gives limited improvements in signal quality.

Generally, most noise reduction techniques with one microphone reduce the perceived noisiness or annoyance for most test subjects. This is a valuable benefit. Hence, it is worthwhile to integrate such an algorithm into a modern hearing instrument to increase the ease of listening.

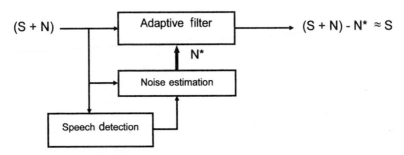

**Figure 5–5.** The principle of spectral subtraction for noise cancelling. Noise is estimated during speech pauses, between syllables and words. S denotes the useful speech signal, N represents the unwanted noise. The algorithm therefore includes a speech detection function. The spectrum of the noise that is estimated during the speech detection pauses is subtracted from the overall spectrum of the noisy signal. The resulting spectrum is an estimate of the useful speech signal alone. *(Courtesy of Phonak AG.)*

The essence of the noise-reduction techniques above lies in the separation of speech and noise. This can be achieved in several possible ways briefly described next:

- ▼ **Speech detection.** Speech pauses can be labelled with speech detection algorithms. The noise spectrum is estimated during these pauses. Because the estimate is derived from past data, the method is sensitive to fluctuations of the noise. If the noise spectrum is changing too quickly over time, the estimate of the current noise spectrum becomes erroneous. This situation often occurs in a group of different competing talkers. Speech detection can be accomplished in different ways. Generally, all detection algorithms identify certain robust features of speech such as voiced parts and plosives.
- ▼ **Temporal envelope.** In some acoustic environments, the noise level changes much more slowly over time than do the amplitude modulations of speech. This provides a lot of useful information. Thus, the minima of the envelope of the noisy speech signal determine the level of the quasi-stationary background noise. For the calculation of the envelope, a time constant of 25 ms appears to be appropriate.
- ▼ **Statistical estimation.** The time characteristic of a speech signal can be described with frequency-dependent level statistics or histograms. The histograms of clean and noisy speech clearly differ from each other, allowing an identification of the noise spectrum after a sufficiently long observation period.

## Comfort in Quiet

At low signal levels, nonlinear hearing instruments usually provide maximum gain. This is acceptable as long as the amplified signals are desirable. In many situations, we are in relatively quiet environments, like living rooms or in an office, where the average background sound level is typically below 45 dB SPL and no verbal communication takes place. AGC amplifiers tend to increase the gain to a maximum, amplifying the background noises to a disturbing level. This behavior is not desired and hearing instrument users will hesitate to wear their instruments or will turn them off.

Obviously, there is a need for noise suppression in situations with background noise only. Under such conditions, the amplification should be reduced automatically to *soft*, mapping the environmental noise level close to the hearing threshold, and thus making it inaudible. A well-designed noise canceling system must react appropriately in quiet conditions with background noise only, as well as in loud environments.

A robust speech/no speech detector is essential for this task. The signal processing entails a complex intelligence to cope with everyday situations. If somebody starts speaking in a quiet environment, the hearing instrument must recover from *soft* and immediately produce the amount of gain required for understanding speech. If the talker stops, the gain has to remain high for a while and should not fall back to *soft* abruptly. Level hysteresis or a long release time for the gain control will guarantee the listener's acceptance and comfort of hearing.

Although a sophisticated automatic system can cope more or less with the scenario described above, the hearing instrument user should be able to interrupt the automatic process in situations where he or she really wants to listen to the background sound. The hearing instrument, however, cannot make this decision for the user.

# BEAMFORMERS

An important application of adaptive algorithms to hearing aids is in the area of beamformers. Whereas a fixed beamformer consists of at least two microphones with fixed directivity, in an adaptive beamformer the microphone directivity characteristics automatically change so that noise coming from different directions can be optimally suppressed.

Because directional microphones are not practical in all arbitrary listening situations, it is important to allow for an omnidirectional microphone response if desired. Fixed and adaptive beamformers are described in more detail in the following sections.

## Time-Invariant or Fixed Beamformers

The simplest form of array processing is the delay and sum method where the microphone signals are weighted, delayed, and subsequently summed to build the array output. The delays are chosen in such a way that the signal from the desired direction is maximally amplified relative to signals incident from other directions. The directionality of the array can be visualized in a polar diagram or be described with the directivity index (DI). Examples are given in Figure 2–12. The directivity index is the ratio of the array output power due to sound from the desired direction and the average array output power due to sound from all other directions.

As an example, consider a simple array consisting of two omnidirectional microphones. If the internal delay of one microphone is equal to the time required for sound to travel from one microphone port to the other, then the polar diagram has a cardioid shape (first-order array). The directivity index of this cardioid is 4.8 dB over a relatively large frequency band and the sensitivity of this array in the target direction decreases by 6 dB/octave for low frequencies. Compared to the conventional directional microphone, the main advantage of the double microphone array is the possibility of switching the directionality on or off electrically just by activating or deactivating one of the two microphones.

An advantage of a digital realization with a digital delay in a dual microphone array over the analog realization of the delay is the easier adjustment of the delay and sensitivity of the two microphones. Also, tolerances of electronic components do not play a role.

## Time-Variant or Adaptive Beamformers

Adaptive beamformers adapt their directional pattern to the current acoustic environment. A fixed time-invariant beamformer is most appropriate in situations where background noises come from many different directions simultaneously, whereas arrays with adaptive processing are better suited for cancelling a limited number of strong directional interferences.

In many situations, it is possible to separate $n$ signals from $n$ different directions with $n$ microphones. Since a particular direction is defined to be the desired direction (usually the front), the adaptive array with $n$ microphones can localize and cancel out background noises from $(n-1)$ different directions. A block diagram of a typical adaptive beamformer is shown in Figure 5–6. The simplest adaptive array would therefore consist of two microphones that can attenuate one noise signal incident from an arbitrary direction.

Adaptive array processing is usually based on two assumptions. First, the desired signal comes from straight ahead and second, the target signal is uncorrelated with all interfering

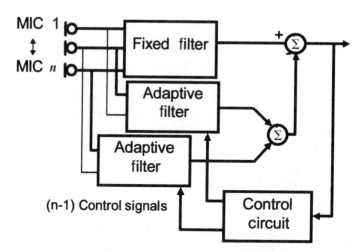

**Figure 5–6.** Block diagram for an adaptive beamformer. The adaptive filters are adjusted by the control circuit and they estimate the direction of incidence of noise signals. The fixed filter increases the SNR for a fixed beamformer. *(Courtesy of Phonak AG.)*

signals. For target misalignment (through head movements) and resonant environments, these assumptions are violated, leading to a decrease in performance.

It should be noted that the sound quality may suffer due to artifacts and distortions during the adaptation process. This effect can be decreased by slowing down adaptation. However, in this case, the beamformer may not adjust rapidly enough to keep pace with a time-varying acoustic environment.

## Mixing Fixed and Adaptive Beamformers

Fixed beamforming is most effective in highly resonant rooms, at parties, or in restaurants where sound comes from many directions simultaneously. Adaptive beamforming is best suited for cancelling single directional interferences (e.g., a passing car or signals arriving from single sources in weakly resonant environments). Consequently, a hybrid of both methods could cover a wide range of situations in which interference reduction is required to increase the intelligibility of a desired talker.

## FEEDBACK CANCELLERS

Feedback is a particularly debilitating problem in hearing aids. Feedback affects not only listener comfort, but also the ability of the fitter to adjust the instrument optimally for the user. The existence of, or potential for, acoustic feedback represents limitations in fitting hearing instruments:

▼ because of feedback, high-frequency amplification is often reduced to a level that is less than desired, resulting in poorer speech understanding.

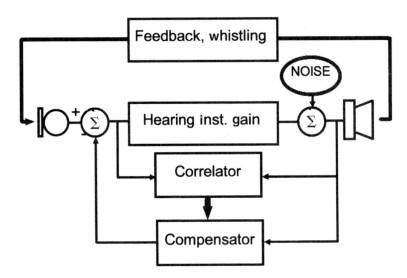

**Figure 5–7.** Structure of an adaptive feedback canceller. *(Courtesy of Unitron Hearing Ltd.)*

▼ although larger earmold vents offer greater wearing comfort, they can only be used in cases where little gain is needed, or with greater depth in fitting, or greater separation between the microphone and receiver.

Feedback happens when the closed-loop system gain reaches values larger than unity and the phase of the feedback signal is 0 degree or an integer multiple of 360 degree (the Nyquist criterion). In digital systems and devices, solutions to the problem are implemented in the form of feedback reduction algorithms.

Feedback canceling techniques and the corresponding theories are well-known, but practical solutions are rare (Hays, 2002; Kates et al., 2002; Kuk, 2002).

Figure 5–7 shows a simple block diagram of a feedback canceller using time-domain processing. The feedback signal is canceled by the output signal from an adaptive compensation filter adjusted to predict the feedback transfer function. This function can be identified using a noise signal from an internal source at the system output. The noise source injects a short duration noise signal into the hearing instrument output and if some amount of correlated noise is found at the input, there is feedback, since this is the only possible signal path. The compensatory filter will then be adjusted, driving the correlation between the input minus the estimated feedback signal and the output noise signal to zero.

It is not ideal, however, to introduce a noise signal into the hearing instrument's signal path because low-noise performance is a crucial design objective. The parasitic noise must therefore be inaudible, thus masked by the useful signal. The weaker the internal noise source, however, the less accurate is the adaptation of the compensatory filter. To work efficiently, this type of feedback suppression algorithms consequently requires a fine-tuned optimization of parameters.

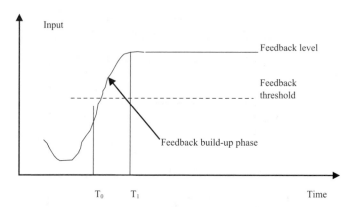

**Figure 5–8.** Stages of feedback development in a hearing instrument from $T_0$ when it is stable while the signal is below the feedback threshold, to onset when it crosses the threshold, to build up above the feedback threshold until $T_1$ when it reaches its saturation level. *(Courtesy of Unitron Hearing Ltd.)*

Alternative approaches use signal-processing strategies in the frequency domain and do not require an internal noise source. The implementation details of this solution are quite complex but it requires less computational effort than the well-known time-domain algorithms.

A fundamental issue with feedback management is the reliable and rapid detection of the onset of feedback. Figure 5–8 shows a stable acoustic condition before time $T_0$. However, during a telephone call, or during meals and other daily activities requiring jaw movements, the feedback path can change so that input signal reaches a critical feedback threshold level at time $T_0$ and by $T_1$ the input has grown to the point where saturation occurs and the instrument is in a feedback condition.

To prevent any audible feedback reaching the hearing aid user's ear it is necessary to detect the onset of the feedback build-up pattern and to suppress the build-up of feedback between $T_0$ and $T_1$ very quickly. Most current feedback detection technologies, for example an antiphase feedback canceller, need about 200 ms to characterize a feedback path. Then it might need another 200 ms to eliminate feedback in the antiphase feedback canceller. Therefore, a short burst of feedback is usually audible before it is canceled. This is perceived as annoying and can, at times, be uncomfortable.

Frequency-domain signal processors split the signal up into multiple bands. Feedback can occur in one or several of these bands. It is, therefore, advantageous to implement independent feedback detectors in each frequency band. These feedback detectors continuously monitor and detect feedback in real-time independently and simultaneously in all individual frequency bands. Ideally, feedback is detected during the build-up stage and cancellation begins before feedback becomes audible.

One example of such an adaptive feedback canceller in a WDRC amplifier is a feedback canceller with a fixed feedback margin. When feedback is detected, the adaptive feedback canceller modifies the system gain around the kneepoint $I_1$ by the fixed feedback margin shown in Figure 5–9. This is done over a very narrow input signal range so that the overall dynamic input signal, such as speech and music, will not be significantly affected.

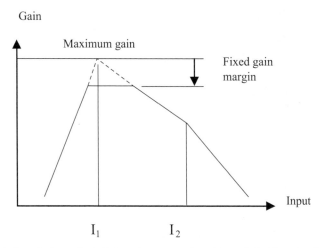

**Figure 5–9.** The gain/input characteristic in a frequency band in a digital hearing instrument. The instrument is in a low-level expansion mode below $I_1$, exhibits maximum gain at $I_1$, at which point it enters a compression mode until $I_2$ after which gain decreases further as input increases due to output limiting. The feedback canceller algorithm dynamically reduces the maximum gain by a fixed margin around $I_1$, when the onset of feedback is detected. The gain is restored when no feedback is detected. *(Courtesy of Phonak AG.)*

The output signal in the particular frequency band with a potential for feedback is reduced depending on how close the signal input is to the kneepoint $I_1$. The maximum gain reduction occurs when the input signal coincides with the kneepoint $I_1$. The gain reduction is adaptively applied and adaptively removed in accordance with the continuous feedback detection decision.

The simplicity of using a fixed feedback margin is also its principal drawback, because it is not necessarily optimized to provide the best performance for all different hearing aids and different degrees of feedback. Sometimes, it might reduce gain more than required. At other times, the feedback canceller might underreact and not cancel the feedback completely.

One solution to this problem is the adaptive feedback canceller. Once feedback is detected during the build-up phase, or even when feedback is already established, this canceller first applies a small feedback margin, such as 3 dB. If the feedback is canceled immediately, it continues to apply the small feedback margin. If the feedback still exists or continues to build up, the feedback margin is adaptively increased until the feedback is completely eliminated.

Modern sophisticated algorithms can provide 10–20 dB feedback suppression, which is sufficient to fit severe hearing losses with vented earmolds or moderate losses with completely open fittings. This improves comfort significantly. It is worth mentioning, however, that sound quality can degrade markedly even before the instrument starts to whistle.

Therefore, feedback suppression enhances sound quality, which is an important benefit of such systems.

## RECRUITMENT COMPENSATION

A healthy cochlea is an active system with approximately 50 to 60 dB amplification (control range) measured at threshold. The amplification is regulated nonlinearly by the external hair cells. The transmission properties of this system can be compared with a compressor. With increasing sound pressure level, the system reduces the amplification continuously (controlled by the outer hair cells). At high sound pressure levels, amplification is reduced to nearly 0 dB.

When the outer hair cells are damaged, cochlear amplification decreases and the regulation process is increasingly lost. Transmission degenerates from a compressive to a linear character. With a hearing loss over 60 dB, the cochlear amplifier (see Figure 5–10) is already inactive and the loss of the inner hair cells brings about a further linear shift of the hearing threshold. A maximum compression factor of 2.5:1 suffices as compensation for the loss of the outer hair cells. A digital hearing instrument can compensate for the loss of the outer hair cells by compressing the incoming signals appropriately. It must be noted that for compensation of recruitment, syllabic compression is necessary. This means extremely rapid activation of the compression (attack time < 10 ms; release time < 50 ms). The disadvantage of such rapid adjustment is distortion in the low frequencies. This problem is overcome in digital instruments

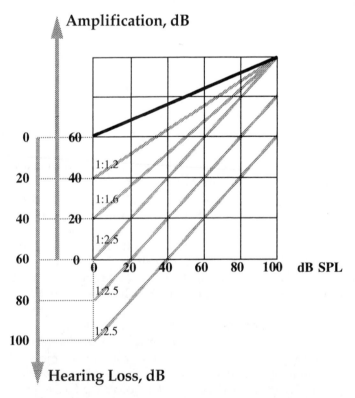

**Figure 5–10.** Characteristic of the cochlear amplifier. *(Courtesy of Phonak AG.)*

where the frequency range to be compressed can be subdivided into various bands, allowing fast attack and release times in the high frequencies and slower ones in the low frequencies where distortions may otherwise occur.

## THE SUMMATION OF LOUDNESS

The sensory cells (one row of inner and three rows of outer hair cells) are arranged along the basilar membrane such that pitch is perceived at a quite specific place. For this reason, twenty-four filter bands have been defined along the cochlea. These are the so-called critical bands. A critical band for loudness is a narrow band of noise, which, when it surrounds a tone of equal loudness, makes the tone just imperceptible. The width of such a narrow band is designated as a bark, so named after the early twentieth century acoustician and physicist Barkhausen. Below 500 Hz, the critical bands are 100 Hz wide. Above 500 Hz, the bands are divided roughly into thirds.

Figure 5–11 shows a simplified diagram of the excitation pattern in various bands (Zwicker, 1982). The form of the filters is identical in all critical bands at first approximation.

A pure tone is the simplest of all signals, constituting just one single spectral line. Nevertheless, a pure tone generates a wide excitation pattern on the basilar membrane, spreading over several critical bands as shown in Figure 5–11. A broad band noise stimulates all critical bands equally. The more critical bands have been stimulated, the greater is the sensation of loudness. For example, if a 1 kHz pure tone at 64 dB SPL and a broadband noise of the same intensity are presented to a listener, the broadband noise will be experienced as 12 dB more intense.

The explanation for this effect lies in the fact that, with broadband stimulation along the basilar membrane, many more nerve cells are simultaneously contributing to the loudness. Spectral components of a sound lying within a critical band add together physically in accordance with their level; components falling in another critical band experience a greater rating, something which is described in psychoacoustics as summation of loudness. However, summation of loudness decreases for the most part with increasing severity of the hearing impairment and even disappears completely in certain patients. This is because the critical bands widen so that fewer are active than is the case with normal hearing persons. To compensate for decreased or absent summation of loudness, it must be assessed at the diagnostic stage.

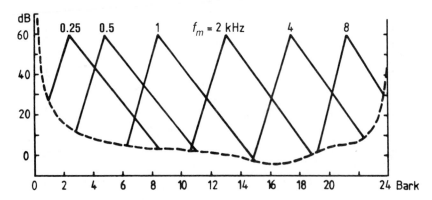

**Figure 5–11.** The critical bands. *(Adapted from Zwicker and Fastl, 1990.)*

At present, selective amplification is determined on the basis of the hearing threshold or with loudness scaling. However, these methods are both based on narrowband stimuli and, thus, do not reflect any summation of loudness. As a result, broadband signals are experienced as being too loud or narrow band ones as too weak. The same problem also arises in the case of maximum output SPL. The maximum output SPL control must depend on the signal spectrum and the summation of loudness so that valuable hearing instrument dynamics do not unnecessarily fall victim to a fitting compromise. The digital hearing instrument can be made to measure the signal spectrum and thus constantly adapt the frequency-dependent amplification and the maximum output SPL control on the basis of total loudness.

## MASKING

In Figure 5–12, the masking curves of a narrowband noise with a center frequency of 1 kHz are shown for various intensity levels. Any pure tone located below such a masking curve will be covered (masked) by the narrowband noise and, thus, not heard. In connection with this, the terms premasking and postmasking are used. Premasking means that a tone below the center frequency of the noise is masked, while postmasking refers to the masking of a signal with a higher frequency than that of the center frequency.

Masking curves are asymmetrical, spreading more on the high-frequency side of the center frequency than on the lower side. As a result of this, a low-frequency sound disturbs speech understanding to a greater extent than does a high-frequency sound because it interferes more with hearing the high-frequency components of speech.

The masking curves are dependent on the level of the masker: with increasing level they become increasingly asymmetrical due to the nonlinear regulating mechanism on the cochlea (through the external hair cells) only being active at low levels and saturated at high levels. The

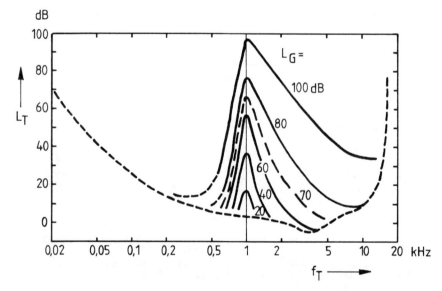

**Figure 5–12.** Masking curves for a person with normal hearing. *(Adapted from Zwicker and Fastl, 1990.)*

masking curves run practically uniformly through all critical bands. In the case of hearing impairment, the critical bands widen, and masking curves flatten out and spread upward at much lower levels than is the case with normal hearing.

What are the possibilities for demasking by means of a hearing instrument? As a result of wider masking curves, a hearing-impaired person's perception of the high-frequency components of the speech spectrum are hampered to an even greater degree by the low-frequency parts of the signal. At present, hearing instruments do not, for the most part, contain any mechanisms for demasking.

Adaptive filters in the bass range or two-channel AGC systems can be somewhat helpful in the case of dominant low-frequency interference. However, the algorithms utilized in these instruments compensate for the upward spread of masking by means of steeply sloping filters in the low frequencies. The frequency response curve of such an instrument is consequently steeper than indicated for the individual hearing loss. Wearers often react negatively because the hearing instruments sound too shrill. In a digital hearing instrument, an adaptive filter demasks the spectra based on a model for normal hearing persons; masked spectral components are amplified as much as possible, while at the same time, compensation for loudness changes occurs. However, if the masking curves for an individual are practically flat, even such a method will not help.

## INTELLIGENT HEARING INSTRUMENTS

There is no accepted definition for intelligent hearing instruments, but they should include at least three fundamental capabilities: auditory scene adaptation, adaptive signal enhancement, and adaptive hearing compensation.

Auditory scene adaptation gives the hearing aid the capability to detect, recognize, and adapt to surrounding environments and sound sources (Bregman, 1990; Moss, 2001). In other words, auditory scene adaptation is the intelligent interface between the hearing instrument and a real-world environment.

Adaptive signal enhancement gives hearing instruments the ability to optimize signal quality and to reduce or eliminate the interference of noise as it exists in the real world. It includes applying adaptive filtering, artificial intelligence, array signal processing, neural networks, and various signal-processing technologies to achieve signal enhancement, noise reduction, or even separation of the signal from noise. Intelligent signal detection, adaptive noise reduction, beam-forming or adaptive beamforming, feedback cancellation, and overlapping signal separation are key technologies used to achieve signal enhancement.

Adaptive hearing compensation can provide significant benefits for people with hearing loss. In its simplest form, it is equivalent to level-dependent compression but digital systems provide an opportunity to extend this technique to multiple frequency bands as required.

Usually, an individual program and functionality is designed for a specific purpose or specific auditory scene. For example, in a normal office environment, an omni-directional microphone that senses the surrounding acoustic signal may be required. A noise reduction (NR) function can also be active in the hearing aid to reduce the effect of background noise in the office. Such background noise usually contains low-frequency noise (lower than 500 Hz), such as computer fan noise, or air-conditioning noise and these noises could be as high as 60 dB SPL. The parameters of a noise reduction function for office environments can be optimized to deliver the best performance by reducing such kinds of office background noise and enhancing the target signal such as speech or music.

A typical change of auditory scene is that a phone rings when the hearing instrument was working in the office environment described above. It may be desirable to switch the instrument to the T-(telecoil) program, the magnetic signal pick-up mode, to provide the best telephone communication without acoustic interference, or to the MT (microphone and telecoil) mode. In the latter case, the telecoil senses the telephone signal and the microphone provides some awareness of acoustic activity in the environment. The noise reduction function may need to adapt to the scene to be more efficient for telecoil noise reduction. Again, in the T-program or MT program, parameters of the noise reduction algorithm may need to be optimized to deliver the best overall performance. Right after the phone conversation, it might be natural to switch back to the omnidirectional program for the normal office environment.

The auditory scene may then switch to a cafeteria with many people engaged in conversations in the usual cafeteria style background noise. It will be difficult to engage in a conversation under these conditions if a high level of speech babble is present in the background. It might be beneficial to switch from the omni-directional program to a program with either an adaptive directional or a fixed directional pattern to listen to a partner's talk and reduce the background speech babble. The noise reduction (NR) function may need to be activated and the parameters of the NR need to be optimized to provide best performance for the conversation. A car ride may follow the cafeteria situation. Now a different directional program may best deal with the driving conditions, specifically a traffic noise reduction function to reduce traffic noise. In addition, some parameters of the NR need to be optimized for the particular traffic noise condition.

In order to adapt to the many acoustic environment changes mentioned above, it is necessary to switch the hearing program or function and even adjust parameters accordingly. It is not convenient, or it may be difficult for the user, to switch hearing programs whenever the environment changes. It is also very difficult for the user to switch functions manually in a timely manner. The user usually has no way to adjust internal parameters, since they are usually predefined for the function and program to optimize the performance for specific acoustic situations. It would be beneficial to automatically detect acoustic environment changes reliably and make intelligent decisions automatically to adapt to such environmental changes. However, the danger is that if detection of the acoustic environment changes is not reliable, the so-called intelligent decisions can be disastrous since unreliable signal detection will lead to incorrect decisions (Buechler, 2001).

Binaural information about acoustic events contains important clues for hearing localization and hearing perception. Integrating binaural information and binaural processing into intelligent hearing aids will benefit the users by providing improved acoustic source localization, acoustic environment adaptation and hearing perception.

Although some digital hearing instruments offer a capability of simple environment adaptation there is still a long way to go to achieve reliable and intelligent adaptation to auditory scene changes. But intelligent and more reliable technologies for acoustic environment adaptation will be the cornerstones for intelligent digital hearing aids of the future. A broad knowledge of signal detection, sound source detection and localization, signal identification, auditory scene analysis, fuzzy logic, artificial intelligence, and so on, will be required to improve hearing instrument performance.

## PROCESSING DELAY

Algorithms provide immense capabilities in a digital hearing instrument but they require a finite time to perform their calculations. Processing delays should be as short as possible but processing delays of 5 to 10 milliseconds are observed in some digital hearing instruments. Short processing delays are particularly important when fitting with a large vent. If the processed signal reaches the ear much later than the signal reaching the ear through the vent, the user can experience an echo effect. Short processing delays are also necessary to ensure that the audio signal and the visual (lip reading) signals are perceived to be simultaneous. Processing delays of approximately 1 millisecond are optimal.

## SUMMARY

1. Digital hearing instruments were made possible in the mid-1990s when digital ICs offered the necessary computational power in a sufficiently small size and could be powered by a hearing instrument battery.
2. Digital technology is an important new tool for improving hearing health care.
3. Digital hearing instruments have a digital signal path.
4. Digital hearing instruments provide more flexible amplification strategies than are available in analog instruments.
5. Digital hearing instruments employ signal-processing strategies to produce a "clean" amplified signal with low noise and low distortion.
6. Digital technology enables the development of hearing instruments with automatic functions, such as auditory scene adaptation, adaptive directional microphones, adaptive noise, and feedback reduction.
7. More powerful and more efficient DSP platforms of small size and with low operating voltage and lower power consumption will be available in the future for the development of intelligent digital hearing instruments.
8. More advanced signal-processing technologies for signal detection, signal extraction, and signal enhancement will continue to be developed.
9. Digital signal-processing hardware and the associated algorithms will continue to improve in quality and performance.
10. Intelligent digital hearing instruments will make it possible to maximize hearing aid benefit by automatic adaptation to changes in the acoustic environment.

## REVIEW QUESTIONS

1.  Digital hearing instruments:
    A. Will lead to much easier fittings                                   A ☐
    B. Use digital signal processing in the signal path                   B ☐
    C. Use time discrete signals                                          C ☐
    D. Have a bandwidth which is at least double the sampling frequency   D ☐
2.  The noise canceller in a digital hearing instrument can:
    A. Improve speech intelligibility in a constant background noise       A ☐
    B. Eliminate the need for directional microphones                     B ☐
    C. Achieve a better speech intelligibility compared to directional
       microphones in speechlike noises                                   C ☐
    D. Can reduce microphone noise                                        D ☐
3.  The sampling frequency of a digital hearing instrument:
    A. Has to be at least 120 MHz                                         A ☐
    B. Is at least twice as big as the bandwidth of the hearing instrument  B ☐
    C. Depends on the hearing instrument microphone                       C ☐
    D. Is independent and has no influence on the current consumption     D ☐
4.  Describe the development that made it possible to use digital signal processors in hearing instrument amplifiers.
5.  Describe the difference between an ASIC implementation of a digital hearing instrument and one using an algorithm-based implementation.
6.  List the most common signal-processing algorithms in use today in digital hearing instruments.

# CHAPTER 6

# Acoustic Path

## INTRODUCTION

The trend in the hearing instrument world is clear. More and more, hearing instruments are electronic, digital, programmable units. With this emphasis on the electronic characteristics of hearing instruments, it is easy to forget that they also have acoustic properties.

Like a musical instrument, if the acoustic quality of a hearing instrument is poor, no amount of complicated electronics can make up for it. In this chapter, it will be demonstrated how a hearing instrument frequency response can often be quite simply changed for better or worse through acoustic modifications to the tubes associated with the microphone, the receiver (angle), or the earmold. These modifications can also be performed to a certain extent by the hearing health care professional.

## ACOUSTIC MODIFICATIONS TO THE MICROPHONE

For a discussion of the types of microphones used in hearing instruments, the reader is referred to Chapter 2.

### MICROPHONE TUBING

The choice of the microphone tubing (length and diameter) determines, to a large extent, the frequency response (see Figures 6–1 and 6–2).

### *Length*

Lengthening the microphone tube causes a shift in the resonance to lower frequencies.

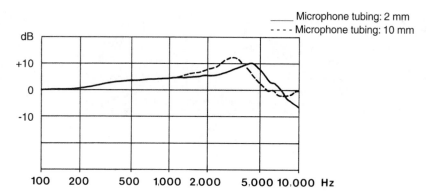

**Figure 6–1.** Microphone frequency response with sound inlet tubes of different lengths. *(Courtesy of Phonak AG.)*

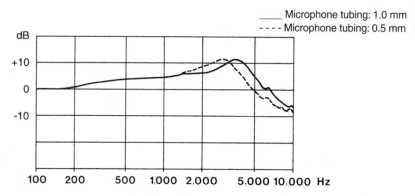

**Figure 6–2.** Microphone frequency response with sound inlet tubes of different diameters. *(Courtesy of Phonak AG.)*

Without going into extensive and complicated calculations to confirm such a trend, it is sufficient to note that this effect is evident from the fundamental relationship between wavelength ($\lambda$), the speed of sound in air ($c$), and the frequency ($f$) of the sound traveling through air: $f = c/\lambda$. As the length of a piece of tubing is increased, the wavelength of the fundamental resonance of the tube becomes longer, and since $c$ is constant, the resonance occurs at a lower frequency.

## Diameter

A reduction of the tubing diameter cuts the high frequencies. The disadvantage of modifying the frequency response in this manner is that it does not diminish noise in the hearing instrument, as is the case when the frequency response is altered electronically.

## ACOUSTIC MODIFICATION FOR THE HEARING INSTRUMENT RECEIVER, EARHOOK, AND EARHOOK TUBING

The manufacturers of hearing instruments offer a variety of receivers in terms of size, output capability, and frequency response. The standard receiver exhibits pronounced resonances, but damped receivers, which suppress the receiver resonances by means of an acoustic filter (damper), are available.

In the case of the undamped frequency response of a behind-the-ear receiver, five typical peaks (resonances) can be identified (see Figure 6–3).

The exact location of the resonance peaks over the whole frequency band depends on the size of the receiver as well as the length and the diameter of the tubing.

Users of hearing instruments with such strong resonances often comment that the sound is unnatural with an unpleasant tonal quality. Damping of these resonances is often a good way to promote user acceptance of the hearing instrument.

The most frequent and simplest acoustic modification to the behind-the-ear unit is changing the hearing instrument hook. The tubing/receiver resonances can now be damped by means of special filters in the hook (see Figure 6–4). The filters are made of a stainless steel or plastic screen and introduce a resistance to the flow of air in the tube. The finer the screen, the greater the flow resistance.

The advantage of damping the resonances to obtain such a flat frequency—apart from a more natural sound—is that a smooth frequency response ensures that no resonance peaks exceed the user discomfort level (UCL). Note that the dynamics of the hearing instrument user are not necessarily reduced by smoothing the response. It is interesting to note that not only the flow resistance of the damping element but also its location in the hook or the earmold is of great importance.

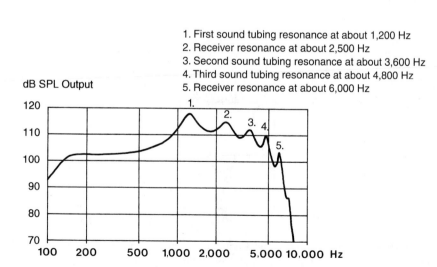

1. First sound tubing resonance at about 1,200 Hz
2. Receiver resonance at about 2,500 Hz
3. Second sound tubing resonance at about 3,600 Hz
4. Third sound tubing resonance at about 4,800 Hz
5. Receiver resonance at about 6,000 Hz

**Figure 6–3.** Resonance peaks in the frequency response of an undamped receiver. *(Courtesy of Phonak AG.)*

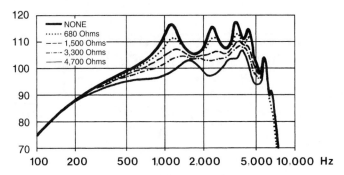

**Figure 6–4.** The effect of damping elements with different acoustic resistance on the resonant peaks in a frequency response curve. *(Courtesy of Phonak AG.)*

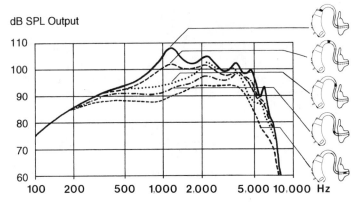

**Figure 6–5.** The effect of an acoustic resistance element (damper), placed at various locations between the receiver sound outlet and the earmold outlet, on the shape of the frequency response of a hearing instrument. *(Courtesy of Phonak AG.)*

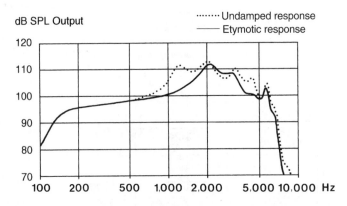

**Figure 6–6.** Transformation of an undamped frequency response (dotted curve) into an eytmotic response (solid curve) by damping the 1,000-Hz resonance in the response with an acoustic resistance damping element. *(Courtesy of Phonak AG.)*

Figure 6–5 shows various frequency responses measured with the same filter. Varying the position of the filter changes the frequency response. If the filter is located near the receiver, the overall response is smoothed slightly. When the filter is moved nearer the earmold, a greater overall damping occurs. There is an especially large reduction of the output at the first tubing resonance. Careful positioning of the correct filter in the hook produces a so-called etymotic frequency response.

## ETYMOTIC FREQUENCY RESPONSE

By damping the resonance peak at 1,000 Hz with a hearing instrument hook, an etymotic frequency response is produced (see Figure 6–6). An etymotic frequency response compensates for the loss of the natural auditory canal resonance.

The susceptibility of damping screens to dirt and humidity is a major disadvantage of using such screens in the hook. In countries with consistently high humidity, the filter screen can become blocked within a few weeks. This is often unacceptable to the user.

## SPECIAL HOOKS

Etymotic Research manufactures specially shaped hooks which, when combined with commercially available behind-the-ear instruments, offer simple and effective solutions for fitting three different types of hearing loss (see Figure 6–7). However, these hooks are costly and rather large, limiting their use to only the more serious cases. Since modern digital hearing instruments offer a wide variety of frequency-shaping possibilities, these shapes can be achieved with electronic filtering as well.

### High-Tone Hook

A high-tone hook makes it possible to alter the response of a broadband hearing instrument such that gain is limited to the high-frequency range, dropping sharply for frequencies below 3 kHz (see Figure 6–8).

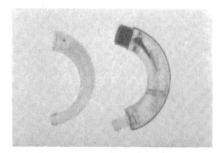

**Figure 6–7.** Standard hook on the left and special frequency shaping hook (from Etymotic Research) *(Courtesy of Phonak AG.)*

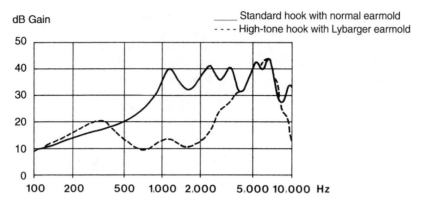

**Figure 6–8.** Low-frequency attenuation with a high-tone hook and a Lybarger nonoccluding dual-diameter earmold bore. *(Courtesy of Phonak AG.)*

### Low-Tone Hook

This hook has been developed for low-frequency hearing losses. The frequency transmission falls sharply after 800 Hz (see Figure 6–9).

### Notch-Filter Hook

The notch-filter hook contains a narrowband stop filter which achieves a response reduction of 20 dB at 2 kHz. The advantage of such a notch filter is that it can be used with a normal earmold. Thus the effect can be immediately tested in the fitting situation (see Figure 6–10).

## ACOUSTIC MODIFICATIONS TO THE EARMOLD

The most important acoustic modification which the hearing health care professional can carry out is an earmold modification. The question now arises as to how and in what frequency range an acoustic modification is possible.

Figure 6–11 clearly shows the frequency ranges that can be affected by earmold venting, damping, and horn bore.

*Important:* As the three ranges only slightly overlap, one or more modifications can be made simultaneously.

## VENTING

A vent is an additional opening in the earmold leading to the outside air. A vent has various effects depending on its size and length:

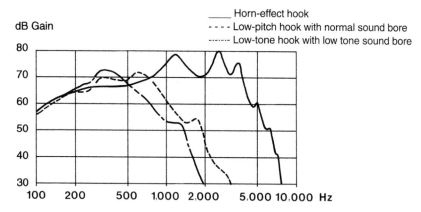

**Figure 6–9.** Frequency response with different hooks and earmold sound bores. *(Courtesy of Phonak AG.)*

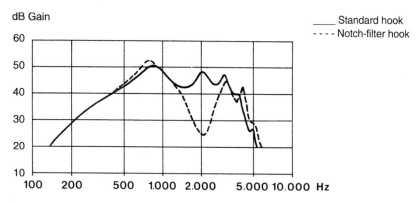

**Figure 6–10.** Frequency response with a notch-filter hook. *(Courtesy of Phonak AG.)*

▼ **Pressure equalization and elimination of the occlusion effect.** Occlusion of the auditory canal causes a considerable increase in perceived loudness due to bone-conducted sound, including sounds made by the wearer (own voice, chewing noises). Some sounds (e.g., vocalization) can be amplified as much as 30–40 dB at around 125 Hz due to ear canal occlusion.

In contrast to a sensation of pressure, which can be relieved by drilling a small additional hole in the earmold, the occlusion effect can only be remedied by means of a fully open earmold (see Figure 6–12). In fact, reducing the diameter of vents prevents the transmission of high-frequency signal components through the vent (see Figure 6–2) although the lower-frequency components can escape from the ear canal. For example, it is possible to achieve attenuation of signals below 750 Hz yet still allow amplification of up to 20 dB at 1 kHz.

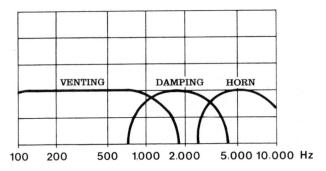

**Figure 6–11.** The effect of venting, damping, and horn bores in the earmold on different frequency regions of the response. *(Courtesy of Phonak AG.)*

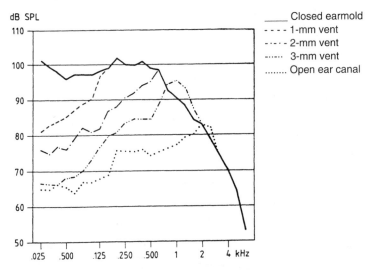

**Figure 6–12.** Influence of vent diameter on the occlusion effect (Courtois et al., 1988). *(Courtesy of GN ReSound A/S.)*

▼ **Damping of the low frequencies.** By enlarging the size of the vent, gain in the low frequencies is lost. The reduction in gain in the lower frequencies is a function of the diameter and the length of the vent (see Figures 6–13 and 6–14).

Avoiding excessive low-frequency amplification can improve speech understanding, especially in low-frequency noise situations. Changes in the low-frequency response of the hearing instrument can be affected either by acoustic or electrical means. Leaving the ear canal open to some extent is an acoustic modification which can result in up to 30 dB less gain at 500 Hz. Although the same effect can also be produced with electronic filters, subjective comparisons with acoustic modifications often show a preference (both with respect to resultant sound quality as well as speech understanding) for the acoustic solution.

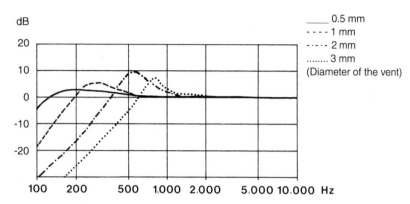

**Figure 6–13.** Low-frequency damping as a function of vent diameter. *(Courtesy of Phonak AG.)*

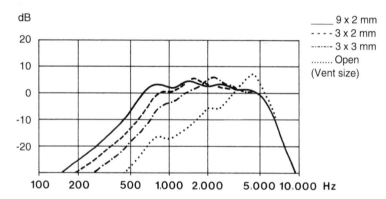

**Figure 6–14.** Low-frequency damping as a function of vent length. *(Courtesy of Phonak AG.)*

## DAMPING

Frequencies in the range from 800 Hz to 4,000 Hz can be attenuated by using acoustic damping elements (acoustic resistances) in the earmold. Today, these damping elements are usually inserted in the hearing instrument hook rather than the earmold (as it is simpler to do) (see Figures 6–4 and 6–5).

## HORN BORE

Progressively increasing the earmold bore diameter increases the transmission of high-frequency components through the earmold (horn effect). Typical earmolds with a horn bore include, for example, the Libby horn and Bakke horn. The effects of various horn bore diameters are shown in Figure 6–15.

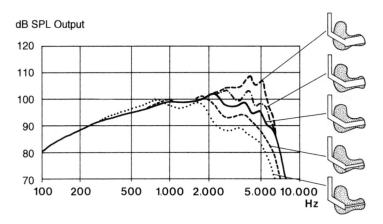

**Figure 6–15.** The effect of different earmold horn bores on frequency response shape. *(From "Earmold Options for Wideband Hearing Aids: by Mead C. Killion, 1981, Journal of Speech and Hearing Disorders, 4–6, p. 16, copyright 1981 by American Speech-Language-Hearing Association. Reprinted by permission.)*

As a rule, the best high-frequency transmission possible is desirable. Problems with horn bores include the relatively large space requirements and the danger of feedback.

# CONTROL OF FEEDBACK

## WHAT IS FEEDBACK?

Figure 6–16 shows how feedback can occur in a hearing instrument.

1. An input signal S1 is introduced to a system and is amplified.
2. An output signal S2 appears. S2 is larger than S1 by the amplification factor.
3. Part of S2 (signal S3) leaks back to the input. This results in a loop where part of the output signal is continually reintroduced as input to the system and amplified.

→ when S3 is greater than S1, there is feedback.

## TYPES OF FEEDBACK

Four different types of feedback can occur in hearing instruments:

1. **Acoustic feedback.** The most important and frequently occurring kind of feedback is acoustic when the sound loop from the receiver leaks back to the microphone. This kind of feedback is often due to a problem with the earmold. The vent may be too large or there is a poor seal between the earmold and the ear canal. It is, however, possible that the feedback is due to internal coupling between the microphone and receiver in the hearing instrument, in which case the repair technician must replace the internal microphone and receiver tubes.

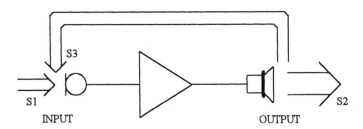

**Figure 6–16.** Schematic diagram of acoustic feedback. *(Courtesy of Phonak AG.)*

2. **Mechanical feedback.** This occurs when the vibrational damping of the microphone and receiver mountings is not adequate. Vibrations which are produced by the receiver are transmitted via the hearing instrument housing and picked up by the microphone and amplified. Hearing instruments with strong amplification in the very low frequencies, mostly at frequencies below 1000 Hz, can exhibit mechanical feedback.
3. **Magnetic feedback.** Magnetic feedback occurs when the induction coil is active. The magnetic field around the receiver is picked up by the induction coil and amplified. Magnetic feedback can appear over the hearing instrument's whole frequency range.
4. **Electrical feedback.** In the case of electrical feedback, the amplifier becomes unstable, most often because of a weak battery. The voltage of the battery decreases and the inner resistance increases, resulting in a low-frequency hum, which is referred to as "motorboating" due to its resemblance to the sound of a running motorboat.

## ELIMINATION OF FEEDBACK

Mechanical, magnetic, and electrical feedback can be considered hearing instrument faults requiring the instrument to be sent for repair by the manufacturer.

To eliminate feedback, the following measures must be taken:

1. Determine the type of feedback (Points 1, 2, 3, or 4 described above).
2. In the case of acoustic feedback, determine whether it is an external (via the earmold) or an internal (in the hearing instrument housing) type of feedback. When the hearing instrument hook opening is closed, the hearing instrument should not whistle. If it does, this means there is internal feedback.
3. Determine the feedback frequency in the case of acoustic feedback.
4. If the feedback appears in the mid-frequencies (1,000 Hz to 2,000 Hz), the following measures can eliminate it:
   ▼ reduce the gain
   ▼ damp by means of a filter in the hook of behind-the-ear units
   ▼ reduce the size of the vent

5.  If the feedback appears at high frequencies (3,000 Hz to 5,000 Hz), the following measures can eliminate it:
    ▾ reduce the high-frequency amplification by means of a high-cut filter or modify the earmold
    ▾ reduce the size of the vent

    See also Chapter 8 "Hearing Instrument Troubleshooting."

## SUMMARY

1.  Acoustic modifications remain an important tool for the hearing health care professional because they solve problems for the patient in a very efficient way during an office visit.
2.  Modifications that eliminate feedback, improve sound quality, or improve user comfort have an immediate beneficial effect.
3.  In BTE instruments, modifications are done on the earmold, earhook, and acoustic tubes.
4.  In ITE instruments, modifications are performed on the shell of the instrument.
5.  Modifications are more difficult to carry out on ITEs and CICs because their shells can be damaged by excessive material removal.

## REVIEW QUESTIONS

1.  **A.** What is the effect of acoustic filters in the hook or in the earmold?
    **B.** How does the frequency response change when the same acoustic filter is used at different places from beginning at the receiver end of the earhook and ending at the end of the earmold?
2.  What is the reason for a damping screen in the earhook?
    **A.** To damp the high frequencies                         A ☐
    **B.** To damp the receiver resonances                      B ☐
    **C.** To reduce the low frequencies                        C ☐
    **D.** To reduce the maximum sound pressure level           D ☐
3.  A vent in the earmold of approximately 0.8 mm changes:
    **A.** The sound pressure level                             A ☐
    **B.** The dynamic range                                    B ☐
    **C.** The feeling of having the ear plugged up             C ☐
    **D.** The low-frequency response                           D ☐
4.  What is the disadvantage of producing a high-frequency reduction with an acoustic modification at the microphone instead of an electronic high-cut?
    **A.** More distortion                                      A ☐
    **B.** Higher current consumption                           B ☐
    **C.** More feedback                                        C ☐
    **D.** Higher equivalent input noise level                  D ☐

**5.** How can the main tube resonance of a BTE be smoothed?
   **A.** With an acoustic filter (damping screen) close to the receiver      A ☐
   **B.** With a very fine mesh, the placement does not make a big difference   B ☐
   **C.** With an acoustic filter (damping screen) at the end of the hook      C ☐
   **D.** An acoustic filter (damping screen) smoothes out only the receiver
   resonances, but not the tubing resonances                                D ☐

# CHAPTER 7

# Accessories

## INTRODUCTION

Many hearing instrument users encounter situations where the amplification their hearing aids provide does not meet their needs. A variety of hearing instrument accessories provide assistance in these cases. A person fitted with an ITE hearing instrument not equipped with a telecoil may have difficulty using the telephone in a work setting and would benefit from having the hearing instrument fitted with a telecoil. The audio input accessory will allow a hard-of-hearing individual to use a remote microphone in noisy surroundings or allow a student to use an FM system in a classroom setting. CROS fittings are not accessories but do make use of the audio input accessory provided on many BTE instruments. FM communications systems have been developed for personal use as well as for classroom settings and other public places and the audio input connections on most BTE hearing instruments allow them to be used as required for short or extended periods of time. Remote controls are used to adjust volume and selected specific functions on their hearing instruments. The chapter concludes with a discussion of hearing instrument batteries.

## INDUCTION COIL

An induction coil (or telecoil) is built into nearly all behind-the-ear units and some in-the-ear units (Figure 7–1). The induction coil provides an input signal to the hearing instrument from magnetic sources. The induction coil is operational when the input selection switch is on the "T" position. This coil picks up electromagnetic signals and converts them into an electrical voltage, which is then amplified by the hearing instrument.

The name "telecoil" derives from the fact that it picks up electromagnetic signals from the telephone, making it possible to use the T setting for telephoning. Unfortunately, the magnetic field radiated from a modern telephone is much weaker than old telephones so that the signal is often too weak to be useful.

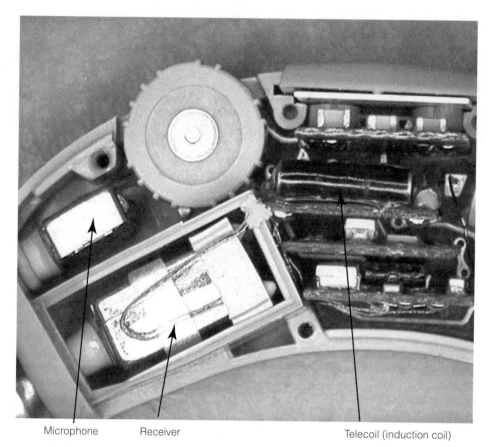

Microphone          Receiver                                    Telecoil (induction coil)

**Figure 7–1.** Interior view of BTE hearing instrument with telecoil. *(Courtesy of Unitron Hearing Ltd.)*

A second purpose of the induction coil in hearing instruments is to receive magnetic fields from special induction loops. Such loop systems are common in churches and public buildings. The advantage of these loop systems is that the hearing instrument receives and amplifies the signal (e.g., the pastor) and not the surrounding noise. (See also Chapter 2.)

## THE AUDIO INPUT

Many behind-the-ear units are equipped with the means for providing an electrical input signal to the hearing instrument amplifier. Since this electrical signal is often produced by a remote microphone, this feature is commonly referred to as an audio input. The usual abbreviation for audio input is "A" or "DAI" for direct audio input.

The audio input has a very specific aim: to pick up an acoustic or audio signal as close as possible to the source and thereby deliver a high fidelity, undistorted signal to the hearing in-

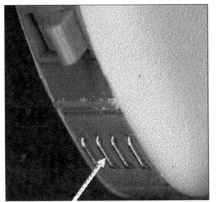
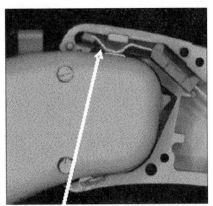

Audio contact system on the hearing instrument | Contact system in the audio boot

**Figure 7–2.** Audio input contact system on a BTE hearing instrument and contact system in the audio input adaptor (boot). *(Courtesy of Unitron Hearing Ltd.)*

strument amplifier. Picking up the signal at or close to the source avoids the attenuation of high-frequency components of speech or music as sound propagates through air and also eliminates ambient acoustic noise from the signal. The audio input connections have also become useful for CROS and BiCROS applications.

All audio equipment (e.g., television, radio) could be connected electrically via a cable connection or acoustically via a microphone placed close to the loudspeaker of the audio or entertainment unit. The audio input consists of electrical contacts to which a plug or an audio shoe can be connected (see Figure 7–2).

Figure 7–3 illustrates three commonly used electrical configurations for connecting the audio input signal to the hearing instrument amplifier. Figure 7–3a connects audio input contacts in parallel with the microphone connections. In this case, the microphone sensitivity can be affected by the device, usually a remote microphone or an FM system receiver, that is connected to the audio input terminals. This may also happen in the situation shown in Figure 7–3b, where the telecoil sensitivity can be affected in a similar way. Figure 7–3c provides separate inputs for the microphone, telecoil, and audio input device and each input can be selected independent of the others. In this case, however, a more complex and usually more expensive switch is required. The three preamplifiers shown in Figure 7–3c may be used to properly match the sensitivities of the three different input devices to the amplifier.

## CONTRALATERAL ROUTING OF SIGNALS (CROS)

Contralateral routing of signals (CROS) is, strictly speaking, not an accessory, but rather a special hearing instrument application. CROS is covered in this section because the audio input accessory system (contacts and the audio boot) are often used to produce a CROS fitting.

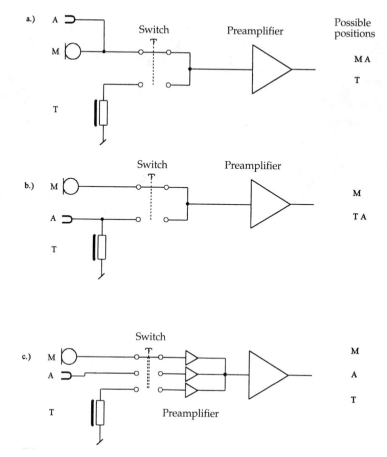

**Figure 7–3.** Connection schemes for different audio input systems. *(Courtesy of Phonak AG.)*

A CROS fitting is usually used when an individual has a unilateral hearing loss. The CROS fitting is used to compensate for the head shadow effect for sounds originating on the deaf side of the head. In practice, a microphone is placed on the deaf side and connected to the hearing instrument amplifier on the opposite ear. An open fitting is often used, depending on the loss in the better ear.

In the case of a particularly severe hearing loss, increased amplification is possible (without feedback) because the microphone is located on the opposite side of the head from the ear canal that receives the amplified sound. Only one ear receives amplification, but information to be heard often comes from the other side (e.g., taxi driver).

A CROS design is most easily implemented in an eyeglass hearing instrument. The microphone is removed from the hearing instrument and attached to the opposite temple bar. The microphone is connected via a thin three-conductor cable to the existing microphone terminals of the amplifier. However, eyeglass instruments are not frequently prescribed, but CROS configurations are available for BTE instruments as well.

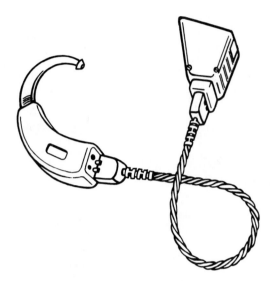

**Figure 7–4.** CROS adaptor with a BTE microphone unit, cord, and audio input adaptor. *(Courtesy of Phonak AG.)*

In BTE instruments, the hearing instrument microphone is removed from the hearing instrument. A CROS adaptor, resembling a small BTE unit and normally containing only a microphone, is placed behind the opposite or contralateral ear and connected to the audio input via a thin cable as shown in Figure 7–4. The cable is routed behind the head.

## BiCROS

When the microphone in the hearing instrument and the microphones on the opposite ear are both active, the system is referred to as a bilateral CROS or a BiCROS system. This means that there are microphones on both sides of the head but only one ear is fitted.

Although the worse ear cannot be fitted, the patient is able to hear sound from both sides of the head.

*Important:* BiCROS is not a binaural fitting.

## THE HANDHELD MICROPHONE

The handheld microphone is designed to allow the hard-of-hearing listener to be closer to the speaker thereby achieving a better signal to noise ratio.

The handheld microphone (Figure 7–5) is connected to the audio input via a cable, enabling better understanding under noisy conditions, especially if the handheld microphone has good directional characteristics.

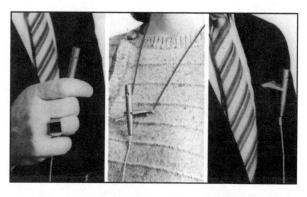

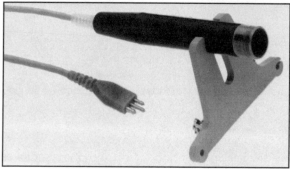

**Figure 7–5.** Examples of handheld, body worn, and tabletop remote microphones. *(Courtesy of Phonak AG.)*

Frequently, the handheld microphone is used when fitting children. For example, a handheld microphone makes it possible for a parent to communicate with their hearing-impaired child as well as to teach speech and language skills without the interference of ambient noises.

A hearing instrument microphone is frequently built into the handheld housing in order to obtain a similar frequency response to that of the microphone in the wearer's hearing instrument.

# FM COMMUNICATIONS SYSTEMS

An FM communications system (FM = frequency modulation) consists of a microphone (frequently a directional microphone), an FM transmitter, and an FM receiver (see Figure 7–6). It is suitable for group amplification systems in schools (i.e., an FM transmitter and several FM receivers) and for personal use. The speaker has an FM transmitter and the hearing-impaired listeners have FM receivers that are all tuned to the frequency of the transmitting microphone. Today's wireless FM systems possess good speech transmission properties. The FM receiver is connected to the audio input of the hearing instrument. The purpose of an FM system is the

**Table 7–1.** Allocated frequency bands in different countries.

| Country | Allocated Frequencies |
|---|---|
| France | 36–39 MHz and 175–176 MHz |
| Germany | 36–39 MHz and 173–175 MHz |
| Switzerland | 36–39 MHz and 174–223 MHz |
| United States of America | 72–76 MHz and 216–217 MHz |
| Canada | 72–76 MHz and 216–217 MHz |

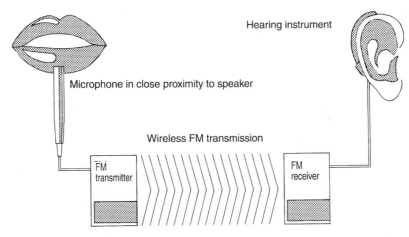

**Figure 7–6.** Operating principles of an FM system. *(Courtesy of Phonak AG.)*

same as for the handheld microphone: to bring the speaker closer to the ear in order to improve signal-to-noise ratio. FM systems work with various transmission frequencies. The transmitting frequencies shown in Table 7–1 are assigned according to country (see Chapter 13 for more details).

If several FM systems are being used simultaneously in different rooms in the same building, different transmission frequencies must be used in the different rooms to avoid interference in adjacent rooms.

*Important:* It is possible to serve many receivers with one transmitter (teacher [transmitter] and pupil [receiver]). However, it is not simple to work with several transmitters and one receiver (different teachers and one student). The receiver will only receive the signal from one transmitter.

## MEASUREMENT OF FM SYSTEMS

Until recently, there have been no universally accepted standards for the measurement of FM systems. This is further complicated by the large number of coupling options, ranging from an integrated FM receiver and BTE hearing aids to induction loop systems to direct auditory input from body-worn systems. Guidelines for the fitting and monitoring of FM systems have been proposed by the American Speech and Hearing Association (ASHA). Although FM systems are dependent upon hearing aids, there are differences that need to be taken into consideration. The most important difference is that the input level of the FM microphone is more intense than the hearing aid microphone because of its placement close to the mouth. This signal is typically 15 to 20 dB higher than the input to the hearing aid microphone of 60 dB SPL at four to five feet. The second issue relates to the different microphone input possibilities. There may be any number of combinations. In addition, the FM microphone may be omnidirectional or directional. The FM system may also have more than one volume control, which may be located on the FM transmitter, the FM receiver, or the hearing instrument.

The two broad areas for consideration are the use of FM as a self-contained system and the FM system used as an accessory to an existing hearing aid. Within these two areas there are three factors that must be evaluated:

1.  Amplification of sounds received from the hearing aid (environmental) microphone.
2.  The amplification of sounds received from the remote or FM microphone.
3.  Evaluation of the FM and hearing aid together.

The basic recommendation of the guidelines is that an input of 80 dB SPL into the remote microphone should give an output that is 10 to 15 dB higher than that produced by an input of 65 dB SPL into the environmental or hearing aid microphone. For measurements noted below, it is assumed that hearing aid performance has been measured to ANSI standards (see Figure 7–7).

**Evaluation of gain in the FM channel for a personal FM system used as an accessory to a hearing aid:**

1.  Measure output into a 2-cc coupler for an input to the hearing aid microphone of 65 dB SPL at a frequency of 1,000 Hz (see Figure 7–8a).
2.  Couple the FM receiver to the hearing aid in the manner that is to be used. If using a standard neck loop, make sure the shape and orientation of the loop, and the distance and orientation of the air in relation to the loop, are the same as in actual use.
3.  Adjust the volume control of the FM receiver so that a 65 dB SPL, 1,000 Hz input to the remote microphone generates the same output from the hearing aid as measured with the local microphone (see Figure 7–8b).
4.  Increase the input to 80 dB SPL. You should find that the output from the hearing aid has increased by at least 10 dB (see Figure 7–8c). If it does not, increase FM gain to give an FM advantage of between 5 and 7 dB (ASHA, 1998).
5.  If the output does not meet the 10 or 15 dB increase you are looking for, then appropriate adjustments should be made in the FM volume control.

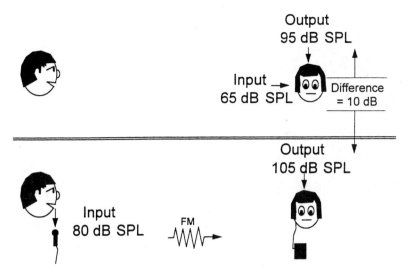

**Figure 7–7.** The goal of an FM system is to increase the speech level from a distant talker by approximately 10 dB in the listener's ear (ASHA, 1998). *(American Speech-Language-Hearing Association. 1998. Guidelines for fitting and monitoring FM systems. Retrieved 02/23/2006 from http://www.asha. org/about/ethics/ref-library.htm  <http://www.asha.org/about/ethics/ref-library.htm>  <exchweb/bin/redir. asp?URL=http://www.asha.org/about/ethics/ref-library.htm>. Reprinted with permission.)*

## ELECTROACOUSTIC CONFIRMATION

**Procedure for confirmation of electroacoustic fitting goals with a 2-cc coupler:**

1. Attach the hearing aid, or the receiver/amplifier of a self-contained FM system, to a 2-cc coupler and place in the test box with the microphone in the calibrated position.
2. Using swept tones or a complex noise, measure output as a function of frequency following standard procedures.
3. Remove the hearing aid, still attached to the coupler, from the test box.
   A. If this is a personal FM system, couple the FM receiver to the personal hearing aid.
   B. If neck loop coupling is being used, make sure the configuration of the loop, and the position and orientation of the aid in relation to the loop, represent real conditions of use (ideally, place them on the user).
4. Place the FM microphone in the test box in the calibrated position. If possible, turn off the local/environmental microphone. If this is not possible, the measurements must be done in a quiet environment. When testing a self-contained FM system in which the environment microphone can be turned off, the receiver/amplifier can remain in the test box.
5. Set all volume controls to their normal use positions.
6. Repeat the output measurements to obtain:
   A. An estimate of gain, as a function of frequency, for a high-input level (80 dB SPL).
   B. An input vs. output curve to obtain an estimate of compression threshold in the FM transmitter (see Figure 7–9).

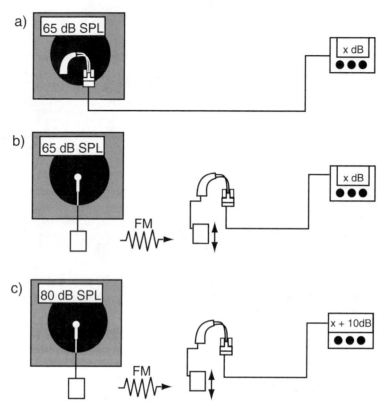

**Figure 7–8.** A suggested procedure for adjusting FM gain in order to preserve a 10-dB advantage: a) using a 1-kHz tone, measure the output for 65 dB SPL input to the local microphone; b) provide 65 dB SPL input to the remote microphone and adjust FM gain to give the same output (the two channels now have equal gain); and c) increase input to 80 dB SPL. If the output increases by 10 dB, the process is complete. *(American Speech-Language-Hearing Association. 1998. Guidelines for fitting and monitoring FM systems. Retrieved 02/23/2006 from http://www.asha.org/about/ethics/ref-library.htm <http://www.asha.org/about/ethics/ref-library.htm> <exchweb/bin/redir.asp?URL=http://www.asha.org/about/ethics/ref-library.htm>. Reprinted with permission.)*

## REAL-EAR MEASUREMENT FOR FM SYSTEMS

When electroacoustic measurements are to be carried out using output measurements in the ear canal, rather than in a 2-cc coupler, the audiologist should follow standard procedures for testing using the local or hearing aid microphone. When testing with the FM microphone, it should be placed as close as possible to the reference microphone.

## PERSONAL FM SYSTEMS

While auditory trainer systems have long been used in classrooms and public places, personal FM systems are gaining in popularity due to improved performance and reduced size. Personal FM systems allow a remote handheld or body-worn microphone to connect over a radio link to a

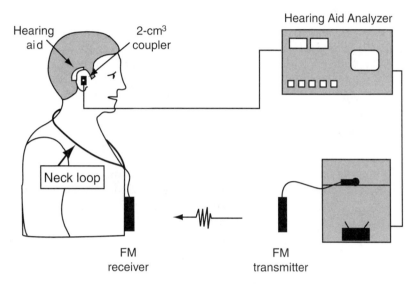

**Figure 7–9.** Suggested arrangement for electroacoustic assessment of a personal FM system that uses neck loop coupling (ASHA, 1988). *(American Speech-Language-Hearing Association. 1998. Guidelines for fitting and monitoring FM systems. Retrieved 02/23/2006 from http://www.asha.org/ about/ethics/ref-library.htm <http://www.asha.org/about/ethics/ref-library.htm> <exchweb/bin/redir.asp? URL=http://www. asha.org/about/ethics/ref-library.htm>. Reprinted with permission.)*

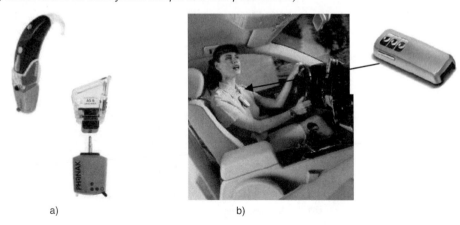

a)          b)

**Figure 7–10.** Components of personal FM systems: a) miniature radio receiver attached to a hearing instrument with an audio adaptor; b) a SmartLink and its application for cell phone use in a car. *(Courtesy of Phonak AG.)*

miniature radio receiver attached to a hearing instrument. The miniature receiver is housed inside a modified audio input adaptor or attaches to a regular audio input adaptor (see Figure 7–10a). While in the past a receiver worked at one frequency, newer models adapt to a range of frequencies automatically.

A new device, SmartLink from Phonak, offers a wide range of convenient features in one package (see Figure 7–10b). It contains a microphone array with adjustable directionality from omnidirectional to a narrow reception angle. This is useful at meetings, for listening to a television, or improving the signal-to-noise ratio in a crowded room. The device is Bluetooth-enabled and communicates with a similarly enabled cell phone for hands-free telephone use. The phone ring is heard in the hearing instrument and the call is enabled by depressing a button on SmartLink. The cell phone is required only to dial numbers for outgoing calls. SmartLink can remotely control the volume and program selection in the hearing instrument and communicates with it via FM to a MicroLink receiver on the hearing instrument.

# REMOTE CONTROL

Remote control of audio and entertainment equipment has long been popular in home electronics. There is hardly a television on the market today which does not have a remote control. Remote controls for hearing instruments also exist (see Figure 7–11). Hearing instrument manufacturers offer different types of remote controls. All remote controls can alter the gain of the hearing instrument. More complex remote controls (and hearing instruments) have additional functions such as:

▾ Switching from M/MT/T
▾ Different user programs
▾ On/Off function
▾ Display

An important difference between the various remote controls is the method of transmission employed. Today, there are four means of transmission in hearing instrument remote controls:

**A.** Infrared
**B.** Radio (AM or FM)
**C.** Ultrasonic
**D.** Inductive

**Advantages and disadvantages of the various transmission systems:**

*Ulrasonic*

▾ Ultrasonic receiver (microphone) is already in the hearing instrument.

▾ Remote control is only possible with line of sight. Otherwise, there is too much interference. → No binaural control is possible.

*Infrared*

▾ Less sensitive to interference. Proven remote control technology.

▾ Remote control works best with line of sight. → Binaural control is possible, but not reliable.

*Radio (AM or FM)*

▾ Good transmission properties, no line of sight necessary. → Binaural control possible.

▾ Sensitive to interference from strong magnetic fields (PC).

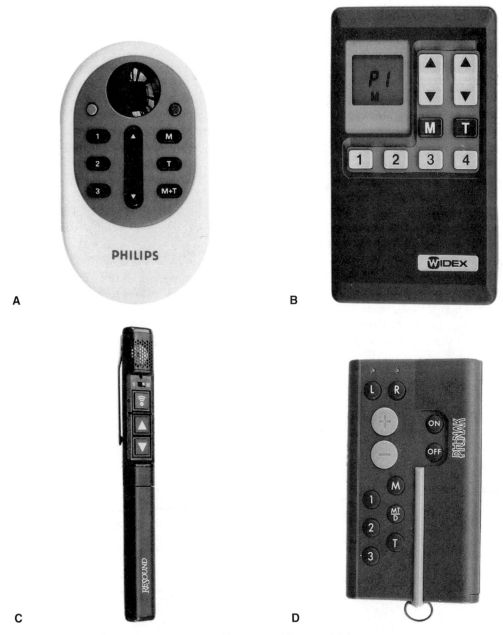

**Figure 7–11.** Different remote controls. *(Courtesy of Phonak AG.)*

*Inductive*

- ▾ Good transmission properties, no line of sight necessary. → Binaural control possible.
- ▾ Sensitive to interference from strong magnetic fields (PC).

# BATTERIES

The battery is a "galvanic voltage source" that supplies electrical power to the hearing instrument.

## CHEMISTRY

A galvanic voltage source consists of two dissimilar metal plates (e.g., a copper and a zinc plate) immersed in an electrically conducting fluid (electrolyte). The chemical reaction between these materials develops a voltage between the two plates (see Figure 7–12).

Positive metal ions pass into the electrolyte from the surface of a metal immersed in the electrolyte so that the remaining metal becomes negatively charged with respect to the fluid. The charge varies depending on the number of the ions released. Precious metals dissolve less rapidly than nonprecious metals. When two dissimilar metal plates are immersed in the same electrolyte, they become charged differently so that there is a potential difference between the two plates. If the plates are connected, the potential difference causes a current to flow between

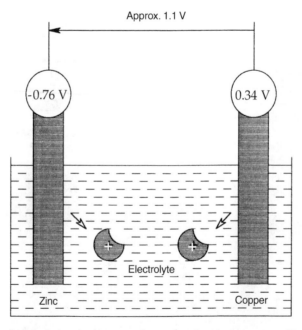

**Figure 7–12.** The chemical and electrical process in a galvanic voltage source. *(Courtesy of Phonak AG.)*

them. Because the precious metal has less negative charge than the nonprecious metal, the precious metal constitutes the positive (plus) pole and the nonprecious metal the negative (minus) pole of the voltage source. A galvanic voltage source is produced in this way. The materials in the voltage source are chosen to produce a specific voltage in accordance with the properties of an electrochemical series.

The electrochemical potentials (in volts) of a variety of materials are listed below:

| Aluminum | − 1.70 V | Tin | − 0.14 V | Carbon | + 0.74 V |
|----------|----------|-----|----------|--------|----------|
| Zinc | − 0.76 V | Lead | − 0.12 V | Silver | + 0.80 V |
| Chrome | − 0.56 V | Oxygen | 0.00 V | Mercury | + 0.85 V |
| Iron | − 0.54 V | Copper | + 0.34 V | Gold | + 1.50 V |

The following is a typical example of an electrochemical series. The zinc-carbon battery is often used in pocket flashlights and other portable electrical appliances. If we consider the electrochemical series we find:

Zinc (− 0.76 V) and carbon (+ 0.74 V) produce an initial voltage of 1.5 V between these two elements.

In the case of hearing instrument batteries, energy density (the highest energy capacity in the smallest space) is of extreme importance. Mercury batteries and silver oxide batteries were in common use in hearing instruments for many years. However, the use of silver oxide cells has diminished because of their high cost and mercury batteries are no longer allowed for environmental and health reasons. Today, the most common hearing instrument batteries are the so-called dry batteries. These differ from those described previously in that the electrolyte has been thickened into a paste. The most popular hearing aid battery today is the zinc-air battery. Fortunately, zinc-air batteries have, by far, the highest energy density of all battery technologies (these batteries are described in more detail later in this chapter).

## SIZE

Five standard battery sizes are used in hearing instruments:

1. "675" → Largest of the batteries used in hearing instruments today. Used in large and powerful behind-the-ear units.
2. "13" → Same thickness as the "675" but smaller in diameter. Used in smaller behind-the-ear units and powerful concha units.
3. "312" → Same diameter as the "13" but thinner. Used in in-the-ear units.
4. "10A" → Same thickness as the "312" but smaller in diameter. Used in small canal units.
5. "5A" → Same diameter on the "10A" but thinner. Used in CIC instruments.

While "675," "13," etc., are the commonly used designations for battery types, the standard labels for these batteries are also included in Table 7–2.

**Table 7–2.** Dimensions of hearing instrument batteries.

| Battery Type | Standard Label | Diameter (max–min [mm]) | Height (max–min [mm]) |
|---|---|---|---|
| 675 | PR44 | 11.6–11.25 | 5.4–5.0 |
| 13 | PR48 | 7.9–7.55 | 5.4–5.0 |
| 312 | PR41 | 7.9–7.55 | 3.6–3.3 |
| 10A | PR70 | 5.8–5.65 | 3.6–3.3 |
| 5A | | 5.8–5.65 | 2.2–2.0 |

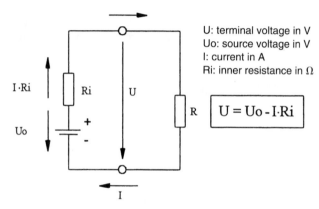

U: terminal voltage in V
Uo: source voltage in V
I: current in A
Ri: inner resistance in Ω

$$U = Uo - I \cdot Ri$$

**Figure 7–13.** Equivalent circuit for a battery. *(Courtesy of Phonak AG.)*

## CIRCUIT TECHNOLOGY

The battery is a voltage source. However, it is not ideal in that it has an internal resistance in series with the voltage source (see Figure 7–13). The internal resistance increases as the battery discharges over time. If the internal resistance becomes too great the voltage across the battery terminals is reduced and negative effects can occur in the hearing instrument (more distortion, humming, etc.). The magnitude of the problem depends on the circuit requirements in the hearing instrument.

## ZINC-AIR BATTERY

The zinc-air battery has a large capacity and no mercury. The battery has several air holes in the case. These are covered by an adhesive plastic tab when the battery is new. When the battery is to be used, the adhesive tab is removed. Air then enters the battery and the chemical process begins; that is, the battery voltage rises to the unloaded initial value of 1.4 V.

Once the air holes are open, the zinc-air battery has a permanent discharge current of about 50 µA, depending on the size of the air holes. The larger the holes, the higher the discharge current.

**Table 7–3.** Battery capacities.

| Battery Type | Capacity (mAh) |
|:---:|:---:|
| 675 | 610 |
| 13 | 290 |
| 312 | 150 |
| 10A | 95 |
| 5A | 55 |

Once a zinc-air battery has been opened, the chemical process cannot be stopped by closing the air holes. The maximum current that the battery can deliver is dependent on the size of the air holes.

The energy capacity of the various types of zinc-air batteries are given in milliampere-hours (mAh) in Table 7–3. These values are useful in calculating the life expectance of a battery in a hearing instrument during normal use. For example, a type 13 battery should last for 193 hours if the instrument draws an average current of 1.5 mA.

Most battery manufacturers give a freshness guarantee for three years for batteries when the tab has not been removed. There will be some drop off over this time, but the percentage should be minimal (probably on the order of 2 to 5% per year) and dependent on storage conditions.

Predicting the shelf life of a battery after tab removal is a very complex issue, but some general statements apply. The life of the cell after tab removal is highly dependent on the temperature and location it is in (whether in use or not). The effects would be different for a user in Asia (hot and humid) versus Arizona (hot and dry) versus Scandinavia (cool and dry). Also, if the cell is stored within the hearing instrument during this period, the effect would be lessened. In general, an elevated temperature will increase the rate of self-discharge and thus reduce capacity. Water vapor transmission into the cell will flood the cathode and/or dilute the electrolyte and thus reduce capacity. The transmission of carbon dioxide ($CO_2$) will react directly with the electrolyte, reduce concentration, and thus reduce capacity.

The effect is also dependent upon cell size. The larger the cell, the more resistant the cell is to the effects mentioned previously. The level of effect is also dependent upon the rate of discharge that the cell will undergo. The higher the discharge rate, the more pronounced the drop-off in performance. Assuming that the cell is in an atmosphere of approximately 25°C and 60% relative humidity, there should be a significant drop-off in performance between one and four weeks. The user retabbing the cell after use will have some impact in extending cell life. However, the extension cannot be guaranteed due to the fact that the adhesive is designed for the first contact to the cell and not for reuse. In addition, the force and accuracy of application will vary between individuals.

### Advantages and disadvantages of zinc-air batteries:

▼ Constant voltage during discharge (see Figure 7–14)
▼ Environmentally friendly
▼ Large capacity

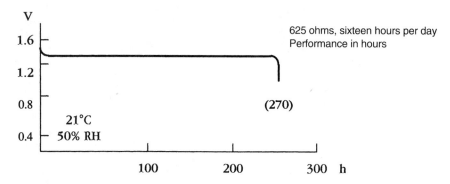

**Figure 7–14.** Discharge voltage of a zinc-air battery over time. *(Courtesy of Phonak AG.)*

▼ Not very long shelf life
▼ Continuous discharge current
▼ Peak current smaller than that of mercury batteries → not suitable for high-performance units

The advantages of zinc-air batteries make it the battery of choice for nearly all hearing aid applications.

## SUMMARY

1. The utility of hearing instruments in difficult situations is much improved by the availability of accessories which may be used on a more or less temporary basis.
2. The telecoil (induction coil) is useful for telephone use in noisy places. Not all telephones produce sufficient magnetic field strength to be used with a telecoil.
3. Telecoils are also used with loop systems installed in private or public places.
4. The audio input accessory is a particularly useful feature in many situations. It allows the connection of a variety of devices such as remote microphones and FM systems to be quickly and reliably connected to the hearing instrument as the need arises.
5. The direct audio input feature is used to provide CROS and BiCROS fittings.
6. Newer personal FM accessories are also equipped with Bluetooth to work with digital cell phones. These devices allow hands-free cell phone operation and eliminate cell phone interference by allowing the cell phone to be used at a distance from the hearing instrument so that interference is essentially eliminated.
7. Remote handheld microphones, FM systems, and personal FM systems move the microphone closer to the sound source to improve the signal-to-noise ratio for the hearing instrument user.

8. Remote controls for hearing instruments permit the user, even those with poor dexterity, to adjust their hearing instruments quickly and discreetly.

9. An active-air (zinc-air) battery discharges once the adhesive tab is removed, even if the battery is not being used.

## REVIEW QUESTIONS

1. Describe advantages and disadvantages of CROS and BiCROS configurations.
2. Which kinds of transmissions are used for hearing instrument remote controls? What are advantage and disadvantages of the different systems?
3. A hard-of-hearing student needs an FM system for school.
   A. What are the required system components?
   B. How is the hearing instrument set to allow the student to understand the teacher and other students?
   C. What has to be taken into consideration?
4. What are the advantages and disadvantages of zinc-air batteries?
5. What is the capacity of a 312 zinc-air battery?
   A. 500 mAh                                              A ☐
   B. 50 mAh                                               B ☐
   C. 312 mAh                                              C ☐
   D. 120 mAh                                              D ☐
6. Which remote control technologies are best suited for binaural control ?
   A. Inductive transmission                               A ☐
   B. Radio transmission                                   B ☐
   C. Infrared transmission                                C ☐
   D. Ultrasound transmission                              D ☐
7. The goals of accessories like a T-coil, handheld microphones, or FM systems are :
   A. Better frequency response                            A ☐
   B. Improve signal-to-noise ratio                        B ☐
   C. Enlarge the dynamic range                            C ☐
   D. Increase the gain                                    D ☐

CHAPTER 8

# Hearing Instrument Troubleshooting

## INTRODUCTION

Hearing instrument dispensers and clinicians return hearing instruments to the manufacturer for repair when problems or malfunctions occur. This chapter presents a number of approaches to diagnosing the fault and suggests possible action that could be taken by the hearing health care professional to perform a portion of the fault diagnosis in order to assist the manufacturer's service technician and, if possible, to resolve the problem in the office without undue inconvenience for the owner of the hearing instrument.

When a hearing instrument is returned as defective to the manufacturer, a number of tests can be performed without having to open the device.

## FEEDBACK

### FEEDBACK IN AN ITE

The causes and remedies for feedback in an ITE instrument can be identified by following the process outlined in Figure 8–1.

### FEEDBACK IN A BTE

The causes and remedies for feedback in a BTE instrument can be identified by following the process outlined in Figure 8–2.

## NO ACOUSTIC GAIN/OUTPUT

Problems with gain and output in a hearing instrument can be identified and resolved by following the steps outlined in Figure 8–3.

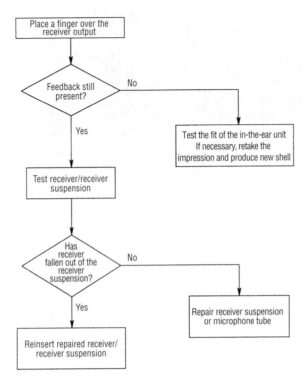

**Figure 8–1.** Flowchart for troubleshooting an ITE hearing instrument with acoustic feedback. *(Courtesy of Phonak AG.)*

# CIC TROUBLESHOOTING

## IN-OFFICE MODIFICATIONS

Successful clinicians and dispensers of CICs realize the increase in fitting time and repeated visits are part of the CIC process. Seventy-five percent of CICs require some modification when fitted on the patient (Voll & Jones, 1998). A few of the most common complaints and modifications are listed below.

### *Discomfort/Pain in Ear*

▼ Identify the area where discomfort is produced with an earlight or otoscope and relieve pressure on this area.
▼ Pressure point may be red.
▼ Match length of the aid to the earlight tip. Place earlight tip to mark in the ear canal and apply gentle pressure. Instruct the patient to report the points of sensitivity. Match those points to the hearing aid to identify the area which needs to be modified.
▼ Modifications to the shell of a CIC should be done conservatively, grinding only small amounts at a time. Overmodification can lead to feedback and occlusion effects.

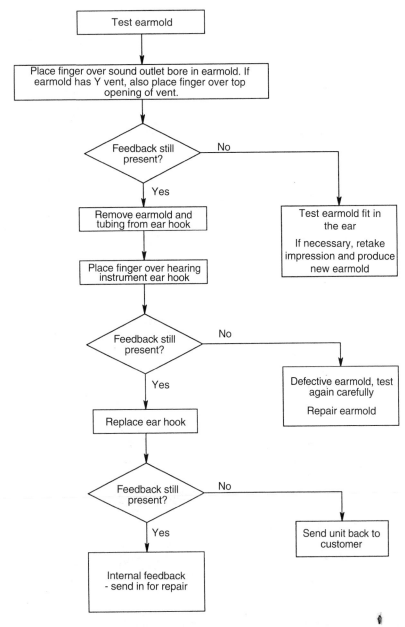

**Figure 8–2.** Flowchart for troubleshooting a BTE hearing instrument with acoustic feedback. *(Courtesy of Phonak AG.)*

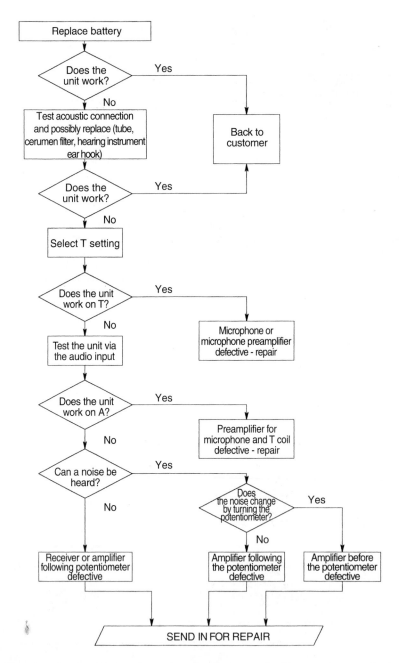

**Figure 8–3.** Flowchart for troubleshooting a hearing instrument with no gain or output. *(Courtesy of Phonak AG.)*

## Occlusion or "Head in a Barrel"

Although reduction of occlusion effects is one of the advantages of CIC instruments, it can also be a problem when the aid is not inserted or properly fitted into the bony part of the canal. Sensitivity, small canal size, or sharp turns may prevent sealing in the bony part of the canal and cause a complaint of occlusion effect.

- ▼ Check that the receiver directs sound towards the eardrum.
- ▼ Check that the vent is clear and unobstructed. Modification may be necessary to redirect the vent away from the canal wall.
- ▼ Make sure the microphone is not obstructed. If it is covered by the tragus or antitragus, it may need to be returned to the manufacturer for repositioning.
- ▼ Check the length of the aid against the impression. Aids that are too short or too tapered may contribute to occlusion effects. If possible, the aid may require that it be remade with a longer canal. If not, it may require further shortening or opening of the vent.
- ▼ Occlusion after wearing the aid for some time: It is possible that the aid is migrating out of the ear. A canal lock can help with retention and holding the aid in place.
- ▼ Counselling for realistic expectations can alleviate efforts spent toward unrealistic goals.

## Feedback

One of the problems that can occur is feedback. Unfortunately, not all fittings are feedback-free initially. Be aware that using a tighter fit to reduce feedback is only a temporary solution. The flexibility of the cartilaginous area of the ear canal will cause the canal to stretch over time, making the problem worse in the long term.

### Microphone/Receiver Placement

- ▼ Verify that the microphone is not covered by the tragus.
- ▼ Compare the shape of the shell to the ear impression. If the angle of the canal is not correct, the receiver may open into the canal wall, causing feedback when the aid is barely on.

### Response-Related Feedback

- ▼ A sharp spike in the REAR can indicate feedback.
- ▼ Dampen with acoustic foam or white (680 ohm) damper in the receiver tube.

### Loose Fit

- ▼ A ring of silicone material or a retention ring can be added around the second bend of the device for a temporary fix.
- ▼ If the patient is not experiencing discomfort, a longer, tighter canal may be required.
- ▼ A canal lock may help hold the aid in place and reduce feedback. The manufacturer will need an impression to add a canal lock.

### Feedback with Jaw Movement

▼ Prevent this problem by taking a good quality deep impression with the jaw half open, thus preventing extremes in jaw movement from creating feedback.

▼ A canal lock can be helpful in holding the aid in place and reducing feedback.

▼ If the jaw movement is visualized at the first bend, it may be possible to recess the faceplate deep enough to avoid the movement.

▼ Movement that is at the second bend can be alleviated by adding a retention ring around the second bend, or building up the anterior wall for a tighter fit.

### Circuitry

Most wearers of CIC hearing instruments do not have a manual volume control. When this is the case, the volume may be adjusted with a screw-set volume control. Compression amplifiers are usually the best choice for CIC instruments with WDRC being preferred. Realize, however, that in quiet environments a WDRC amplifier will amplify the ambient noise, causing the wearer to perceive a "hissing" noise in quiet. This is especially common in patients with normal or near-normal low-frequency thresholds. For these individuals a compression limiting amplifier is recommended.

The ideal amplifier for CIC instruments is a programmable circuit. Since the size of a CIC restricts the number of controls that can be put on the instrument, programmability has many advantages. Some programmable CICs also include multiple memories, allowing the wearer to adjust the gain and/or frequency response for a variety of listening situations.

▼ Lack of volume control adjustment may suggest a stronger preference for compression amplifiers as opposed to linear/peak clipping amplifiers.

▼ Mild to moderate sloping losses: wide dynamic range compression amplifier.

▼ Ski-slope losses: compression limiting amplifier.

▼ Programmable and/or multimemory instruments offer increased adjustability for dispensers and control for wearers.

## CIRCUIT AND MICROPHONE NOISE

Circuit noise is the "hissing" or broadband noise that is always present to some degree. Although it is called "circuit noise," it is primarily caused by the microphone. Occasionally, hearing aid wearers will complain that they hear the circuit noise, especially in quiet settings. There are two possible sources for this noise:

1. Noise from the hearing instrument and/or microphone
2. Ambient noise (computer, air conditioner, etc.)

To identify the source of the noise, place the hearing aid in the patient's ear and lightly (do not press it into the microphone opening) cover the microphone opening with a small amount of putty. If the noise goes away, then the source is ambient noise. If the noise is still there or gets louder, it is microphone noise.

## REDUCING THE NOISE

An environmental noise source can be suppressed by reducing the hearing instrument gain in that frequency range. Beware of reducing the speech intelligibility, too. Sometimes just identifying the source of the noise and counselling the patient appropriately will eliminate the problem. This is often the case with WDRC circuits that provide a lot of gain for soft sounds.

If the source of the noise is the hearing instrument microphone, there are several options. It is possible that the microphone is defective and requires repair by the manufacturer. A measure of equivalent input noise in the test box should help to identify when this is the case. In some instances, adjusting the frequency response can help to eliminate the noise. Either reducing low-frequency gain (to reduce the amplification in that region) or increasing low-frequency gain (to mask the microphone noise) can be effective.

Many modern instruments offer a low-level expansion feature with an adjustable threshold. Increasing the threshold will reduce the noise (internal and external), but can also reduce the intelligibility of soft speech.

## OCCLUSION EFFECT

Occlusion is caused by the enhancement of low-frequency vibrations of a person's voice when the ear canal is blocked by the hearing instrument. When we speak, we produce about 140 dB SPL in the back of the mouth on closed vowels such as /i/ and /u/. The resulting vibration of the flesh and mandible causes the wall of the ear canal to vibrate. When a shallow seal is used, the trapped sounds of the wearer's own voice can produce 100 dB SPL or greater in the ear canal at low frequencies. This is 20–30 dB more than when the ear is unoccluded.

Zwislocki demonstrated that terminating the tip of an earplug in the bony portion of the ear canal reduces the likelihood of occlusion. The possibility of using deep-canal hearing aid fittings to address complaints of occlusion has been discussed by many researchers.

Normally, a large vent is used to reduce occlusion effect. A large vent is not possible in a small CIC instrument. The best way to combat occlusion in a CIC fitting is to seal the canal tip deep into the bony portion of the canal. A small vent is also used to relieve pressure, but it has little effect on frequency response or occlusion effect.

## INTERFERENCE ISSUES AND DIGITAL MOBILE TELEPHONES

This topic is discussed in detail in Chapter 13.

## SUMMARY

1. A number of hearing instrument faults can be diagnosed and corrected by the hearing health care professional.
2. Flowcharts for troubleshooting BTE and ITE hearing instruments that exhibit feedback, lack of output, and gain can be followed to diagnose performance problems.
3. Simple methods exist for correcting circuit and microphone noise problems.
4. Discomfort problems can be eliminated by removing material from the shell or earmold.
5. The occlusion effect can often be reduced with simple corrective measures.
6. Resolving problems when the hearing instrument user visits the clinic or the dispenser's office saves time.

## REVIEW QUESTIONS

1. What kind of feedback can occur in hearing instruments?
2. **A.** A customer sends a BTE for repair. The hearing instrument has no output signal. What kind of failures create such a defect? (at least five answers)
   **B.** A customer sends a BTE for repair. The instrument creates feedback (whistling). What kind of failures creates such a defect? (at least two answers)
3. A CIC user complains that he feels his head is in a barrel when he speaks. List three things that should be checked to find the root cause for this effect.
4. A CIC user complains about discomfort or pain in his ear. What is the recommended procedure for alleviating such a problem?
5. What are two reasons that could initiate a complaint that the hearing instrument sounds noisy?
6. How can hearing aid noise be reduced?
7. What is the recommended procedure when a hearing instrument malfunction cannot be corrected in the office?

# CHAPTER 9

# Hearing Instrument Measurements and Standards

## INTRODUCTION

The first hearing instrument assessment tool was the human ear. A trained ear can, in fact, determine the quality of a hearing instrument quite fast and accurately, and a hard-of-hearing individual can also quickly decide if the sound quality of the hearing instrument is acceptable. However, selecting and fitting a hearing instrument for a specific hearing loss requires much more information than a sound quality assessment. A technical specification that describes the instrument's measured electroacoustic performance characteristics is required; such specifications are also a necessary part of the mandatory medical device registration process in many countries.

Standards have been developed to establish measurement and specification methods as well as tolerances for hearing instrument performance parameters. These standards are developed by working groups consisting of technical experts that are active in the field of hearing instrument research, design, and prescription. The two major standards organizations are the American National Standards Institute (ANSI) and the International Electrotechnical Commission (IEC). They produce voluntary standards that are often mandated by national organizations and regulatory bodies. ANSI standards are mandated primarily in North America and Australia while IEC standards are mandated by many EU and international counties. Both ANSI and IEC standards are subjected to a five-year review cycle to ensure they keep pace with changing technology and business cycles.

The ANSI S3.22 standard and IEC 60118 series of standards prescribe measurement methods for the specification of hearing instrument characteristics. Both have similar objectives, but there are some important differences. ANSI S3.22 specifies the use of a coupler with a 2 cubic centimeter (2-cc) cavity for electroacoustic measurements. While the IEC standard also specifies the 2-cc coupler for measurements for quality control and delivery purposes, it in addition specifies the use of an ear simulator for the purpose of performance specification. Coupler measurements produce different results than measurements made at the user's tympanic membrane, but have the advantage of being easily controlled and reproduced. Requirements for sound fields, couplers, and specific measurement methods of these standards, as well as other applicable standards, are discussed in this chapter.

The main standards in use today for characterizing hearing instruments are listed at the end of this chapter.

# SOUND FIELD REQUIREMENTS

## FREE FIELD MEASUREMENT

The data obtained measuring a hearing instrument in a normal room will be confounded by the reflection of sound from the walls. No two rooms are likely to be alike, so that such reverberation would make comparisons with data obtained elsewhere impossible.

Hearing instruments must, therefore, be measured in free field conditions. A free field is a sound field free from the reflective effects of boundaries. The ideal measurement environment is an anechoic chamber, but such rooms are large and expensive. A more economical solution is to use small sound-treated boxes. These are sufficiently free of reflection in the hearing instrument frequency range (100 Hz to 10 kHz) to make them appropriate for measurement of hearing instruments. Figure 9–1 shows two examples of sound boxes. The first is manufactured by B&K in Denmark and the second, by Frye Electronics, in the United States. Many different sound box designs are commercially available in different sizes and price ranges. These

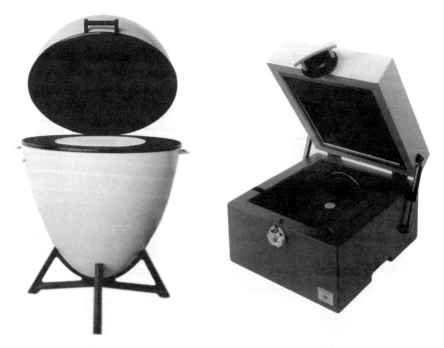

**Figure 9–1.** Sound boxes from B&K and Frye Electronics. *(Courtesy of Brüel & Kjær and Frye Electronics, Inc.)*

boxes usually contain a built-in loudspeaker to produce calibrated sound levels, provisions for a measurement microphone and coupler, as well as a power supply for the hearing aid. Small, inexpensive sound boxes are commonly used in manufacturing and clinical settings.

## LINEAR LOUDSPEAKER FREQUENCY RESPONSE (COMPARISON METHOD)

Any nonlinearity in the loudspeaker frequency response in the sound box causes errors in the measurement of the hearing instrument frequency response. Therefore, the frequency response of the loudspeaker must be flat (+ 1 dB) between 100 Hz and 10 kHz.

It is unusual for a loudspeaker (in the normal price range) to offer such an accurate frequency response, so the variations in the loudspeaker's frequency response are compensated for electronically.

This is accomplished by the arrangement shown in Figure 9–2. A calibrated free field microphone (commonly referred to as a control microphone) is installed in the sound box symmetrically opposite the test point to measure the sound pressure at what is usually referred to as the reference point. Whenever the sound pressure diverges from the reference value (e.g., 60 dB SPL), the electrical input to the loudspeaker amplifier is rapidly adjusted so that the sound pressure at the control microphone again matches the reference value. This is referred to as the comparison method.

Figures 9–3 and 9–4 show typical frequency responses for the test box loudspeaker with and without electronic compensation.

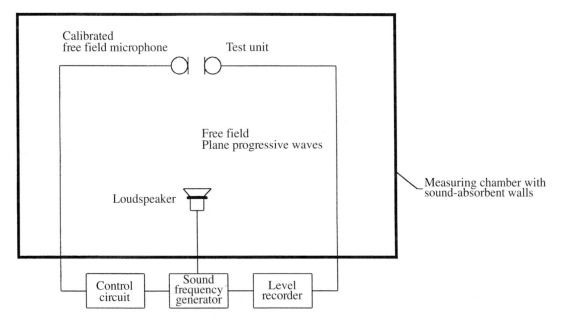

**Figure 9–2.** Equipment schematic for calibrating controlled sound box measurements. *(Courtesy of Phonak AG.)*

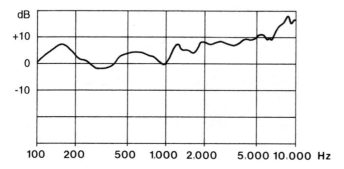

**Figure 9–3.** Frequency response of a loudspeaker in a sound box without electronic compensation for the loudspeaker response (response is normalized to 0 dB at 1 kHz). *(Courtesy of Phonak AG.)*

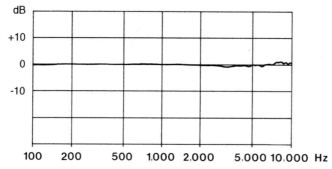

**Figure 9–4.** Frequency response of a loudspeaker in a sound box with electronic compensation for the loudspeaker response (response is normalized to 0 dB at 1 kHz). *(Courtesy of Phonak AG.)*

The substitution method is an alternate method of achieving a linear frequency response in the sound box.

## THE SUBSTITUTION METHOD

This method is particularly suited for clinical use by hearing healthcare professionals. Only one microphone is required for the substitution method. It differs from the comparison method in that the electrical input to the loudspeaker amplifier needed to achieve the desired sound pressure is determined in advance of measuring the hearing instrument. Prior to measuring any hearing instruments, the loudspeaker frequency response is determined with the measuring microphone at the test point. This curve is stored and the microphone is removed. During subsequent measurements the hearing instrument is placed at the test point and the electrical input to the loudspeaker amplifier is manipulated so as to "flatten out" the stored curve. Thus, if the stored curve has a 5-dB notch at 3 kHz, then the electrical input to the loudspeaker amplifier is increased so as to give a 5 dB more intense signal at this frequency. Likewise, a 7-dB spike at 6 kHz would be compensated for by a corresponding decrease in the input to the loudspeaker amplifier, resulting in a 7 dB less intense signal at this frequency. In this way, a flat sound field is achieved at the test point.

# HEARING INSTRUMENT COUPLER AND EAR SIMULATOR

Ideally, a hearing instrument would be measured in situ, or as worn in the ear, to assess its actual performance. However, this would be costly and, due to the nonstandard nature of human ears, any meaningful comparison of results would be impossible. Thus, analyses of hearing instruments are made using standardized couplers and "artificial ears." These coupling devices have been designed to approximate the acoustic characteristics of an average ear.

A microphone is inserted at one end of the coupling device and the sound outlet of the earmold or ITE instrument is connected to the other end. The microphone diaphragm takes the place of the tympanic membrane and the device's volume represents the residual volume and acoustic impedance of the occluded ear canal. The microphone measures the sound levels the receiver delivers into the coupling device.

In 1959 a coupler with a volume of 2 cc was specified for hearing instrument measurements (IEC 126 standard). In spite of the fact that this 2-cc volume is approximately 50% larger than the volume of the average ear canal, and possibly twice as large as the residual volume of the ear canal when occluded with a hearing instrument, it has remained the coupler of choice for quality control and delivery purposes. In its favor are simplicity of construction and repeatability in measurement results over time.

Artificial ears or ear simulators take into account the equivalent volumes or loading of the receiver of the hearing instrument with the same average frequency-dependent impedance of the human ear in the hearing frequency range. This ensures that the sound pressure, which the measuring microphone picks up, agrees with the average value present at the eardrum (IEC 711 standard).

## THE 2-CC COUPLER

An electroacoustic coupler with a cavity of 2 cc is used in place of the human ear for the measurements described above. At one end of the cavity is a capacitor microphone. It transforms sounds into electrical signals that are supplied to the measuring instruments. The method for mounting the hearing instrument on the coupler is modified according to the type of hearing instrument (e.g., behind-the-ear or in-the-ear).

Figure 9–5 shows how the coupler and a behind-the-ear unit are connected via tubing. This tubing should have a length of 25 mm and an inner diameter of 2 mm.

For an in-the-ear instrument, where the receiver is in the ear canal, the connection is made as shown in Figure 9–6. Typical hearing instrument curves as measured with the 2-cc coupler are shown in Figures 9–7, 9–8, 9–9, and 9–10.

The average human ear has a volume considerably smaller than 2 cc. As a consequence, measurements made in the 2-cc coupler differ markedly from those made in the ear, particularly at frequencies higher than 1 kHz.

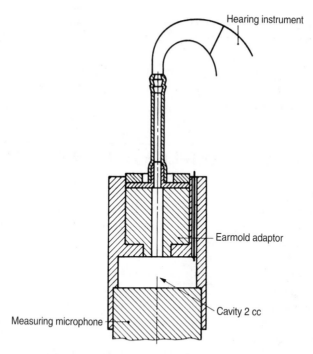

**Figure 9–5.** A 2-cc coupler for BTE hearing instrument measurements. *(Copyright © 1973, IEC, Geneva, Switzerland. www.iec.ch)*

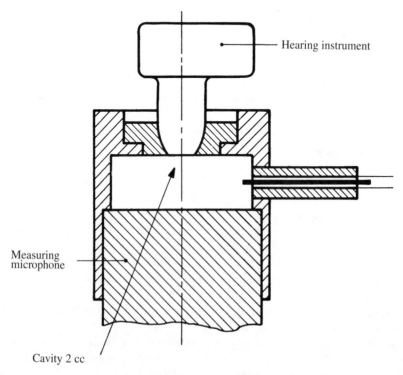

**Figure 9–6.** A 2-cc coupler for ITE hearing instrument measurements. *(Copyright © 1973, IEC, Geneva, Switzerland. www.iec.ch)*

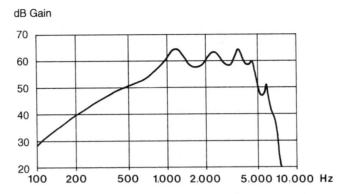

**Figure 9–7.** The gain response of a BTE hearing instrument measured in a 2-cc coupler. *(Courtesy of Phonak AG.)*

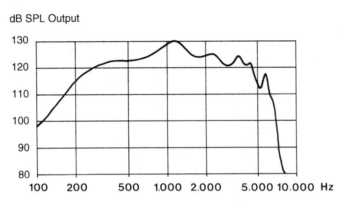

**Figure 9–8.** The maximum output response of a BTE hearing instrument measured in a 2-cc coupler. *(Courtesy of Phonak AG.)*

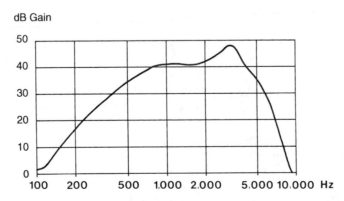

**Figure 9–9.** The gain response of an ITE hearing instrument measured in a 2-cc coupler. *(Courtesy of Phonak AG.)*

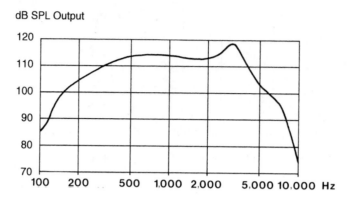

dB SPL Output

**Figure 9–10.** The maximum output response of an ITE hearing instrument measured in a 2-cc coupler. *(Courtesy of Phonak AG.)*

In this case, the SPL measured in the 2-cc coupler will be too low compared to real-ear measurements. This was the impetus behind the 1981 issuance of the IEC 711 standard for a better coupler.

Since the acoustic properties of this new coupler more closely approximated those of the human ear, it was called an ear simulator. It is manufactured by Brüel and Kjær (B&K) in Denmark.

Although the ear simulator has been on the market for a long time, there are some countries (e.g., the United States) that still use the 2-cc coupler (ANSI, S3.22 standard). The reasons for the continued worldwide use of a 2-cc coupler (among hearing health care professionals) include the reproducibility of results, ease of use, relative economy, and its durability.

## THE EAR SIMULATOR FROM B&K (B&K EAR SIMULATOR)

In 1971, the members of the working group "Artificial Ear for Insert Earphones" in the IEC (International Electrotechnical Commission) ratified the following required properties for an ear simulator:

▼ The materials used should be mechanically stable and easy to manufacture.
▼ The simulator should have a geometrical similarity to the ear canal.
▼ The measurable frequency range should be 80–6,000 Hz, extendible, if possible, to 10 kHz.
▼ The acoustic impedance should be the same as the corresponding mean value of the human ear.
▼ The acoustic properties of the different kinds of hearing instruments measured with the ear simulator should correspond to the mean value measured at the real eardrum.

In the late 1970s, Brüel and Kjær (B&K) developed an ear simulator that was selected by the IEC as the standard for hearing instrument measurements. In 1981, this was incorporated into the new IEC standard.

The B&K ear simulator is primarily intended for the measurement of hearing instruments that are coupled to the ear via tubing, earmolds, and so on. It has therefore been designed to fulfill the requirements of the proposed IEC and ANSI standards for an ear simulator for measuring hearing instruments.

The ear simulator closely reproduces the physical parameters of the human ear, presenting the hearing instrument under test with an impedance approximating that of the real human ear. The ear simulator consists of a main housing into which are assembled a number of rings forming annular volumes of air connected to the main cavity of the housing by air passages. The main canal volume is similar in shape and volume to that of the human ear and provides a similar acoustic impedance to the hearing instrument being tested. The capacitor microphone is screwed directly into the housing of the ear simulator. The ear simulator, like the 2-cc coupler, can also be modified to suit different hearing instruments. The various adaptors supplied with the ear simulator allow simple mounting of all types of hearing instruments.

Figures 9–11, 9–12, and 9–13 show the methods for mounting the various types of hearing instruments to the ear simulator with the adaptors provided.

## COUPLER CALIBRATION

Accuracy in hearing instrument measurements requires occasional calibration of the ear simulator (or 2-cc coupler). This can be done most easily using the B&K pistonphone. The pistonphone is connected directly to the ear simulator and provides a stable 250-Hz signal of 124 dB SPL. The measuring instrument must be calibrated with this 124-dB SPL signal. Figure 9–14 shows an ear simulator with the pistonphone connected.

## RESPONSE DIFFERENCES BETWEEN THE 2-CC COUPLER AND EAR SIMULATOR

The ear simulator was developed to simulate the complex auditory canal more closely than the 2-cc coupler. Ear simulator measurements correspond better on average with real-ear measurements than those made in the 2-cc coupler. It must be stressed, however, that the ear simulator is an instrument, and that the measurements obtained with it can only be approximately related to an individual ear. The ear simulator is particularly suitable for comparing one hearing instrument with another, although this is also possible with the 2-cc coupler.

For the hearing health care professional, it is often necessary to determine whether the hearing instrument was measured with the ear simulator or with the 2-cc coupler to avoid confusion.

Figures 9–15 and 9–16 show the gain and output saturation pressure levels of a behind-the-ear unit measured with an ear simulator and with a 2-cc coupler.

Figure 9–17 and 9–18 show the gain and output saturation pressure levels for an in-the-ear unit measured with an ear simulator and with a 2-cc coupler.

It is clear from the comparative measurements that the sound pressure level in the ear simulator is up to 10 dB higher than in the 2-cc coupler. The larger volume of the 2-cc coupler gives a difference of about 4 dB in the low frequencies; the larger difference in the high frequencies comes from a bandstop function of the 2-cc coupler around 12 kHz. One of the main

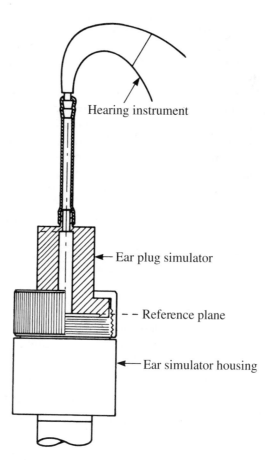

**Figure 9–11.** Ear simulator for BTE hearing instruments. *(Courtesy of Brüel & Kjær, 1981.)*

advantages of the ear simulator is that the results obtained for high frequencies are more similar to real-ear measurements than are those obtained with a 2-cc coupler. There are also differences in measurements dependent on hearing instrument type (BTE, ITE, etc.).

## HEARING INSTRUMENT MEASUREMENTS IN THE SOUND BOX ACCORDING TO IEC

Maximum acoustic gain, reference test gain, maximum output sound pressure level, and so on are all specific data for a hearing instrument that can be measured in a sound box. This section describes the procedures and necessary instrumentation for performing such measurements. The basis for these measurements is the IEC 118-0 standard (with B&K ear simulator). Obtain-

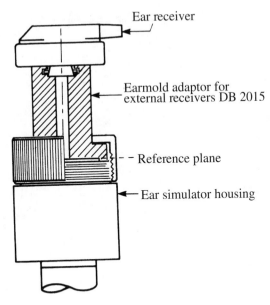

**Figure 9–12.** Ear simulator for a button receiver. *(Courtesy of Brüel & Kjær, 1981.)*

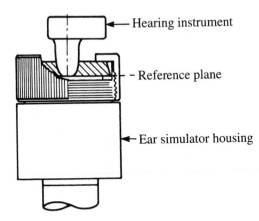

**Figure 9–13.** Ear simulator for an ITE hearing instrument with an earmold. *(Courtesy of Brüel & Kjær, 1981.)*

ing measurements in accordance with other standards and with other couplers (2 cc) will be covered later in this chapter in the section on measurement standards.

The equipment for measuring the acoustic properties of a hearing instrument is shown in Figure 9–19. The sound box has sound-absorbent walls in order to maintain free field conditions. An audio frequency generator drives a loudspeaker, which is also located in the sound

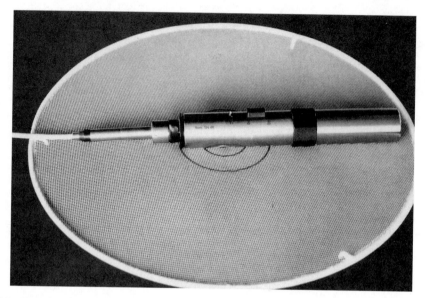

**Figure 9–14.** Ear simulator calibration with a pistonphone. *(Courtesy of Phonak AG.)*

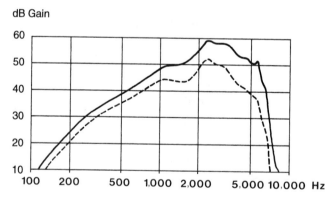

**Figure 9–15.** Gain response of a BTE measured with an ear simulator (solid line) and a 2-cc coupler (dashed line). *(Courtesy of Phonak AG.)*

box. With this set-up, it is possible to use either the substitution or the comparison method as described at the beginning of this chapter. The comparison method will be utilized in the example. The hearing instrument microphone and the control microphone are near to one another and are symmetrically arranged with respect to the axis of the sound source. The control circuit, which is regulated by the control microphone, automatically maintains the desired sound pressure level at the measuring point while the frequency is altered. The hearing instrument is connected to the ear simulator.

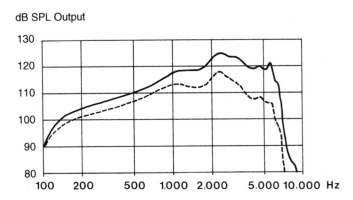

**Figure 9–16.** OSPL90 response of a BTE measured with an ear simulator (solid line) and a 2-cc coupler (dashed line). *(Courtesy of Phonak AG.)*

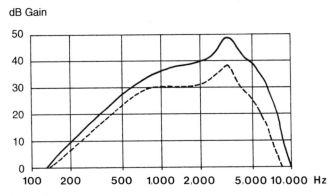

**Figure 9–17.** Gain response of an ITE measured with an ear simulator (solid line) and a 2-cc coupler (dashed line). *(Courtesy of Phonak AG.)*

The pressure microphone in the ear simulator measures the output sound level and transmits the measured value to the level recorder. The level recorder and the frequency changes of the generator run synchronously. The response curve is usually displayed and hard copies can be produced.

## EXPLANATION OF TERMS

In order to measure the hearing instrument accurately in the sound box and to enable comparison with other measurements (e.g., a data sheet), it is necessary to be familiar with certain terms.

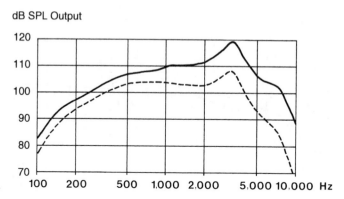

**Figure 9–18.** OSPL90 response of an ITE measured with an ear simulator (solid line) and a 2-cc coupler (dashed line). *(Courtesy of Phonak AG.)*

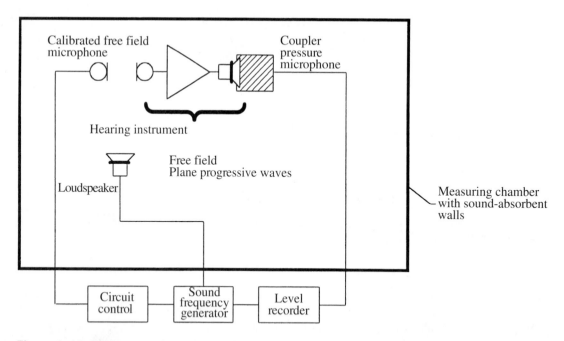

**Figure 9–19.** Equipment schematic for hearing instrument measurements in a controlled sound box. *(Courtesy of Phonak AG.)*

## Acoustic Gain

The difference between the output sound pressure level developed in the ear simulator by the hearing instrument and the input sound pressure level measured at the test point.

## Full-on Acoustic Gain

The acoustic gain under essentially linear input/output conditions obtainable from the hearing instrument measured with the gain control at maximum (full-on) and at stated settings of the other hearing instrument controls.

## Maximum Saturation Sound Pressure Level

The maximum value of a saturation sound pressure level frequency response curve produced in the ear simulator.

## Output SPL for an Input SPL of 90 dB SPL (OSPL90)

The sound pressure level produced in the ear simulator with an input sound pressure level of 90 dB SPL, the gain control being in the full-on position and the other controls set for maximum gain. The abbreviation for this term is OSPL90 (or OSPL90 frequency response curve).

## Reference Test Frequency

The frequency at which the setting of the gain control is made in relation to OSPL90 to obtain a reference test position of the gain control. The reference test frequency is normally 1,600 Hz. For certain hearing instruments, a higher reference test frequency is more appropriate (so-called high-tone hearing instruments). In this case, 2,500 Hz is used as the reference test frequency, and this should be clearly stated in the reported measurement results.

## Reference Test Gain Control Position

The setting of the hearing instrument gain control that provides an output sound pressure level in the ear simulator of $15 \pm 1$ dB less than OSPL90 for an input sound pressure level of 60 dB SPL at the reference test frequency. If the gain available will not permit this, full-on gain control position of the hearing instrument should be used.

## Reference Test Gain

The acoustic gain of the hearing instrument at the reference test frequency with the setting of the gain control set to the reference test gain control position.

## Basic Frequency Response Curve

The frequency response curve obtained at the reference test gain setting with an input sound pressure level of 60 dB SPL.

## OUTPUT SPL FREQUENCY RESPONSE FOR AN INPUT OF 90 DB SPL (OSPL90)

The purpose of this test is to determine the sound pressure level obtained in the ear simulator when using an input of 90 dB SPL and the gain control in the full-on position as a function of frequency (see Figure 9–20).

---

### *Test Procedure*

1. Turn the gain control full on and set other controls to the required positions.
2. Adjust the input sound pressure level to 90 dB SPL at a suitable frequency.
3. Vary the frequency of the sound source over the recommended frequency range from 200 Hz to 8,000 Hz, keeping the input sound pressure level constant at 90 dB SPL. Record the sound pressure level in the ear simulator.

---

## FULL-ON ACOUSTIC GAIN FREQUENCY RESPONSE

The purpose of this test is to determine the full-on acoustic gain obtainable with the hearing instrument. The output sound pressure level in the ear simulator is measured at full-on gain control setting with an input below the hearing instrument's saturation sound pressure level (see Figure 9–21).

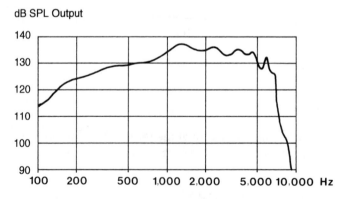

**Figure 9–20.** OSPL90 response curve. *(Courtesy of Phonak AG.)*

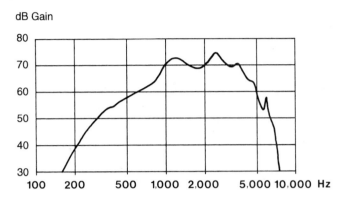

**Figure 9–21.** Full-on acoustic gain frequency response curve. *(Courtesy of Phonak AG.)*

---

## *Test Procedure*

1. Turn the gain control full on and set other controls to the required positions.
2. At a suitable frequency, set the input sound pressure level so that it is below the hearing instrument's saturation sound pressure level, where the relationship between the level of the input and output is essentially linear. Such conditions are considered to exist if at all frequencies within the range of 200 Hz to 8,000 Hz, a change of the input sound pressure level of 10 dB causes a change of recorded output level of 10 +1 dB. The input sound pressure level must be reported.
3. The frequency response with full-on gain is measured by varying the frequency of the sound source over the recommended frequency range of 200 Hz to 8,000 Hz, keeping the input sound pressure level constant.
4. The full-on acoustic gain is plotted as a function of frequency and may be reported for a specific frequency.

---

## BASIC FREQUENCY RESPONSE

The purpose of this test is to measure the frequency response of a hearing instrument without acoustic (feedback) or mechanical (vibration) problems (see Figure 9–22).

→ **Note:** If one compares the shape of the full-on acoustic gain frequency response with the basic frequency response, then acoustic or mechanical problems can be identified. The more similar the shapes of the curves are, the more stable the hearing instrument.

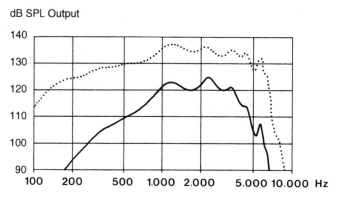

dB SPL Output

**Figure 9–22.** Basic frequency response curve (solid line) and the OSPL90 curve (dotted line). *(Courtesy of Phonak AG.)*

---

### Test Procedure

The basic frequency response is measured as follows:

1. Adjust the gain control to the reference test gain position (i.e., with an input sound pressure level of 60 dB SPL). The gain should be adjusted so that the output sound pressure level at 1,600 Hz is about 15 + 1 dB lower than the OSPL90 value at 1,600 Hz. The gain reduction should be at least 7 dB. If it is not possible to reduce the gain more than 7 dB with the volume control, the reference test gain will be 7 dB below maximum gain.
2. The other controls should be set to positions that give the broadest frequency range.
3. Vary the frequency of the sound source over the recommended frequency range of 200 Hz to 8,000 Hz, keeping the input sound pressure level at 60 dB SPL.
4. Plot the ear simulator sound pressure level as a function of frequency, as shown in Figure 9–22.

---

## BATTERY CURRENT

The purpose of this test is to determine the current consumption of the hearing instrument in operation.

→ **Note:** One method of realizing Item c on the next page is to bypass the current measuring instrument with an 8,000-μF capacitor. However, the capacitor should not shunt the battery or the power supply.

---

### Test Procedure

With the gain control in the reference test gain position, measure the battery current at the reference test frequency with an input sound pressure level of 60 dB SPL. The direct-current measuring system must have the following characteristics:

a.  An accuracy of ± 5% at the value of current measured.
b.  A dc resistance not exceeding (50/I) ohm with the current being measured in mA.
c.  An ac impedance not exceeding one ohm over the frequency range of 20 Hz to 5,000 Hz.

---

## NONLINEAR DISTORTION

The purpose of this test is to determine the degree of the amplitude nonlinearity in the sound output under specified conditions. The amplitude nonlinearity can be described in terms of harmonic distortion and intermodulation distortion.

### Harmonic Distortion

Harmonic distortion occurs when any part of the hearing instrument does not respond in proportion to the input signal. Harmonic distortion products are frequencies in the output of a hearing instrument which are integer multiples of the input frequency (fundamental). At high frequencies, the harmonic distortion products may fall outside the frequency range of the receiver. Therefore, nonlinearity is not sufficiently indicated by measurement of harmonic distortion at high frequencies. However, for the lower frequency range, the amount of harmonic distortion gives a reasonable indication of the hearing instrument's nonlinearity.

### Intermodulation Distortion

Intermodulation distortion occurs when the input is a signal composed of at least two frequencies. Such distortion products are frequencies in the output of the hearing instrument which are not in the input, but are sum and difference tones of the input frequencies. Determination of intermodulation distortion gives a better indication of nonlinearity in the high frequencies than measurement of harmonic distortion. Intermodulation distortion will not be addressed further here. The measurement of harmonic distortion will be discussed in the following section.

### Measurement of Harmonic Distortion

Harmonic distortion is measured using a pure tone input signal having the frequency $f$. The frequencies of the harmonics are then $nf$, where $n$ is an integer.

Total harmonic distortion (THD) is defined as the ratio of the output sound pressure of the harmonics to the output sound pressure of the total signal and can be expressed either as a percentage or in decibels. The total harmonic distortion is given by the formula

$$\%THD = 100\sqrt{\frac{p_2^2 + p_3^2 + p_4^2 + ... + p_n^2}{p_1^2}} \qquad (a)$$

or by the formula

$$\%THD = 100\sqrt{\frac{p_2^2 + p_3^2 + p_4^2 + ... p_n^2}{p_1^2 + p_2^2 + p_3^2 + p_4^2 + ... + p_n^2}} \qquad (b)$$

where $p_1$ is the sound pressure of the fundamental frequency of the signal in the ear simulator and $p_2$, $p_3$, $p_4$, ..., $p_n$ are the sound pressures of the second, third, fourth, ..., and $n$th harmonics in the coupler. Note that the $p$ values are sound pressure values (expressed in micropascals) not SPL values expressed in dBs.

Formula (a) is the basic formula for percentage total harmonic distortion and is preferred when measurements are made on individual harmonics and the fundamental. Formula (b) has been used in previous hearing aid standards and is preferred when using test equipment that filters out the fundamental and determines the total value of the remaining harmonics. The two formulas give almost identical results up to 20% THD and will differ by less than 1.3% at 30% THD. For THD values greater than 30%, formula (a) should be used. In any event, for most hearing aids, including harmonics above the third harmonic will not significantly increase the total value for harmonic distortion.

## Test Procedure

1. Adjust the gain control of the hearing instrument to the reference test gain position. The position of other controls must be reported; preferably these should be set to give the broadest bandwidth.
2. Vary the frequency of the sound source over the frequency range of 200 Hz to 5,000 Hz with an input sound pressure level of 70 dB and analyze the output signal for levels at the harmonic frequencies $nf$ or record the total harmonic distortion content. The bandwidth of the filter should be stated. For continuous recording, the sweep rate should be such that the response does not differ by more than 1 dB from the steady-state value at any frequency. In the event that the response curve rises 12 dB or more from the SPL of the fundamental to that of the second harmonic for any test frequency, distortion tests at that frequency may be omitted.
3. Plot the harmonic distortion as a function of the frequency of the sound source and/or versus the input sound pressure level. Figure 9–23 shows a harmonic distortion measurement in which the second and third harmonics are individually measured and plotted as a function of frequency ($f$). When, as in the example, the total harmonic distortion at a certain frequency also has been calculated, then the percentage of distortion for the individual harmonics can be obtained by applying the formula.

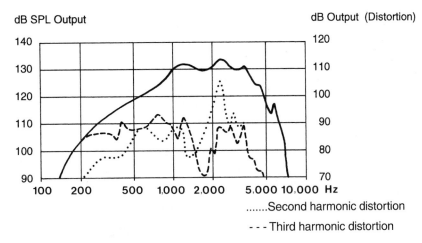

**Figure 9–23.** Basic frequency response curve (solid line) and the second harmonic (dotted line) and third harmonic (dashed line) distortion curves. *(Courtesy of Phonak AG.)*

The curves in Figure 9–23 show the results of a typical distortion measurement. The dB SPL output is essentially the response of the hearing aid to the fundamental frequency input component. The test apparatus also extracts the second and third harmonic components in the output signal possibly caused by an amplifier or transducer nonlinearity. The frequency response and the distortion products are plotted on a dB scale. Many people are more familiar with distortion expressed in percents than in dBs. How does one do the conversion? What is the harmonic distortion for the second harmonic component in percentage? How great is the harmonic distortion for the third harmonic component in percentage? How great is the total harmonic distortion in percentage?

The conversion from distortion expressed in dB and distortion expressed in percentage can be performed by using formula (a). Since only the second and third harmonics are shown in Figure 9–23, formula (a) given previously reduces to

$$\%THD = 100\sqrt{\frac{p_2^2 + p_3^2}{p_1^2}} = 100\sqrt{\left(\frac{P_2}{P_1}\right)^2 + \left(\frac{P_3}{P_1}\right)^2}$$

Distortion is a function of frequency and Figure 9–23 shows that at 2 kHz the second and third harmonics are 36 dB and 51 dB below the fundamental. Then the percentage of second and third harmonic distortion can be derived from the expression

$$\% \text{ second harmonic distortion} = 100 \times inv\left[log\frac{-36}{20}\right] = 1.58\%, \text{ or } \frac{P_2}{P_1} = 0.0158$$

and

$$\% \text{ third harmonic distortion} = 100 \times inv\left[log\frac{-51}{20}\right] = 0.28\%, \text{ or } \frac{P_3}{P_1} = 0.0028.$$

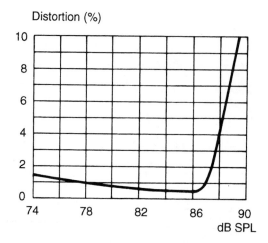

**Figure 9–24.** Total harmonic distortion measured as a function of the input sound pressure level at 1,000 Hz. *(Courtesy of Phonak AG.)*

The amount of total harmonic distortion at 2 kHz can be derived by using formula (a)

$$\%THD = 100 \times \sqrt{(0.0158)^2 + (0.0028)^2} = 1.60\%$$

These are tedious calculations, but they are performed automatically in modern test equipment.

Figure 9–24 shows the harmonic distortion represented as a function of the input sound pressure level. When the harmonic distortion is plotted in this manner, the frequency at which it was measured must be reported.

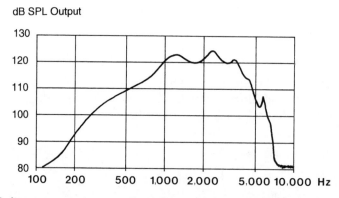

**Figure 9–25.** Basic frequency response used to estimate the equivalent input noise of a hearing instrument. *(Courtesy of Phonak AG.)*

> ## *Test Procedure*
>
> 1. Adjust the gain control of the hearing instrument to approximately the reference test position. A precise adjustment of the gain control is not strictly necessary. The position of the trimmers must be stated in the test report. Here again, the trimmers should be positioned so that the hearing instrument gives the broadest frequency response.
> 2. Measure the output sound pressure level $L_S$ in the ear simulator at the reference test frequency with a pure tone input sound pressure level $L_1 = 60$ dB.
>    *Note:* For hearing instruments with an automatic gain control (AGC), an input sound pressure level of 60 dB may be too high and should be reduced to a level which ensures essentially linear input/output conditions. If this is the case, the input sound pressure level should be stated.
> 3. Switch off the sound source and measure the sound pressure level $L_2$ in the ear simulator. This is the internally generated noise. To ensure that the noise in the ear simulator and the ear simulator microphone system is adequately low, the measured noise should decrease by at least 10 dB when the hearing instrument is turned off.
> 4. Calculate the equivalent input noise level $L_N$ as follows:
>    $L_N = L_2 - (L_S - L_1)$
>    where:
>    $L_2$ is the sound pressure level in the ear simulator as measured in step 3.
>    $L_S$ is the sound pressure level in the ear simulator at the reference test frequency as measured in step 2.

## EQUIVALENT INPUT NOISE LEVEL

The equivalent input noise level is a measure of the internally generated noise. EINL is derived by subtracting the instrument's gain at the reference test frequency from the noise level measured at the output of the instrument with no input signal in the sound box. It is imperative that the ambient noise in the test space be negligible when measuring equivalent input noise level.

In the output curve shown in Figure 9–25, the constant output level above 8,000 Hz is likely to be noise. If this measured output is not filtered, $L_2$ is 81 dB SPL. The gain at the reference test frequency is 120 dB SPL − 60 dB SPL = 60 dB. It is to derive a quick estimate of EINL:

$$L_N = L_2 - (L_S - L_1) = 81 \text{ dB SPL} - (120 \text{ dB SPL} - 60 \text{ dB SPL}) = 21 \text{ dB SPL}$$

This type of calculation is, at best, only a very rough estimate of EINL. The test procedure described must also be used with caution. While it is a convenient way to derive a single number for noise in the instrument, it provides no information about how noise in the instrument varies with frequency. The standard does provide a third-octave band analysis method which does provide such information but the method is much more complex.

It is difficult to conduct accurate and meaningful noise measurements even for simple compression systems, but the fact that signal level influences the gain of the instrument can be taken into account. However, such features as multiband compression, low-level expansion, noise reduction, feedback suppression, and adaptive processing of all types further influence the noise performance of a hearing instrument in very complex ways. It is recommended that these features be disabled, if possible, while performing the EINL measurement and that the conditions of measurement are clearly stated.

## INDUCTION COIL MEASUREMENT

This measurement is described in IEC 60118-1 (1995) and Amendment 1 (1998). Note that recent IEC publications use a modified numbering procedure. The 1995 revision of IEC 118-1 was issued as IEC 60118-1: 1995

To measure an induction coil in a hearing instrument, a current loop must be utilized which can supply a magnetic field of 10 mA/m. The magnetic field strength must remain constant within the frequency range of 100 Hz to 10 kHz. The field strength of 10 mA/m corresponds to an acoustic sound pressure level of 50 dB SPL. The gain control is adjusted to maximum when performing this measurement.

### Instrumentation Setup

Figure 9–26 shows the setup for measuring the induction coil of a hearing instrument.

The induction coil frequency response should be as close to the acoustic frequency response curve as possible. Some countries have standards that allow the induction coil frequency response to differ widely from the acoustic frequency response. In Scandinavian countries, where the use of the induction coil is widespread (through loop systems in nearly all public buildings), the standards for induction coil frequency response are quite strict. Switzerland, on the other hand, has no provisions concerning the deviation of the induction coil frequency response from the acoustic frequency response.

Figure 9–27 shows a comparison between the acoustic frequency response and the induction coil frequency response for a particular hearing instrument. It can be clearly seen that the induction coil is less sensitive at low frequencies compared to the microphone. The reason for this is to be found in the physics of inductivity.

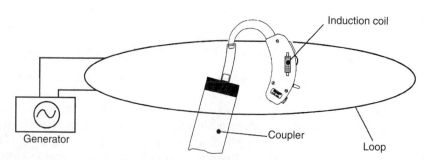

**Figure 9–26.** Equipment schematic for an induction coil measurement. *(Courtesy of Phonak AG.)*

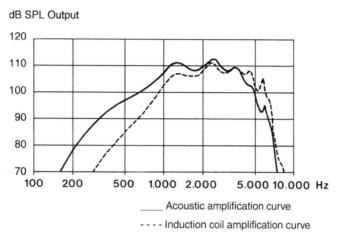

dB SPL Output

_____ Acoustic amplification curve

- - - - Induction coil amplification curve

**Figure 9–27.** Frequency response curves of a hearing instrument measured in the microphone mode with an acoustic input and in the induction coil mode with a magnetic input. *(Courtesy of Phonak AG.)*

→ The voltage that is induced in a coil is frequency dependent; that is, the higher the frequency, the higher the induced voltage.

## MEASURING INSTRUMENTS WITH AUTOMATIC GAIN CONTROL (AGC) CIRCUITS

A standardized method of testing hearing instruments of any type with automatic gain control (AGC) circuits was published in IEC 118-2 (1983) and IEC 118-2 Amendment 1 (1993). This standard includes devices which have compression and/or limiting properties with respect to the envelope of the input signal as well as devices that control the long-term average output level.

1. AGC is used to achieve compression. Put another way, the dynamic range of the output sound signal is reduced in order to preserve the integrity of the input waveform.
2. AGC circuits are often used for limiting gain instead of peak clipping (PC).

A limiting effect occurs when the shape of the input/output function flattens out at higher input levels. Output limitation is mainly used as a means of protecting the ear against excessively high output levels.

## EXPLANATION OF TERMS

### Automatic Gain Control (AGC)

A means by which the gain of a hearing instrument is automatically controlled as a function of the magnitude of the envelope of the input signal or other signal parameter.

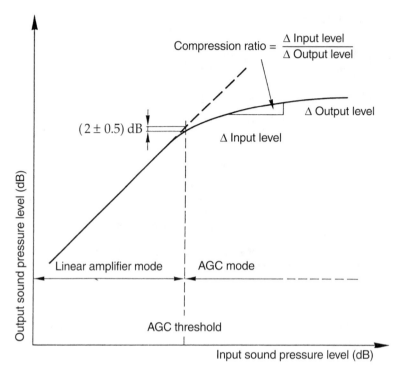

**Figure 9–28.** Steady-state input/output graph of an AGC hearing instrument. *(Copyright © 1983, IEC, Geneva, Switzerland. www.iec.ch)*

## Steady-State Input/Output Graph

The graph illustrating the output sound pressure level as a function of the input sound pressure level for a specified frequency, both expressed in dB on identical linear scales (see Figure 9–28).

## Lower AGC Limit or AGC Threshold

The input sound pressure level at which there is a reduction in the gain of 2 dB ± 0.5 dB with respect to linear gain (see Figure 9–28).

## Compression Ratio

Under steady-state conditions, the ratio of the difference between two input sound pressure levels and the corresponding difference in the output sound pressure levels, both expressed in dB (see Figure 9–28).

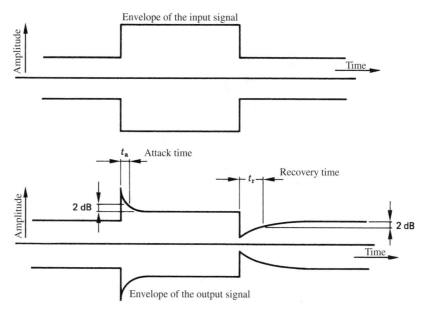

**Figure 9–29.** Dynamic response of an AGC hearing instrument (bottom trace) to the input signal shown in the top trace. *(Copyright © 1983, IEC, Geneva, Switzerland. www.iec.ch)*

## Dynamic Output Characteristics

The output sound pressure envelope as a function of time when a pure tone input signal of a standard frequency and level is modulated by a square envelope pulse with a standard pulse amplitude (see Figure 9–29).

## Attack Time

The time interval between the abrupt increase in the input signal level and the point when the output sound pressure level from the hearing instrument with the AGC circuit stabilizes to within ± 2 dB of the elevated steady-state level (see Figure 9–29).

## Attack Time for the Normal Dynamic Range of Speech

The attack time when the initial input sound pressure level is 55 dB SPL and the increase in input sound pressure level is 25 dB.

## Recovery Time

The time interval between the abrupt reduction in the steady-state input signal level after the AGC amplifier has reached the steady-state output under elevated input conditions, and the point at which the output sound pressure level from the hearing instrument stabilizes again within ± 2 dB of the lower steady-state level (see Figure 9–29).

## Recovery Time for the Normal Dynamic Range of Speech

The recovery time when the initial input sound pressure level is 80 dB SPL and the decrease in input sound pressure level is 25 dB.

# METHODS OF MEASUREMENT

## Steady-State Input/Output Graph

Graph showing the relationship between input sound pressure level and output sound pressure level. The gain control of the hearing instrument is adjusted to its maximum setting. A 1,600 Hz pure tone input is delivered with an SPL of 40 dB and the output SPL measured. The output SPL is plotted on a graph as a function of the input SPL. The input sound pressure level is then increased in steps of 5 or 10 dB up to 100 dB SPL. At each step, the output SPL is measured and plotted on the graph (see Figure 9–28).

## Dynamic Output Characteristics

The gain control is set full-on. A 1,600 Hz (or 2,500 Hz where appropriate) pure tone signal is delivered at 55 dB SPL. An adjustable gain control located after the AGC loop must be adjusted in such a manner that overload of the hearing instrument is avoided.

This signal is modulated by a square envelope pulse increasing the input level by 25 dB. The pulse length must be at least five times longer than the attack time being measured. If more than a single pulse is applied, the interval between two pulses must be at least five times the longest recovery time being measured.

*Note:* The loudspeaker employed for the measurement of dynamic output characteristics must be sufficiently free of transient distortion to ensure that any effect on test results is negligible. The output signal is monitored on a device such as an oscilloscope.

## Example of an AGC Measurement

1. Attack time at an abrupt increase from 55 to 80 dB SPL (see Figure 9–30 for an oscilloscope plot of the envelope drawing shown in Figure 9–29).
2. Recovery time at an abrupt decrease from 80 to 55 dB SPL (see Figure 9–31 for an oscilloscope plot of the envelope drawing shown in Figure 9–29).

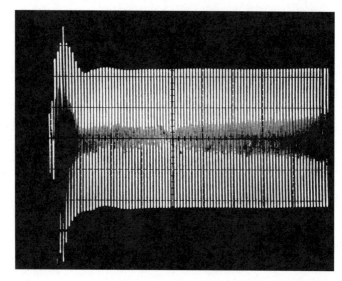

**Figure 9–30.** Oscilloscope trace for the measurement of the attack time of an AGC hearing instrument. The horizontal axis is 5 ms/major division, giving an attack time of approximately 5 ms. *(Courtesy of Phonak AG.)*

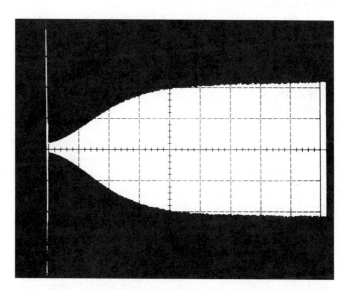

**Figure 9–31.** Oscilloscope trace for the measurement of the release time of an AGC hearing instrument. The horizontal axis is 50 ms/major division, giving a release time of approximately 200 ms. *(Courtesy of Phonak AG.)*

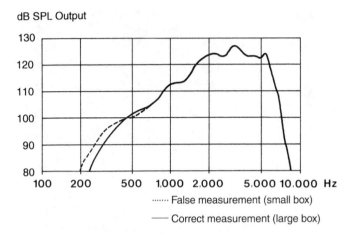

dB SPL Output

...... False measurement (small box)

—— Correct measurement (large box)

**Figure 9–32.** Frequency response curve for a hearing instrument with a directional microphone obtained in a sound chamber that is too small and one that is large enough to give an accurate result. *(Courtesy of Phonak AG.)*

## MEASUREMENT OF HEARING INSTRUMENTS WITH DIRECTIONAL MICROPHONES

In contrast to hearing instruments with omnidirectional microphones, for which the position of the hearing instrument in the measuring box does not play a major role, hearing instruments with a directional microphone require a special measuring arrangement.

1. To obtain valid results, hearing instruments with directional microphones must be measured in free field. If testing is performed in too small a chamber (e.g., in a normal sound box), then false results are obtained in the low frequencies ($<500$ Hz). Figure 9–32 illustrates false results in the low frequencies when the sound box is too small.
2. The front and rear microphone ports must lie on the loudspeaker axis. The axis of the control microphone (using the comparison method) must lie in the reference plane (see Figure 9–33). Figure 9–34 shows a correct arrangement for a hearing instrument with a directional microphone in a sound box with the sound source (loudspeaker) in the box cover. If a sound box has a loudspeaker beneath the test plane then the instrument must be turned 180°.
3. If a hearing instrument with a directional microphone is incorrectly arranged in the sound box (e.g., not facing the sound source), then a damping of the measured signal will occur. The measured gain of the hearing instrument will be lower than the actual value.

It is interesting to observe the directional characteristics of a hearing instrument with a directional microphone. To do this, the instrument is placed directly in front of the sound source (0°) for the first measurement. Subsequent measurements are performed after rotating the instrument by 90° so the sound originated from the side, and by 180° so the sound originates from directly behind the instrument. Figures 9–35 and 9–36 show the result of such measurements.

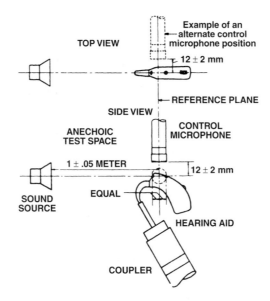

**Figure 9–33.** Hearing instrument orientation for measuring the directional response in accordance with ANSI S3.22 Standard. *(Reprinted from ANSI S3.22-2003 American National Standard Specification of Hearing Aid Characteristics, © 2003 with the permission of the Acoustical Society of America, 35 Pinelawn Road, Suite 114E, Melville, NY 11747.)*

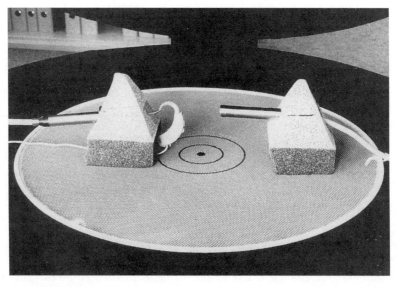

**Figure 9–34.** Positioning a hearing instrument for a directional response measurement in a sound box. *(Courtesy of Phonak AG.)*

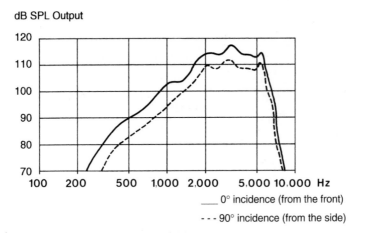

**Figure 9–35.** Frequency response curves of a directional hearing instrument measured at 0° incidence to the loudspeaker and at 90° incidence to the loudspeaker. *(Courtesy of Phonak AG.)*

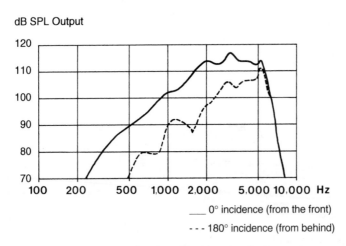

**Figure 9–36.** Frequency response curves of a directional hearing instrument measured at 0° incidence to the loudspeaker and at 180° incidence to the loudspeaker. *(Courtesy of Phonak AG.)*

## MEASUREMENTS ON KEMAR

KEMAR is the Knowles Electronics Mannikin of Acoustic Research. Although the ear simulator can predict the performance of a hearing aid and allow for comparisons between hearing instruments, some factors change when a hearing aid is placed on the head. For these measures, KEMAR is a valuable tool. The applicable standards for KEMAR measurements are IEC 60118-8 and ANSI S 3.25.

The results measured in a sound box provide no information regarding the type of hearing instrument and the effects of different microphone positions, nor the effect of shadowing of the sound by the head and body. Neither is the effect of the ear canal resonance taken into account when testing is carried out in a coupler (or ear simulator).

An anthropometric mannequin has been developed to enable accurate and reproducible measurements which are representative of results obtained from real ears. This mannequin has been proven especially useful for the design of hearing instruments.

The mannequin is constructed with two pinnas fabricated of a flexible plastic and two ear simulators located at the ends of tubes representing median ear canals. In addition, the mannequin has a torso and arms extending to the waist, which enables inclusion of sound diffraction around the body when measuring.

This KEMAR mannequin was developed by Knowles Electronics. The head and torso dimensions of KEMAR are based on the average size of more than 4,000 men. The median values used for construction of the pinnas and ear canals were derived from a study of twelve men and women.

Figure 9–37 shows KEMAR's head and part of its torso. KEMAR is mounted on a turntable which is used when measuring polar responses. In the bottom photograph, the placement of the B&K ear simulator can be seen inside KEMAR's head. To allow flexibility for research purposes, the pinnas can be changed (e.g., replaced by smaller ones) and the head turned with respect to the body.

## THE EAR CANAL RESONANCE OF KEMAR

Figure 9–38 shows the open ear canal resonance of KEMAR. There is a distinct resonance of about 17 dB at 2.5 kHz. In order to measure this open ear canal resonance, KEMAR is placed in a free field and the sound pressure at the ear drum is measured via the ear simulator.

## IN SITU MEASUREMENTS AND INSERTION GAIN

With a BTE or an ITE hearing instrument fitted on KEMAR, it is possible to measure the SPL produced by the instrument at the end of the ear canal via the ear simulator. This measurement is called *in situ gain*.

The ear canal resonance is lost by occluding the ear canal with an earmold or in-the-ear hearing instrument. Therefore, the hearing instrument must compensate for this loss. In other words, showing the effective gain of the hearing instrument requires that the open ear canal resonance be subtracted from the in situ gain. This "effective amplification" is called *insertion gain*.

These definitions are applicable not only to KEMAR measurements but also to hearing instrument fitting.

In situ gain − open ear canal resonance = insertion gain

Figure 9–39 shows the three curves for a hearing instrument measurement on KEMAR. The measurements are made with an in-the-ear hearing instrument.

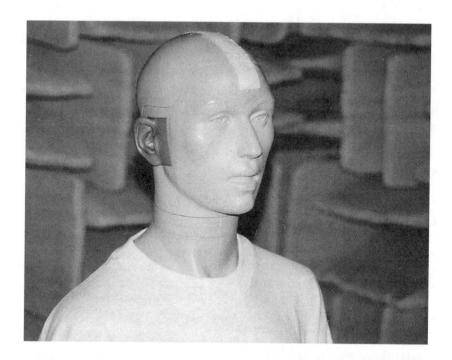

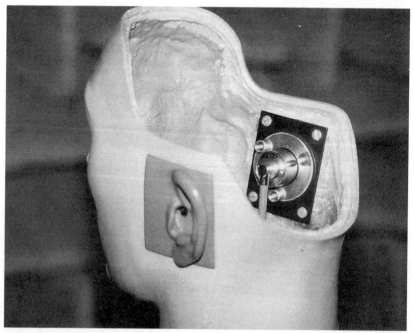

**Figure 9–37.** KEMAR measurement mannequin (top picture) and a view of the ear simulator for the right ear. *(Courtesy of Knowles Electronics.)*

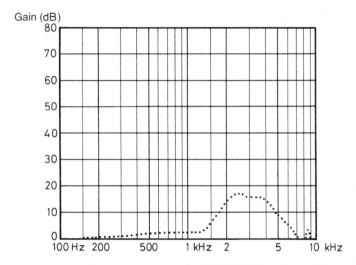

**Figure 9–38.** The open ear canal resonance curve for KEMAR. *(Courtesy of Phonak AG.)*

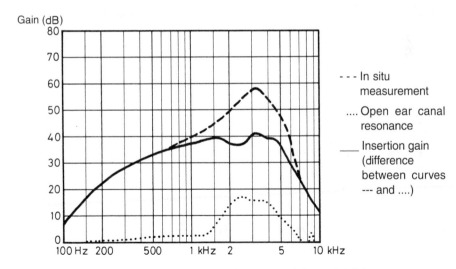

**Figure 9–39.** Insertion gain measured on KEMAR. *(Courtesy of Phonak AG.)*

## MEASUREMENT OF A POLAR RESPONSE

With KEMAR on a turntable, it is possible to determine the directional characteristics of a hearing instrument. It is also possible to measure the influence of the head (head shadow) on a hearing instrument with an omnidirectional microphone.

### Measurement Procedure

With the hearing instrument in place on KEMAR, a pure tone signal (e.g., 500 Hz, 1,000 Hz, or 2,000 Hz) is presented, initially at 0° incidence. As KEMAR is turned once around its own axis, the sound pressure (amplification) is recorded as a function of the angle of rotation. Such a curve is called a polar response, or polar plot.

Figure 9–40 shows a diagram of a polar response of KEMAR's right ear without a hearing instrument. The influence of the head and pinnas at different frequencies and from different directions can be observed.

→ **Note:** High frequencies are affected more strongly by sound diffraction around the head than low frequencies.

Figure 9–41 shows a polar response of a behind-the-ear unit with a directional microphone. We can see that sound coming from behind is attenuated by up to 20 dB. The main effect (suppression of noise) of hearing instruments with a directional microphone is to attenuate sound from behind.

# SOUND BOX MEASUREMENTS ACCORDING TO ANSI

## ANSI S3.22 STANDARD (2003)

The ANSI S3.22 standard (2003) is the latest revision of the ANSI standard for the "Specification of Hearing Aid Characteristics." It is developed by a working group of the Acoustical Society of America (ASA) standards secretariat under the sponsorship of the American National Standards Institute (ANSI). This ANSI standard and the IEC 118 series of standards are widely used today. The ANSI standard specifies measurements to be made with a 2-cc coupler. ANSI terminology will be briefly explained in this section. All measurements in the examples were made with PICONET 231X BTE hearing instrument. (Try to carry out these measurements in your sound box.)

### Saturation SPL for 90 dB Input SPL (OSPL90)

With the gain control of the hearing instrument full on and an input sound pressure of 90 dB SPL, the output sound pressure is determined from 200 to 5,000 Hz (see Figure 9–42).

### HF-Average OSPL90

The maximum output sound pressure level with full-on gain at three frequencies (1,000/1,600/2,500 Hz) are added and the sum divided by three. The sound pressure level so obtained is called the HF-average OSPL90. HF-average OSPL90 from the curve in Figure 9–42: 112 dB SPL.

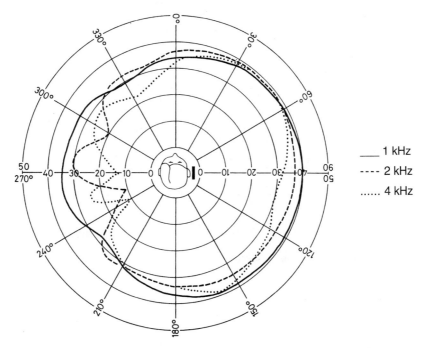

**Figure 9–40.** Polar response measured on KEMAR's right ear without a hearing instrument. *(Courtesy of Phonak AG.)*

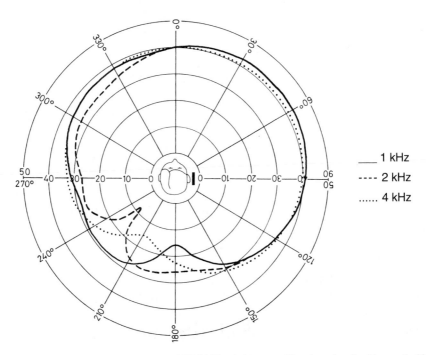

**Figure 9–41.** Polar response measured on KEMAR's right ear with a hearing instrument. *(Courtesy of Phonak AG.)*

187

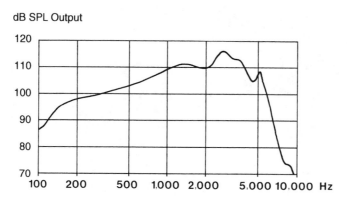

**Figure 9–42.** OSPL90 response. *(Courtesy of Phonak AG.)*

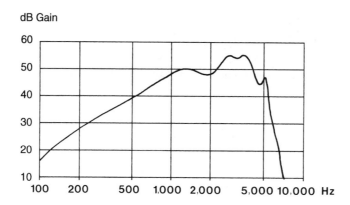

**Figure 9–43.** Full-on gain response. *(Courtesy of Phonak AG.)*

## Full-On Gain

With the gain control of the hearing instrument set at full on and an input sound pressure of 60 dB SPL, full-on gain is recorded as a function of frequency. If a 60 dB input SPL overloads the hearing instrument, then an input of 50 dB SPL is used (see Figure 9–43).

## HF-Average Full-On Gain

The average of the full-on gain at the frequencies 1,000/1,600/2,500 Hz. HF-average full-on gain from the curve in Figure 9–43: 50 dB.

## Reference Test Position of the Volume Control

With an input sound pressure of 60 dB SPL, the volume control is adjusted so that the average (1,000/1,600/2,500 Hz) of the output sound pressure level is 17 dB lower than the HF-average OSPL90. Reference test position from the curve Figure 9–44: 95 dB SPL.

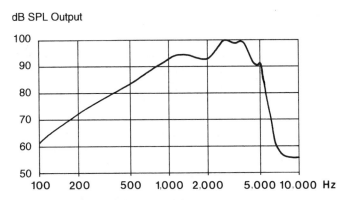

**Figure 9–44.** Frequency response at reference test gain. *(Courtesy of Phonak AG.)*

## Reference Test Gain

The average of the gain of a 60 dB SPL input at 1,000/1,600/2,500 Hz with the volume control set at the reference test position. Reference test gain from the curve in Figure 9–44: 35 dB.

## Frequency Range

A frequency response curve is obtained with the volume control in the reference test position and the average output SPL of 1,000/1,600/2,500 Hz is determined. A horizontal line is drawn on the graph 20 dB below this average value. The points at which the line intersects the frequency response curve indicate the frequency range. Frequency range from the curve in Figure 9–44: 230 Hz-6,000 Hz.

## Induction Coil Sensitivity (SPLITS Curve)

The hearing instrument is set to the "T" (telecoil input) mode and placed in a sinusoidal alternating magnetic field having an rms magnetic field strength of 31.6 mA/m. The gain control is set in the reference test position, and the hearing instrument is oriented to produce the greatest coupler sound pressure level.

HFA-SPLITS: Average the SPLITS values at 1,000 Hz, 1,600 Hz, and 2,500 Hz.

HFA-SPLITS: As shown in Figure 9–45: 95 dB SPL.

→ **Note:** SPLITS stands for sound pressure level in telephone simulator.

## Battery Current

The battery current is determined with the hearing instrument adjusted to the reference test position. The battery current is measured at this position with an input sound pressure level of 65 dB SPL/1,000 Hz. Battery current of the unit: 1.55 mA.

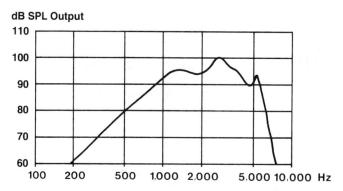

**Figure 9–45.** Induction coil output (SPLITS curve). *(Courtesy of Phonak AG.)*

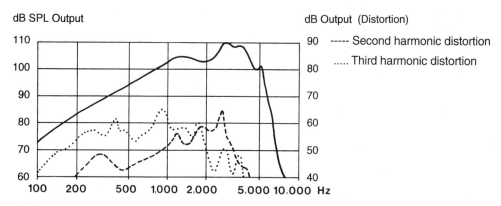

**Figure 9–46.** Basic frequency response and harmonic curves. *(Courtesy of Phonak AG.)*

## Equivalent Input Noise Level

The equivalent input noise level $L_N$ is measured with the volume control in the reference test position. It is calculated as follows:

$$L_{av} = \text{average dB SPL output at } 1{,}000/1{,}600/2{,}500 \text{ Hz}$$

$$L_2 = \text{noise level of the unit in the reference test position}$$

$$L_N = L_2 - (L_{av} - 60) \text{ dB}$$

Equivalent input noise level from the curve in Figure 9–44: 21 dB SPL.

### Harmonic Distortion

The volume control is adjusted to the reference test position and the input sound pressure level increased to 70 dB SPL. The harmonic distortion is measured at 500, 800, and 1,600 Hz, or the values can be taken from the distortion measurement curves shown in Figure 9–46.* In the event the specified frequency response curve rises 12 dB or more between any distortion test frequency and its second harmonic, distortion tests at that frequency may be omitted.

Total harmonic distortion at 500 Hz: < 2%

Total harmonic distortion at 800 Hz: < 2%

Total harmonic distortion at 1,600 Hz: < 1%

* Distortion measurements at 1,600 Hz are performed with a 65 dB SPL input on a PICONET 231X hearing instrument.

# REAL-EAR MEASUREMENTS

Sound box and in situ mannequin measurements are usually the preferred methods for characterizing hearing instrument performance during product development, to produce technical specifications, and to generate performance data for regulatory purposes. Standardized couplers eliminate the variability of the human ear canal from these measurements so that these test methods produce accurate and repeatable results.

In the clinical environment, on the other hand, hearing health care professionals work with people. Coupler data is an acceptable starting point for the hearing instrument selection and fitting process, but it is only a starting point. Fine-tuning is required. It is useful for the clinician to obtain an objective real-ear measurement for a number of reasons. First, it is used to verify the fitting by determining that sound pressure levels at the tympanic membrane are consistent with the predicted values and that no undue irregularities are evident in the response. A real-ear response is a permanent record of the instrument's performance at the time of fitting and serves as a reference for resolving performance problems during follow-up office visits.

Real-ear measurements began as a laboratory tool in the 1940s. But it was the development of miniature microphones and soft probe tubes during the 1980s that made real-ear probe tube systems a clinical reality (Mueller et al., 1992). A real-ear system consists of a thin, flexible tube connected to a microphone, equipment to produce a sound field, a reference microphone, a PC or a microprocessor, and a video terminal to record and display the probe microphone signal. Real-ear probe tube equipment is available as an optional feature with most hearing instrument measurement systems.

Real-ear measurements are performed for a number of different configurations. The patient is subjected to a calibrated sound field usually one meter in front of the loudspeaker. The probe tube is inserted into the ear canal with the end of the tube approximately 6–8 mm from the tympanic membrane. The ear is unoccluded to obtain an open ear response. For an aided response, the probe tube is placed along the wall of the ear canal with the earmold or ITE shell inserted into the ear in the usual manner. If a vent is available, the probe tube may be threaded through the vent.

Real-ear measurements should be performed in an audiometric booth but an office can be a suitable space if the noise floor is more than 10 dB below the level of the sound field signal. A number of responses are usually measured by the real-ear probe tube method.

The real-ear unaided response (REUR) is a measure of the open ear canal resonance. The real-ear aided response (REAR) is the sound pressure level produced in the residual ear canal volume by the hearing instrument. The real-ear insertion response (REIR) is derived by subtracting the REUR from the REAR. This operation is usually performed automatically by the test equipment and the result is shown on the video monitor. The real-ear insertion gain (REIG) is equivalent to the REIR.

The real-ear saturation response (RESR) is measured with a sound field of 90 dB SPL. The real-ear occluded response (REOR) is measured with the hearing instrument turned off to determine the attenuation of the instrument or earmold and the transmission of the vent if one is provided.

Finally, the real-ear method can be used to determine the real ear-to-coupler difference (RECD). REAR is measured first with a 60 dB SPL free field signal. Next, the output of the hearing instrument in a 2-cc coupler is measured with the same input level and identical hearing instrument settings. RECD is calculated by subtracting the coupler output from the REAR. An individual's RECD can be used to select an instrument with a suitable 2-cc coupler gain in order to achieve a required real-ear insertion gain (REIG).

# OTHER MEASUREMENTS: DI, AI, COHERENCE

The following is a description of measurements that are often used to describe hearing aid function. Although they are not a part of any published standard, they are terms which are found in increasing frequency in the literature.

*Directivity index* (DI) is an important tool to describe the quality of a directional system.

The *Articulation index* (AI) is a valuation of speech intelligibility. Although several methods of measuring AI can be found, the one described here is the most common.

*Coherence measurement:* Coherence is a composite measure of distortion and noise. Specialized equipment is necessary to measure coherence. ANSI S3.42 (1992), *Testing Hearing Aids with a Broad-Band Noise Signal,* describes the coherence as "a number ranging from 0 to 1 showing to what degree the output from a hearing aid is correlated to the input. Coherence for a random noise test signal is reduced by nonlinearity and by system noise."

## DIRECTIVITY INDEX (DI)

The directivity index (DI) is expressed in dB and defines the amount by which a directional microphone attenuates sounds in a diffuse sound field, compared to an omnidirectional microphone. According to this definition, the directivity index of an omnidirectional microphone is 0 dB.

The implementation of a diffuse sound field is very complicated. The exact measurement of the directivity index is therefore rather time-consuming and costly. Provided that the spatial directivity pattern is symmetrical, which is normally the case for microphones in free field conditions, and to a first-order approximation—this is the case with KEMAR—the measurement of the directivity index can be simplified to the measurement of the polar response pattern, as described in the section on measurement of a polar response earlier in this chapter.

The directivity index can be calculated from the polar response data at each frequency:

$$DI = -10 \log \left\{ \sum_{i=1}^{n} (P_i)^2 \cdot \left| sin\left( \frac{2\pi}{n} \cdot i \right) \right| \cdot \frac{\pi}{2n} \right\}$$

where

▼ $P_i$ is the sound pressure level at the angle of incidence $2\pi/n$ compared to the sound pressure level at 0° azimuth
▼ $n$ is the number of points measured

Measurements and calculations according to the equation above have been made initially with KEMAR's open ear in order to define a basis for comparison. It should be noted, however, that KEMAR can be used with none, one, or two neck rings, and different ear sizes, with each setup yielding different directivity patterns.

The directivity index of an open ear is very similar to the open ear frequency response, being rather flat (−1 to −2 dB) up to 1.6 kHz, where the response rises steeply to about 2.5 dB, falling steeply again above 4 kHz (see Figure 9–47).

Due to the head shadow effect, the directivity index of a BTE with an omnidirectional microphone worn by KEMAR does not necessarily yield exactly 0 dB, as defined for the ideal free field condition (See the section in Chapter 2 on the directional microphone.)

When compared to the open ear, on the other hand, the omnidirectional instrument reduces KEMAR's open ear directivity index by about 2.5 dB at the high frequencies. However, the directional mode of the PICONET 232X AZ Multimicrophone Technology (MMT) fully compensates for the loss of directivity at high frequencies. Overall performance of this

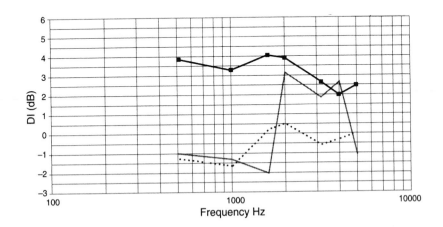

**KEMAR 1 neck ring, large ear**
**PICONET 232X AZ Omnidirectional**
**PICONET 232X AZ Directional**

**Figure 9–47.** The directivity index as a function of frequency for different measurement conditions. *(Courtesy of Phonak AG.)*

sophisticated directional microphone is superior to that of the open ear, especially in the low-frequency area, where environmental noises often reach high levels.

## THE ARTICULATION INDEX (AI)

The articulation index is a number that represents the ability to understand speech in noisy surroundings. The AI can be calculated with the hearing loss and the hearing instrument frequency response. All frequencies that are amplified with the hearing instrument above the hearing threshold (and so can be heard) will increase the AI. The important frequencies for understanding speech are described in the frequency importance function.

These AI measurements describe what can be understood in a noisy environment. It is sometimes difficult to interpret the signal-to-noise ratio (SNR) in practical terms and to estimate its real benefit for communication. One way to interpret the value of SNR improvements is via the articulation index (AI), which has been found to be a useful measure to calculate and quantify speech intelligibility (Pavlovic, 1987).

The articulation index is a weighted sum of the signal-to-noise ratios in specific frequency bands, mostly one-third octave bands, where the weights are described by the frequency importance function. The frequency importance function takes into account the fact that not all frequencies are equally important for speech discrimination. The importance of particular frequency bands is variable across different languages and speech material used, be it sentences or syllables. In order to allow global, general analysis of conversational speech, Pavlovic (1987) has defined a theoretical average frequency importance function, where the frequencies around 2 kHz are considered to be most important for speech discrimination (see Figure 9–48).

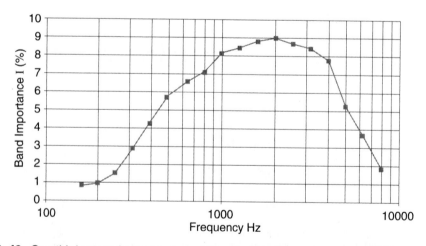

**Figure 9–48.** One-third octave frequency importance function for average speech (Pavlovic, 1987). The relative weights of the specific bands are expressed in percentages and sum to 100%. *(Courtesy of the American Institute of Physics.)*

| SNR in dB | -12 | -9 | -6 | -3 | 0 | 3 | 6 | 9 | 12 | 15 | 18 |
|---|---|---|---|---|---|---|---|---|---|---|---|
| AI | 0 | 0.1 | 0.2 | 0.3 | 0.4 | 0.5 | 0.6 | 0.7 | 0.8 | 0.9 | 1.0 |
| Speech intelligibility | Poor | | Insufficient (for some situations bearable) | | Sufficient to satisfactory | | | Good | | Very good | |

**Figure 9–49.** Average speech intelligibility rating for normal hearing subjects (adapted from Lazarus et al. [1985]).

**The articulation index can be calculated by applying the following equation:**

$$AI = \Sigma\, I_i \cdot \frac{(SNR_i + 12)}{30}$$

where $I_i$

▼ is the frequency importance value of band $i$, according to Figure 9–48
▼ $SNRi$ describes the signal-to-noise ratio of band $i$
▼ $AI$ is expressed in percent or from $0 \ldots 1$

The equivalence between SNR and A1 and the correlation between these measures and speech intelligiblity are shown in Figure 9–49.

In 1990, Mueller and Killion published an easy method for calculating the articulation index, which they called the "count-the-dots" method. The method is based on the observation that higher frequency components of speech are more important to speech understanding than lower frequency components. Therefore, the number of dots at specific audiometric frequencies grows with increasing frequency until the number again declines somewhat above 4 kHz. One hundred dots cover the long term speech spectrum, so that if all 100 dots appear above the hearing threshold, the AI is 1.0. The distribution of the dots is shown in Figure 9–50a. The vertical axis represents hearing level and the horizontal axis shows the standard audiometric frequencies. Figure 9–50b shows an unaided audiogram. Forty dots fall below the line of the audiogram resulting in an AI = 0.4. The same process is repeated with the aided audiogram to obtain an estimate of the improvement provided by the hearing instrument.

## COHERENCE MEASUREMENT

The description on the following page is from ANSI S3.42 (1992).

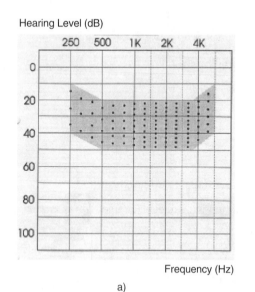

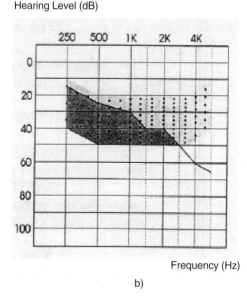

**Figure 9–50.** Count-the-dot method for determining the articulation index. a) Shows the distribution of dots according to their importance for understanding speech; forty dots are audible for the unaided audiogram in b). *(Reprinted from* The Hearing Journal, *Vol. 43, No. 9, pages 14–17, with the permission of Lippincott, Williams, and Wilkins.)*

## Coherence with Cross Spectrum Analysis

The cross-spectrum method of FFT analysis characterizes the hearing aids for an arbitrary input test signal, and can be used to predict the hearing instrument output in response to a particular input, or to determine the input signal that will generate a particular output signal. The validity of the results depends on the degree of linearity and on the noise level of the hearing aid under test. A way to check on the degree of linearity and on the noise level is with the coherence function.

$$coherence \ \gamma^2(f) = \frac{[G_{AB}(f)]^2}{G_{AA}(f) \cdot G_{BB}(f)}$$

where

$$0 \le \gamma^2(f) \le 1$$

$G_{AB}$: The cross spectrum indicates the degree to which the same signal frequencies are mutually present in the input and output of the hearing instrument. It is computed by multiplying the complex conjugate of the Fourier transform of the input signal to the hearing instrument by the Fourier transform of the output signal from the hearing instrument.

$G_{AA}$: The auto-spectrum of the input signal to the hearing instrument in the frequency domain.

$G_{BB}$: The auto-spectrum of the output signal to the hearing instrument in the frequency domain.

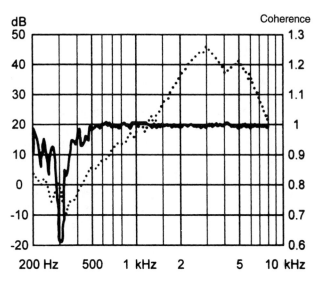

**Figure 9–51.** Coherence measurement (solid line). The gain response of the hearing instrument is shown on the dotted line. *(Courtesy of Phonak AG.)*

If the coherence = 1, the hearing instrument under test is perfectly linear and noise-free. If the coherence = 0, there is no linear relationship at all between the input to the hearing instrument and the output from the hearing instrument. The reduction in coherence can be caused by noise, nonlinear distortion, or the presence of both in the hearing instrument at the same time.

Coherence is a measurement that describes the transfer function of a system (hearing instrument). Unwanted parameters such as noise and distortion are quantified. The coherence measurement is independent of the input signal, as long as all frequencies are stimulated. For a coherence measurement the input signal can be speech, music, or any broadband noise. The result of the coherence measurement is between zero and one. The closer the signal to one the better the system (see Figure 9–51).

## ELECTROMAGNETIC COMPATIBILITY (EMC)

EHIMA (European Hearing Instrument Manufacturers Association) commissioned a project in 1993 designed to develop a standardized test protocol and test equipment to measure the immunity of hearing instruments to cellular phone emissions. In addition, recommendations for immunity levels (expressed as an input related interference level [IRIL]) were published as a basis for further consideration by IEC committees responsible for generating applicable standards.

The EHIMA study suggested that an upper limit of 55 dB IRIL should not be exceeded in a hearing aid used in a noisy environment when a GSM (Global System for Mobile operating at 800–960 MHz) phone is used at a distance of 2 m. This requirement applied for any direction, with GSM cell phones transmitting at a power level of 2 W. The same IRIL applies to

DCS1800 phones operating at 1.4–2 GHz and transmitting at a power level of 1 W. The recommendation for quiet situations was 45 dB IRIL. Accordingly, the hearing aid is placed in a uniform field with a field strength of 3 V/m in the corresponding GSM frequency range and 2 V/m in the DCS1800 frequency range, to calculate the IRIL. It is recommended that measurements are performed over the full range from 0.8 MHz to 2,000 MHz. This allows predictions for compatibility with both current and future systems.

Two standards, IEC 60118-13 and ANSI C63-19, specify measurement methods and acceptance levels for hearing instrument immunity to high-frequency electromagnetic fields originating from digital cellular telephone systems. Although these devices operate primarily in two bands (800–960 MHz and 1.4–2 GHz), small segments of voice data are compressed into data packets and sent in short bursts from the handset to a base station. The base station communicates with the handset in a similar way. The wires in a hearing instrument act as small antennas for these radio transmissions. While the MHz and GHz frequencies cause no problem, the data burst repetition rate, which is in the audio frequency band, is one source of the interference problem. A second source is due to audio band power modulation in the cell phone. The cell phone draws more power from the battery every time a data burst is sent than when it is receiving data. This current modulation causes a pulsation of the magnetic field in the vicinity of the handset, which the hearing instrument's telecoil can pick up.

IEC 60118-13 prescribes the use of a gigahetz transverse electromagnetic (GTEM) test chamber. This is a pyramid-shaped metal chamber available in different sizes, but a model 1.5 m high is well suited for hearing instrument work. A hearing instrument is placed in the GTEM cell, and electric fields of a prescribed magnitude and modulation are produced for the measurement. An input related interference level (IRIL) is measured for the hearing instrument. Two different measurements are described. The first is bystander interference measured at low field levels (3 V/m in the low-frequency band and 2 V/m in the high-frequency band). This measurement determines if the hearing aid user would experience interference from a cell phone being used at a distance of two meters from the hearing aid user. A second measurement is intended to assess hearing aid immunity when using a cell phone with the hearing aid. In this case, much higher fields are used (75 V/m for the low-frequency band and 50 V/m for the high-frequency band). The latest revision of IEC 60118-13 was published in December 2004.

ANSI C63.19 was published in 2001. This standard prescribes equipment and procedures for measurement of emission from wireless devices (e.g., cell phones) and immunity of hearing aids to electromagnetic radiation. A small dipole antenna is used to measure emissions and to produce electric and magnetic fields for the measurement of hearing instrument immunity. While the dipole method is more difficult to carry out than the GTEM method, it does measure immunity to magnetic as well as electric radiation. C63.19 is undergoing revision to also include the GTEM method from IEC 60118-13 as a normative method.

Refer to Chapter 13 for additional discussion about interference issues.

## RELEVANT STANDARDS

Table 9–1 lists the hearing aid standards that are commonly used during hearing instrument design and performance verification.

**Table 9–1.** Hearing Instrument Standards.

| | Number | Title | Revision |
|---|---|---|---|
| 1 | ANSI S3.22 | Specification of Hearing Aid Characteristics | 2003 |
| 2 | IEC 118 | Hearing aids—Part 0: Measurement of electroacoustic characteristics | 1983 |
| 3 | IEC 118 | Hearing aids—Part 1: Hearing aids with induction pick-up coil | 1995 Amendment 1–1998 |
| 4 | IEC 118 | Hearing aids—Part 2: Hearing aids with automatic gain control circuits | 1983 Amendment 1–1993 Amendment 2–1997 |
| 5 | IEC 118 | Hearing aids—Part 3: Hearing aid equipment not entirely worn on the listener | 1983 |
| 6 | IEC 60118 | Hearing aids—Part 4: Magnetic field strength in audio-frequency induction loops for hearing aid purposes | 1981 Amendment 1–1998 |
| 7 | IEC 118 | Hearing aids—Part 5: Nipples for insert earphones | 1983 |
| 8 | IEC 60118 | Hearing aids—Part 6: Characteristics of electrical input circuits for hearing aids | 1999 |
| 9 | IEC 60118 | Hearing aids—Part 7: Measurement of the performance characteristics of hearing aids for quality inspection for delivery purposes | 2005 |
| 10 | IEC 60118 | Hearing aids—Part 8: Methods of measurement of performance characteristics of hearing aids under simulated in situ working conditions | 2002 |
| 11 | IEC 118 | Hearing aids—Part 9: Methods of measurement of characteristics of hearing aids with bone vibrator output | 1985 |
| 12 | IEC 118 | Hearing aids—Part 10: Guide to hearing aid standards | 1986 |
| 13 | IEC 118 | Hearing aids—Part 11: Symbols and other markings on hearing aids and related equipment | 1983 |
| 14 | IEC 118 | Hearing aids—Part 12: Dimensions of electrical connector systems | 1996 |
| 15 | IEC 60118 | Hearing aids—Part 13: Electromagnetic compatibility (EMC) | 2004 |

*(Continued)*

**Table 9–1.** Hearing Instrument Standards *(continued)*.

| | Number | Title | Revision |
|---|---|---|---|
| 16 | IEC 60118 | Hearing aids—Part 14: Specification of a digital interface device | 1998 |
| 17 | ANSI S3.7 | Methods for Coupler Calibration of Earphones | 1995 |
| 18 | IEC 126 | IEC reference coupler for the measurement of hearing aids using earphones coupled to the ear by means of ear inserts | 1973 |
| 19 | IEC 711 | Occluded-ear simulator for the measurement of earphones coupled to the ear by ear inserts | 1981 |
| 20 | ANSI S3.35 | Method of Measurement of Performance Characteristics of Hearing Aids under Simulated Real-Ear Working Conditions | 2004 |
| 21 | IEC 6086-2 | Primary batteries—Part 2: Physical and electrical specifications | 2000 Amendment 1–2001 Amendment 2–2004 |
| 22 | ANSI S3.42 | Testing Hearing Aids with a Broad-Band Noise Signal | 1992 |
| 23 | ANSI S3.5 | Method for Calculation of the Speech Intelligibility Index | 1997 |
| 24 | ANSI C63.19 | American National Standard for Methods of Measurement of Compatibility between Wireless Communication Devices and Hearing Aids | 2001 |

# THE REGULATORY ENVIRONMENT

The preceding discussion has dealt with the technical requirements for hearing instrument design and performance. It was pointed out that the standards are mandated by different countries and this is done for the purpose of hearing instrument approval, or homologation, in the individual countries.

Hearing instruments are classified as medical devices and a number of requirements apply to their manufacture and distribution. The European Union requires hearing instruments to comply with the essential requirements of the Medical Devices Directive for safety and performance. Manufacturers are required to attain specific levels of quality system compliance and adherence to the technical standards listed above, in order to be able to apply the CE marking to the product. This certification is required for the medical device to be sold in EU countries. A similar requirement exists in the United States in that the FDA has required hearing instrument manufacturers to comply with the Good Manufacturing Practices guidelines. More recently, hearing instruments have been declassified and manufacturers no longer have to meet this requirement, although all hearing instrument models offered for sale in the United States require FDA registration. This is, in fact, the case in most countries around the world.

## SUMMARY

1. ANSI S3.22 and the series of IEC 60118-18 standards are the principal standards that establish measurement and specification methods for hearing instrument performance parameters.
2. ANSI S3.22 recommends the use of a 2-cc coupler and a sound box for hearing instrument measurements.
3. ANSI S3.35 is a standard for characterizing hearing instrument performance in situ on a mannequin.
4. The IEC 60118 series of standards is a voluntary standard that is mandated in Europe and in most other countries in the world.
5. IEC 118-0 recommends the use of an ear simulator and a sound box for the measurement of hearing instrument characteristics.
6. IEC 60118-8 describes in situ hearing instrument measurement methods on a mannequin.
7. The revisions of IEC 118 documents published since 1995 are published as IEC 60118 standards.
8. IEC 60118-8 recommends the use of a 2-cc coupler and a sound box for measurement of hearing aid characteristics for quality inspection and delivery purposes.
9. Neither the ear simulator nor the 2-cc coupler data simulate the performance of a hearing instrument in an actual ear.
10. Current mandated standards specify the use of sinusoidal test signals. Such test signals are well suited for instruments with linear amplification but not well suited to characterize performance of nonlinear devices such as AGC instruments and digital devices

that contain other nonlinear processing. Noise reduction and feedback reduction circuits can produce measurement artifacts. Current measurement standards recommend the instrument be set to linear operation or that nonlinear features be disabled during testing.

11. Nonlinear instruments are more effectively characterized with test signals that are more representative of real use conditions, such as speech signals. It is expected that many of the standards in force at this time will be revised in the coming years to enable a more effective characterization of complex, nonlinear digital hearing instruments.

12. Published IEC and ANSI standards describe methods for determining hearing instrument and cell phone compatibility.

## REVIEW QUESTIONS

1. In a polar response measured at 1,000 Hz/2,000 Hz/4,000 Hz without a hearing instrument, which curve was measured at each frequency? Give an explanation.

2. A frequency response curve of a hearing instrument was measured with a 2-cc coupler. Draw the curve if this instrument is also measured with a B&K ear simulator.

3. What are the advantages of KEMAR measurements compared to coupler measurements?

4. Draw the insertion gain. (Show an in situ measurement and an open ear resonance [REUG]).

5. What is the harmonic distortion if the difference between the frequency response curve and the second harmonic distortion is 20 dB? $[x]_{dB} = 20 \cdot \log(x)$

   A. 10%     A ☐
   B. 0.01     B ☐
   C. 20%     C ☐
   D. 0.05     D ☐

6. What kind of curve is this?

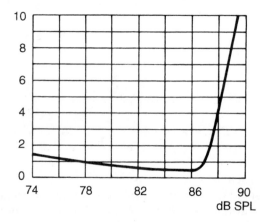

    **A.** Distortion                               A ☐

    **B.** Battery discharge             B ☐

    **C.** Volume control curve     C ☐

    **D.** Speech test               D ☐

**7.** What is correct?

    **A.** Max. gain is: 68 dB SPL     A ☐

    **B.** The insertion gain is measured in dB     B ☐

    **C.** The threshold of the AGC is at 60 dB     C ☐

    **D.** Distortion is −30 dB     D ☐

**8.** Sound box measurements with a coupler are valid:

    **A.** For objective measurements of different hearing instruments     A ☐

    **B.** For a production test of hearing instruments     B ☐

    **C.** For fine-tuning of a fitting     C ☐

    **D.** Due to real-ear measurements, couplers are no longer needed     D ☐

# CHAPTER 10

# Digital Mechanics

## INTRODUCTION

All hearing instruments need to be comfortable when worn for an extended period of time. This imposes somewhat conflicting requirements on the shell manufacturing process. On the one hand, the fit to the ear must be tight enough to prevent unintentional feedback. On the other hand, the fit cannot be so tight that it creates discomfort. In short, the fit needs to be anatomically correct. This, of course, applies to both ITE and BTE instruments. In the former, the critical part is the shell and in the latter the earmold needs to fit well.

Approximately 80% of all hearing aids produced in North America are of the in-the-ear type, and the trend in Europe and other markets is an increasing proportion of sales that are also of the ITE types of products. In spite of its popularity, these products have been traditionally manufactured using a complex, labor-intensive, custom process.

The process begins with an impression of the pinna and ear canal. The shell or earmold is then reproduced from this impression in a number of steps. Traditionally, the outer shape of the instrument is manufactured by casting a shell from the impression. This process incorporates the manual steps of cutting the ear impression, grinding it down, and filling voids with wax.

The traditional shell-making processes has depended in large part on the polymerization of acrylic shell material using an investment cast of the original impression. Polymerization is performed in an environment of controlled temperature and pressure or through the use of UV radiation. In either case, the shell-making process is reasonably accurate, but it is an expensive, manual process. The process and materials used to fabricate the shell have improved to the point where anatomically correct shells can be routinely fabricated. The hearing aid is completed by building the electronic components into the shell and closing the instrument with a faceplate.

The hearing aid is delivered to the dispenser, who in one or more sessions adjusts the instrument to the individual needs of the user. While many of these adjustments consist of fine-tuning the amplification circuitry to restore the individual's hearing loss, modifications or remaking of the hearing aid shell is frequently done to achieve a perfect solution. Problems with fit and lack of comfort account for 19% of the reasons behind people's rejection of their hearing instruments.

Much effort has been put into developing a more accurate and more automated computer-based process in which the shell is produced from a three-dimensional numerical model of the impression. But, regardless of the process, a good fit can be achieved only if the initial impression accurately duplicates the anatomical details of the ear and the ear canal.

## PARTS OF THE OUTER EAR AND DIMENSIONS

An important consideration in the fabrication of custom ITE hearing instruments is the fit rate one can achieve. Is the finished instrument small enough to fit into all ears regardless of their size or will only 80% of all orders, for example, be successfully completed? There is considerable variability in the size of the outer ear and the ear canal from one person to another. It is useful to know if all necessary components can be built into the available space. Furthermore, a number of useful options, which influence the size of the finished instrument, are usually available for custom products.

For that reason, it is useful to know when the order and the ear impression are sent to a manufacturer if the instrument can indeed be built as requested. For example, severe-to-profound hearing losses require a larger receiver than does a mild-to-moderate loss. If the ear canal is small, the receiver cannot be placed in the canal portion of the shell, and must be placed in the concha portion of the instrument where it is likely to interfere with the battery compartment. If a directional instrument is requested, the hearing aid must have space for two omnidirectional microphones instead of one. There must be sufficient faceplate area to accomplish this. Telecoils, trimmers, programming socket, and larger batteries all consume space and impact the fit rate of a custom instrument.

It is preferred that these decisions be made before the construction of the hearing instrument begins. Manufacturers used to rely on gauges and experience to determine if an instrument with all the requested options can be produced. The availability of computer-based modeling techniques now makes these predictions more reliable.

Modeling techniques require precise dimensional information and a great amount of data was generated in a number of studies that eventually led to the development of the Knowles Electronics Mannikin for Acoustic Research (KEMAR). Some of these dimensions are defined in Figure 10–1 and the relevant data are given in Table 10–1.

Table 10–1. Typical dimensions of the concha (from Burkhard & Sachs, 1975).

| Dimension | Units | Overall | Male | Female |
| --- | --- | --- | --- | --- |
| Concha length | cm | 2.63 ± 0.24 | 2.73 ± 0.23 | 2.53 ± 0.20 |
| Concha breadth | cm | 1.80 ± 0.22 | 1.88 ± 0.21 | 1.72 ± 0.21 |
| Length of lower part of concha | cm | 1.68 ± 0.17 | 1.74 ± 0.16 | 1.62 ± 0.16 |
| Concha depth | cm | 1.29 ± 0.10 | 1.29 ± 0.12 | 1.29 ± 0.08 |

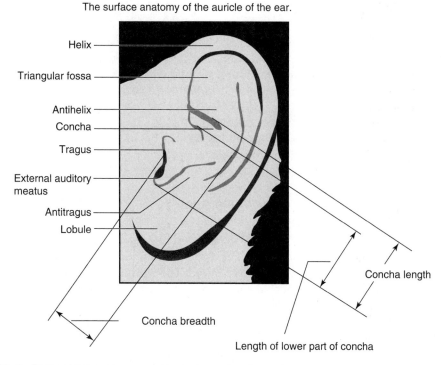

The surface anatomy of the auricle of the ear.

Helix

Triangular fossa

Antihelix

Concha

Tragus

External auditory meatus

Antitragus

Lobule

Concha length

Concha breadth

Length of lower part of concha

**Figure 10–1.** Parts of the outer ear and typical concha dimensions.

The mean and standard deviation for several dimensions given in Table 10–1 provide important information to the manufacturer about the maximum size of a faceplate layout or a modular ITE insert. This type of information allows the manufacturer to make use of mass-production techniques and prebuild faceplate assemblies and modular inserts using the maximum amount of automation and thereby minimizing the final cost of the product.

It is reasonably safe to assume that the size of the human ear for a large group of people follows a normal distribution. This means that for 68.3% of people in this group concha length is within one standard deviation of the mean, and for 99.6% concha length is within two standard deviations of the mean. The same holds true for concha breadth and depth. It is a relatively straightforward calculation to determine the maximum dimensions of a modular faceplate insert if the manufacturer wishes to achieve, for example, an 80% fit rate with that product. It is also possible to predict the impact that adding an additional component in a fixed position has on the fit rate.

The same reasoning applies for canal and CIC instruments. Knowledge of critical dimensions will allow the manufacturer to design products for the best cosmetics and maximized fit rate.

# THE EAR IMPRESSION

A high-quality ear impression is mandatory for a successful hearing instrument fitting. This means that the impression must be not only anatomically correct when it is taken, but the impression material must be resistant to moisture, shrinkage, and any other influence it may be exposed to during shipment to the hearing instrument manufacturer. A two-part silicone material meets these requirements.

Figure 10–2 shows a good ear impression. Note that the impression clearly shows the locations of the first and second bend in the canal portion of the impression as well as the tragus position and the contours of the helix and concha.

# DIGITAL MECHANICAL PROCESSING

A new shell manufacturing process, which can be called digital mechanical processing (DMP), starts with digitizing the shape of the ear. Using laser scanning technology, a three-dimensional data set that replicates the ear impression is generated. The digitized image of the ear is also analyzed, filtered, and treated by dedicated software. By this process, an optimized virtual shell is created. As the shape information now resides in a digitized format, it can be stored, evaluated, compared, and analyzed, with the objective of creating an optimal anatomic fit. As a first benefit, this process makes it possible to accurately reproduce the shape of the instrument, and to store the data for building exact duplicates in case of damage or loss.

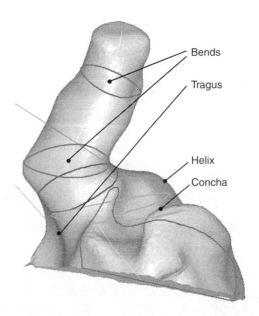

**Figure 10–2.** Ear impression showing the concha, the bends in the canal, the location of the tragus, and the helix.

By making controlled, rule-based refinements of the instrumentís outer shape, the fit to the anatomy of the ear can be greatly improved. A tight, but comfortable, seal in the soft cartilaginous part of the ear canal is necessary to acoustically isolate the inner outlet of the sound transmitter from the outer openings of the microphones. This acoustical seal is required to allow maximum amplification before the onset of feedback. Controlled shape trimming of the inner end of the instrument avoids irritation of the sensitive skin in the deeper, bony part of the ear canal. Simulation of insertion and removal, and ultimately of the dynamics of the ear canal during jaw movements when speaking or chewing, will be vital to reduce the need for modifications and thereby the number of return visits in deploying a tailor-made hearing instrument.

## THREE-DIMENSIONAL LASER SCANNING

The impression of the ear is measured using lasers (see Figure 10–3). Specially created high-end optics are used to scan the impression taking 100,000 data points with a precision in the micron range. By viewing the impression from various positions and angles, the shape—including undercuts and hidden areas—is reconstructed perfectly.

## HEARING INSTRUMENT DESIGN

The electronic impression model is used to design the hearing instrument by placing all the necessary components into the preferred location in the ear canal (see Figure 10–4). The modeling software contains all the necessary components required to construct the instrument. The orientation of the faceplate cut and the length of the instrument are defined in this way. This visualization technique is useful to also detect any potential interferences between components. If the components cannot be properly placed in the canal, the instrument cannot be built.

The software enables a number of electronic detailing functions to be carried out during the design of the instrument. Examples of faceplate tapering and canal extensions are shown in Figure 10–5. It may be useful to extend the canal up to the second bend in order to reduce occlusion

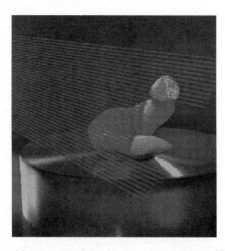

**Figure 10–3.** Three-dimensional laser scanning of an ear impression. *(Courtesy of Phonak AG.)*

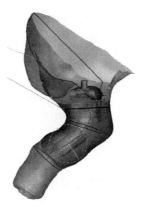

**Figure 10–4.** Electronic visualization of a canal instrument in the ear. *(Courtesy of Phonak AG.)*

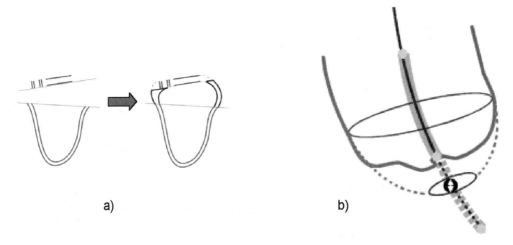

a)

b)

**Figure 10–5.** Electronic detailing: a) faceplate tapering and b) canal extension. *(Courtesy of Phonak AG.)*

effects. In that case, it is essential to ensure that the receiver opening is oriented in a plane perpendicular to the center line of the ear canal. This can be visualized with this modeling software.

The position and appearance of the completed hearing instrument design can be viewed in the ear canal before proceeding to the actual manufacturing phases of the production process (see Figure 10–6). At this time, final adjustments can be made to the faceplate or eartip orientation by modifying the data in the design file.

A further feature of the modeling software is the ability to show how the instrument appears in the user's ear. This feature allows the health care practitioner to set realistic expectations for the user (see Figure 10–7).

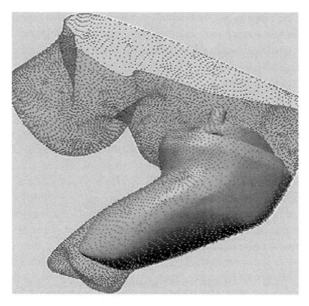

**Figure 10–6.** Location of the finished instrument in the ear canal. *(Courtesy of Phonak AG.)*

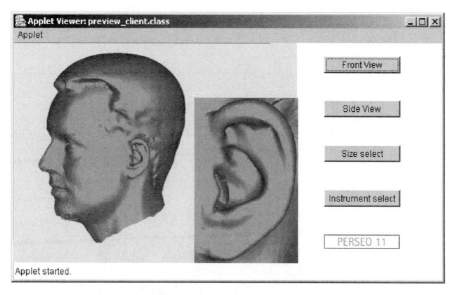

**Figure 10–7.** Demonstration of the cosmetic appearance of the finished instrument in the user's ear. *(Courtesy of Phonak AG.)*

# SHELL FABRICATION

When all the requirements for the instrument are met, the electronic design of the hearing instrument is complete and the instrument can be fabricated. The final part of the shell-making process is also a departure from the traditional acrylic shell fabrication method.

Two somewhat different technologies are used to turn the virtual model back into real parts: selective laser sintering using pigmented polyamide powder and stereolithography using colored acrylic resins. In both methods, the shell is built up as the laser beam traces out successive layers to either sinter (melt and fuse together) the powder or polymerize the liquid resin (see Figure 10–8). As each layer is completed, the shell is further submerged by the small amount required for the next layer.

Vents, the sound bore, serial number, and the exact opening details required for modular instruments (see Figure 10–9) can all be produced in the shell during this production phase. In contrast, stereolithography uses a liquid material that the laser solidifies in successive layers.

Both technologies exhibit different trade-offs in meeting the requirements for accuracy, mechanical stability, surface finish, biocompatibility, and production speed.

Small details of miniature features and dimensional process control could be easier achieved with stereolithography. The sintered polyamides prove to be highly superior in surface properties and in mechanical stability, especially after stress testing (temperature/humidity

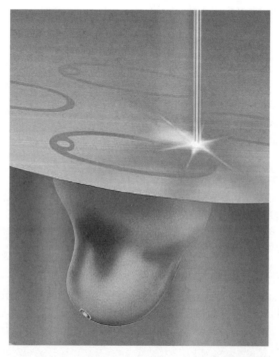

**Figure 10–8.** Sintering or polymerizing with a laser beam. *(Courtesy of Phonak AG.)*

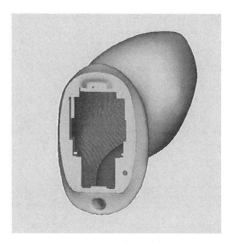

**Figure 10–9.** Complete laser-sintered shell assembly for a modular canal instrument. *(Courtesy of Phonak AG.)*

cycling, sweat, and UV light exposure). Therefore, selective laser sintering is, at times, the preferred manufacturing process.

## SURFACE FINISH

The outer surface of the shell is only slightly smoothed in order to preserve the exact shape and intricate details of its structure and an innovative surface finish has been developed for laser-sintered shells. The surface retains a slightly pebbled texture that ensures a firm and consistent retention in the ear canal, while the low-friction polyamide surface allows smooth insertion and removal. This type of surface finish compares well with the traditional glossy acrylic shell finish.

## FUTURE DIRECTIONS

The hearing instrument industry has developed a vital competence for building custom-made devices that meet the requirements of an individual user. This industry relies on short turnaround times and frequent and close communication between dispensing professionals and the manufacturer. The value of new technologies will be measured by their impact on shorter production times and improved communication.

Production times can be significantly reduced if the impressions are scanned at the dispensing site. Orders can then be transmitted electronically, eliminating the time for mailing the impressions to the manufacturer. The elimination of the variability inherent with manual impression taking is likely to be the next frontier. The challenges are to scan not only the static shape of the ear canal, but to also measure in real-time its dimensional changes during jaw movements.

Because of high equipment costs, current fabrication processes produce shells in relatively large batches. Batch processing is not a preferred method in a build-to-order industry. The use of multiple machines of smaller size can reduce response times dramatically. Reducing the size and cost of current equipment would also encourage multiple manufacturing sites to better service smaller local markets.

It is expected that innovations in materials technology, particularly flexible materials that are compliant to soft tissue in the ear canal, will improve the performance of hearing instruments and be more comfortable to wear for extended periods of time.

## SUMMARY

1. Digital mechanical processing (DMP) allows the manufacturer to design the product and decide if it can be built as ordered before any production work starts.
2. The application of DMP in the fabrication of hearing aid shells demonstrates an innovative implementation of technologies such as 3-D scanning, free-form modeling, and direct manufacturing using rapid prototyping equipment.
3. The digitization of free-form objects and the controlled manipulation of mechanical devices in virtual space opens new opportunities in designing devices that interact with the human anatomy.
4. DMP of hearing instruments optimizes the ITE production process from beginning to end, starting from the human ear and finishing with a perfect fit hearing solution. This chain of technologies brings greatly improved quality to ITE instruments.
5. This technology is the beginning of a digital journey into mechanics and acoustics. The residual volume with the instrument in place can be determined and used to predict gain and output increases for the 2-cc coupler data taken from technical specifications.
6. DMP is at its beginning but it already translates into improvements in precision, efficiency, and customer satisfaction.
7. It will provide the basis for groundbreaking e-commerce opportunities for hearing instruments.

## REVIEW QUESTIONS

1. Name two reasons for rejecting a hearing instrument.
2. Describe the properties of a good ear impression.
3. Explain the term *digital mechanical processing*.
4. Name some advantages of working with a three-dimensional electronic version of an ear impression.
5. Name two technologies that can be used to produce shells for custom hearing instruments.

# CHAPTER 11

# Fitting, Verification, and Outcome

## INTRODUCTION

A number of different components of hearing loss (attenuation, abnormal growth of loudness, and binaural loss) were discussed in Chapter 5. Each component requires characterization and several tools exist. The audiogram is routinely used to measure the amount of signal attenuation that exists in the impaired ear. Abnormal growth of loudness, or recruitment, is often measured by using some form of loudness scaling. Binaural loss can be assessed by measuring the binaural intelligibility difference, and finally, the speech reception threshold provides information about frequency discrimination.

Successful hearing aid fittings start with a characterization of the hearing deficiency. The following sections describe some of these measures.

## FITTING

### AUDIOGRAM

The audiogram provides the information required to begin the fitting process. The audiogram indicates the levels at which tones of specific frequency are just audible. The standard audiometric frequencies are 125, 250, 500, 1,000, 2,000, 4,000, and 8,000 Hz. Hearing level is measured over a range of −10 to 120 dB. The completed audiogram shows an individual's hearing threshold over a frequency range from 125 to 8,000 Hz.

There is no consensus on varying degrees of hearing loss. However, the categories shown in Table 11–1 are often used.

Hearing threshold level (HTL) values at the audiometric frequencies are used in fitting formulas to calculate the hearing instrument gain required to restore normal loudness for normal speech.

**Table 11–1.** Hearing loss categories.

| Hearing Level (dB) | Degree of Hearing Loss |
|:---:|:---:|
| 0–20 | No functional loss |
| 20–40 | Mild loss |
| 40–60 | Moderate loss |
| 60–80 | Severe loss |
| 80–110 | Profound loss |

**Table 11–2.** Fitting formulas.

| Frequency (Hz) | NAL-R (Target Gain) X = 0.05 (HTL500 + HTL1k + HTL2k) | POGO (Target Gain) | Berger (Target Gain) |
|:---:|:---:|:---:|:---:|
| 250 | X + 0.31 HTL250-17 | HTL250/2-10 | |
| 500 | X + 0.31 HTL500-8 | HTL500/2-5 | HTL500/2.0 |
| 750 | X + 0.31 HTL750-3 | HTL750/2-3 | HTL750/1.8 |
| 1,000 | X + 0.31 HTL1000+1 | HTL1000/2 | HTL1000/1.6 |
| 1,500 | X + 0.31 HTL1500+1 | HTL1500/2 | HTL1500/1.6 |
| 2,000 | X + 0.31 HTL2000-1 | HTL2000/2 | HTL2000/1.5 |
| 3,000 | X + 0.31 HTL3000-2 | HTL3000/2 | HTL3000/1.7 |
| 4,000 | X + 0.31 HTL4000-2 | HTL4000/2 | HTL4000/1.9 |
| 6,000 | X + 0.31 HTL6000-2 | HTL6000/2 | HTL6000/2.0 |

## Classical Prescription Fitting Formulas

Different methods are used to predict the required gain and maximum extent of the hearing instrument from the measured audiometric data. This calculated gain is called the target gain. The target gain should amplify normal speech to the most comfortable level (MCL) of the hearing instrument user. Different formulas have been developed to predict the right gain. In Table 11–2, three well-known fitting formulas are described.

- ▼ Berger et al., 1988
- ▼ POGO (Prescription Of Gain and Output) (McCandless and Lyregaard, 1983)
- ▼ NAL-R (National Acoustic Laboratory, Australia)

The Berger and POGO formulas are quite easy to understand and they are given in Table 11–2. The NAL formula is more complicated and it is described in detail on the next page.

## NAL-R

In 1986 Byrne and Dillon presented an updated version of the NAL fitting formula. In this second version, the real-ear gain of a particular frequency is partly dependent on the hearing threshold slope. The NAL-R formula for calculating the necessary insertion gain (IG) for mild-to-moderate hearing losses is:

1. Calculate: X = 0.05 (HTL500 + HTL1k + HTL2k)
2. Insert X in Table 11–2.

Where HTL500 denotes the hearing threshold level at 500 Hz, HTL1k denotes the hearing threshold level at 6,000 Hz, etc.

## NAL-RP

In an additional revision, Byrne, Parkinson, and Newall (1991) adapted the NAL procedure to severe-to-profound hearing losses. In essence, this modification for severe-to-profound hearing losses allows a relatively greater overall gain and a flatter frequency response than NAL-R does for mild-to-moderate hearing losses.

The calculation is the same as for NAL-R when the average hearing loss at 0.5, 1, and 2 kHz are equal or better than 60 dB. The factor X is determined as follows:

$$X = 0.05 \times (HTL500 + HTL1k + HTL2k)$$
$$\text{when } (HTL500 + HTL1k + HTL2k) \leq 180 \text{ dB.}$$

When hearing losses exceed 60 dB, X changes as follows:

$$X = 0.116 \times (HTL500 + HTL1k + HTL2k)$$
$$\text{when } (HTL500 + HTL1k + HTL2k) > 180 \text{ dB.}$$

When the hearing thresholds level at 2 kHz exceed 95 dB, the correction factors listed in Table 11–3 must be added to the gain already calculated.

**Table 11–3.** Modifications to NAL fitting formula for severe-to-profound hearing losses.

| 2 kHz HTL | Frequency (Hz) | | | | | | | | |
|---|---|---|---|---|---|---|---|---|---|
| | 250 | 500 | 750 | 1k | 1.5k | 2k | 3k | 4k | 6k |
| 95 | 4 | 3 | 1 | 0 | −1 | −2 | −2 | −2 | −2 |
| 100 | 6 | 4 | 2 | 0 | −2 | −3 | −3 | −3 | −3 |
| 105 | 8 | 5 | 2 | 0 | −3 | −5 | −5 | −5 | −5 |
| 110 | 11 | 7 | 3 | 0 | −3 | −6 | −6 | −6 | −6 |
| 115 | 13 | 8 | 4 | 0 | −4 | −8 | −8 | −8 | −8 |
| 120 | 15 | − | 4 | 0 | −5 | −9 | −9 | −9 | −9 |

Fitting formulas predict the target gain for a specific hearing loss. The formulas are derived by averaging results for hundreds of individuals with similar audiograms.

It is important to realize that the target gain is always an average value and can be used for an excellent start for the fitting; but because it is an average value, the individual value can be different, and so it is necessary to fine-tune the gain of the hearing instrument for each individual fitting.

To obtain a more precise target gain for the hearing instrument, a more precise hearing loss assessment procedure has to be performed. This procedure loudness scaling is described later in this chapter. Although the loudness scaling procedure adds time in the diagnostic phase of the fitting, the end result is a more precise fit, requiring fewer modifications.

## NAL-NL1

The NAL-NL1 (nonlinear version 1) method attempts to maximize speech intelligibility while maintaining overall loudness of speech at any level to that perceived by a normal hearing person (Dillon, 2001). The calculations are quite complex and are often used in the form of a "dll."

The term *dll* stands for dynamic link library, a library of executable functions or data, that can be incorporated in a manufacturer's fitting software. Using dlls is a convenient way to incorporate such complex calculations because, as improvements are made to the fitting formula, a revised dll can be loaded in the next revision of the fitting module.

## DESIRED SENSATION LEVEL (DSL) [i/o]

The DSL [i/o] prescription method was originally described by R. C. Seewald et al. and again by Cornelisse et al. in 1995 as a tool for pediatric fittings. The goal of DSL is to make speech sufficiently audible to allow speech perception, without discomfort, for all degrees of hearing loss. It relies on the fact that speech must be amplified to a sufficient sensation level in order to maximize intelligibility, but that this sensation level decreases as hearing loss increases. Clearly, hearing aids for children, who are developing language skills, must go beyond providing mere audibility of speech. Amplified speech must be sufficiently audible so as to be intelligible.

The target sensation level is paired with a maximum output level target which is sufficiently elevated above the aided speech spectrum to ensure headroom for the peaks of the long-term average speech spectrum. These maximum output targets are designed to limit the output of the hearing aid before the UCL is reached.

DSL attempts to make accurate comparisons between adult and pediatric data by converting all numbers to dB SPL with common reference values. This attention to acoustic detail has become an integral part of the DSL method. In particular, application of the real ear to coupler difference (RECD) measurement is used as the primary means of converting audiometric data to coupler or real-ear data. The method accurately predicts the real-ear performance of a hearing aid, and is now informally known as the "coupler approach."

The current version of the DSL method is based on an algorithm called the "input/output formula" ([i/o]), which is essentially loudness-based. It can be used with linear, wide dynamic range compression, or curvilinear compression hearing aid circuitry, but all will amplify average speech to the same sensation levels.

DSL [i/o] and periodic upgrades are, like the NAL fitting formulas, also available in the form of a "dll."

For more information on the DSL method, please contact (519)661-3901, or DSL@audio. hhcru.uwo.ca.

## LOUDNESS SCALING

### *Purpose and Target*

Loudness scaling is a method to measure the complete hearing range between hearing threshold and uncomfortable level (UCL) (Kiessling et al., 1998). It is called auditory field audiometry when the patient is scaling the whole auditory field with narrowband test signals. The auditory field is the audiologically important frequency range between 125 Hz and 8,000 Hz and from hearing threshold to UCL.

For hearing losses where the origin lies in the middle or inner ear, altered loudness perceptions for all infant levels are the main part of the hearing loss problem. With inner-ear damage, one often observes near-normal loudness sensation well above threshold in spite of a significant loss at the hearing threshold. This fact is taken into account by the fitting formulas (POGO, Berger), which calculate the target gain for the most comfortable level (MCL) from the hearing threshold. Unfortunately, these estimates are not precise, because there is only a loose connection between hearing threshold and MCL.

The advantage of loudness scaling is that the MCL is not predicted, it is measured. It gives much more precise audiological data for fitting modern hearing instruments with nonlinear signal processing than threshold-based audiometry.

Auditory field audiometry measures the frequency-dependent individual loudness-growth function. The loudness-growth function is the relationship of loudness and sound pressure level. The individual loudness-growth function can be determined by measuring sound pressure levels covering the whole dynamic range and the corresponding loudness at a certain frequency.

### *Method*

The test should have at least four test frequencies: 500 Hz, 1,000 Hz, 2,000 Hz, and 4,000 Hz. The sound pressure level and the order of presentation should be selected by the hearing health care professional (or with an adaptive algorithm) depending on the measurements that have already been done. The pressure levels of the different frequencies should be selected between hearing threshold and UCL in a way that scaling data exists for all loudness ranges. The order of presentation should be designed so that no similar test signals succeed each other.

Before loudness scaling can be started, the patient must be well informed about the task. The patient uses a categorical scale. A simple version of a categorical scale has five response steps: very soft, soft, medium, loud, and very loud. A more precise loudness scale should have more than five response steps. Figure 11–1 shows a suitable scale with 5 + 2 categories and eleven response steps.

→ **Note:** Loudness scaling should always be done monaurally.

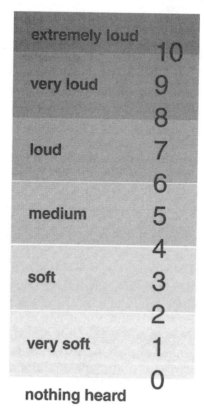

**Figure 11–1.** Loudness scale with 5 + 2 categories and eleven response steps. *(Courtesy of Phonak AG.)*

## Analysis of Results

The results of sound pressure level/loudness are plotted and entered in a graph. The comparison of the results with the reference (the average loudness growth of normal hearing) shows the level-dependent hearing loss and also the required gain. Figure 11–2 shows a loudness-growth function of a hearing-impaired subject with a sensorineural hearing loss.

The sound pressure level in dB SPL is plotted on the horizontal or the x-axis and loudness is plotted on the vertical or the y-axis. It is easy to see that the loudness-growth function of the hearing-impaired subjects is below and steeper compared to those with normal hearing. The hearing loss is a function of the input level and becomes smaller for higher input signals.

The results in Figure 11–3 show that at each frequency there is a hearing loss with different recruitment. The hearing loss is higher at higher frequencies. Multiband digital hearing instruments are well suited to compensate for these types of losses.

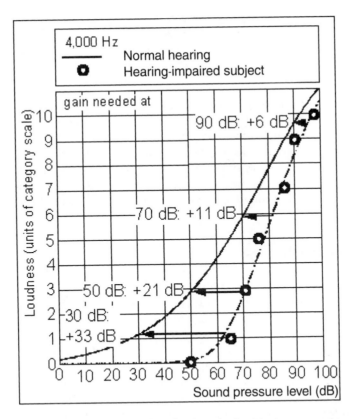

**Figure 11–2.** Loudness-growth function of a hearing-impaired subject compared to a loudness-growth function for a nonimpaired ear at 4,000 Hz. The horizontal difference between the two curves gives the required gain for the hearing impaired. It is marked by an arrow at 30, 50, 70, and 90 dB SPL. *(Courtesy of Phonak AG.)*

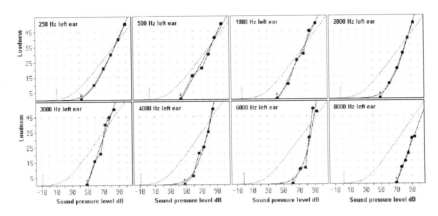

**Figure 11–3.** Results of monaural loudness scaling with sensorineural hearing loss. The eight graphs show the eight individual loudness-growth functions at 250 Hz, 500 Hz, 1 kHz, 2 kHz, 3 kHz, 4 kHz, 6 kHz, and 8 kHz compared to a reference function. The individual hearing threshold is marked with an "s." The hearing threshold for normal hearing is marked with a vertical line above the corresponding level. *(Courtesy of Phonak AG.)*

# VERIFICATION

Following the assessment, selection, and fitting of the hearing instruments there remain two very important steps to complete the fitting process. The verification procedure is done to determine if the appropriate electroacoustic parameters such as gain, output, frequency response, and compression characteristics of the hearing instrument have been met compared to the fitting goal. The more common types of verification procedures are: speech intelligibility in quiet and noise, sound-quality judgments, loudness ratings (soft, normal, loud, etc.), functional gain, and probe microphone measurements using fitting targets.

# OUTCOME MEASURES

Increasingly, third-party payers, government agencies, insurance companies, and other health authorities require some form of measurement that confirms benefit for the end user or patient. Medically effective and economic treatment will grow in importance as new treatments and new technology continue to drive up the cost of hearing health care. Typically, outcome measures are subjective questionnaires rating the "before" and "after" treatment. The following is a list of some of the more common outcome measures: Hearing Handicap Inventory for the Elderly (HHIE, Newman and Weinstein, 1998), Profile of Hearing Aid Benefit (PHAB, APHAB, Cox and Gilmore, 1990), Client-Oriented Scale of Improvement (COSI), and Patient Satisfaction Data. The value of outcome measures goes beyond the individual being fitted with hearing instruments. Outcome measures provide the dispensing professional with a valuable feedback mechanism for confirming the overall fitting process and takes into account not only objective measures but also lifestyle information.

This type of information can be obtained from different assessment scales. These scales are derived from standardized questionnaires and attempt to measure the degrees of difficulty individuals have in everyday listening situations. They are now also available in electronic form and are often included as a module in fitting software packages. Some of the more common assessment scales are:

APHAB (abbreviated profile of hearing aid benefit)

HHIE (hearing handicap inventory for the elderly)

COSI (customer oriented scale of improvement)

They provide a subjective rating of the perceived disability or handicap (without and with a hearing aid) and of the efficacy of amplification.

## APHAB

APHAB was developed by Robyn Cox. Twenty-four items are scored in four subscales: ease of communication (EC), reverberation (RV), background noise (BN), and aversiveness (AV). Some examples of items are:

▼ It is hard for me to understand what is being said at lectures or church services (RV)
▼ The sounds of construction are uncomfortably loud (BN)
▼ When I am in a crowded grocery store, talking with the cashier, I can follow the conversation (EC)

The questions are rated on a seven-point scale from never to always.

## HHIE/HHIA

Barbara Weinstein developed HHIE in 1982 to quantify emotional and social consequences of hearing losses in adults at age of sixty-five years. The Hearing Handicap Inventory for Adults (HHIA) was subsequently developed for younger adults. Each contains twenty-five items, while a screening version contains ten items. The list includes social-situational items and emotional items. Some examples are:

▼ Does a hearing problem cause you to feel embarrassed when you meet new people?
▼ Does a hearing problem cause you difficulty when in a restaurant with relatives or friends?

The questions are rated on a three-point scale: yes, sometimes, and no.

## COSI

Dillon et al. (1999) developed COSI at the National Acoustics Laboratories in Australia. It is different because the clients write the questionnaire by choosing five listening situations where they feel they need help, and then rank the importance of these situations. At a follow-up, these scenarios are compared to the situation before rehabilitation. The final ability to hear in these situations is also rated. Because the client is involved in every aspect of administering this rating scale, COSI ensures that the client acknowledges the disability and COSI also manages expectations.

## SUMMARY

1. Fitting, verification, and outcome measures are necessary elements of the hearing health care process.
2. Hearing instrument selection by threshold-based information provided by the audiogram is still the most common method in use today.
3. The extensive use of digital instruments with nonlinear amplification strategies and additional signal enhancement algorithms, requires that current assessment and prescriptive methods advance beyond their present state.

## REVIEW QUESTIONS

1. Name three commonly used fitting formulas.
2. What value of hearing levels are considered to be a moderate and profound losses?
3. What is the difference between the NAL-RP and the NAL-R fitting formulas?
4. How does DSL attempt to make accurate comparisons between adult and pediatric data possible?
5. How does DSL convert audiometric data to coupler or real-ear data?
6. How does loudness scaling differ from threshold audiometry?
7. List three commonly used verification methods.
8. List three outcome measures.

# CHAPTER 12

# Audiology and Psychoacoustics

## INTRODUCTION

This chapter presents a very basic introduction to audiology and psychoacoustics. The chapter also discusses the principle of the decibel and the rules for safe exposure to noise.

## HEARING AND UNDERSTANDING

Hearing and understanding are two different aspects of the perception of acoustic signals. For an acoustic signal, like a voice, to be intelligible, it obviously must be audible. If a signal is not audible, it cannot be understood. However, it does not work the other way around. The mere fact that we are able to hear a sound does not imply that we can also understand it. "Intelligibility," then, is dependent on recognition of the sound signals. To illustrate this, imagine you are sitting on a park bench and that a couple of people are sitting on another bench some distance away, talking. You can hear quite clearly that they are talking, but you do not understand what they are saying. There is, then, a distinct difference between audibility and intelligibility. Nevertheless, the two terms are frequently used synonymously. How often, in an acoustically demanding situation such as a busy restaurant, have you found yourself saying: "I'm sorry, I can't understand you," when what you really mean is: "Sorry, you were talking too quietly for me to hear what you were saying which is why I didn't understand." We often find ourselves speaking very loudly to people with hearing impairments, believing they must be able to understand that someone is talking to them and what is being said. And they do understand that someone is saying something, but unfortunately not always what it is they are saying.

So what is the reason behind the fact that individuals with a hearing problem often fail to understand what they have heard? Is it possible for a signal to be audible but not intelligible? In the case of a foreign language that we did not master, it is simply a case of being unable to decipher a linguistic code using the available acoustic information. In the case of an inner-ear hearing disorder, the problem is similar (but has completely different causes): affected individuals are very often unable to decipher the sound signals using the available acoustic information.

To understand the effects of a hearing impairment, it is necessary to look at the way in which the ear functions.

## THE STRUCTURE AND FUNCTION OF THE HUMAN EAR

The ear consists of three main parts (see Figure 12–1):

▼ the outer ear, or the auricle, consists of the pinna on the outside of the head, the auditory or ear canal. The ear canal is terminated by the tympanic membrane or eardrum
▼ the middle ear is filled with air and consists of the eardrum and the ossicles: malleus, incus, and stapes
▼ the inner ear, or the cochlea, which is filled with fluid, converts mechanical vibrations into electrical signals

Sound signals (noise, speech, music, etc.) reach the eardrum at the end of the auditory canal. These changes in air pressure at the eardrum are extremely small but the eardrum is so sensitive that the small forces the pressure variations exert on the eardrum cause it to move a significant distance.

However, it takes less force to push on air in the outer and middle ear than on the fluid in the cochlea. The small forces felt at the eardrum are, on their own, not sufficiently strong to

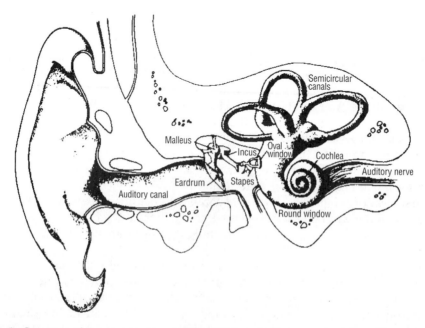

**Figure 12–1.** Structure of the human ear: auricle, middle ear, inner ear, cochlea. *(From Moore [1995], Perceptive Consequences of Cochlear Damage [Oxford University Press].)*

push the fluid in the cochlea. The middle ear serves to amplify the forces exerted by the eardrum on the malleus in two ways. First, there is a hydraulic multiplication of force due to the difference in eardrum and oval window areas (approximately 50 and 3 mm$^2$, respectively). The force exerted on the large area of the eardrum is transmitted to the smaller area of the oval window providing a multiplication in force by a factor of nearly seventeen. Secondly, the configuration of the ossicles provides additional amplification. The malleus is longer than the incus, forming a basic lever between the eardrum and the stapes. Since the total energy (energy = force × distance) in the system is conserved, the malleus moves a greater distance and the incus moves a smaller distance with greater force.

In this way, the outer ear and the middle ear efficiently convert sound waves into vibrations and deliver them to the oval window of the cochlea. The pressure applied to the eardrum is amplified by a factor between twenty and twenty-five when it reaches the cochlea, where it is transformed into electrical signals the brain can understand as distinct information.

The cochlea is the most complex part of the ear (Dallos and Popper). Physically, it is a fluid-filled chamber resembling the shell of a snail, approximately 5 mm high, with just under three revolutions. If the cochlea were to be unwound, it would be approximately 35 mm long.

The cochlea is divided into three parallel sections stretching the length of the cochlea from the oval window. Figure 12–2 shows a cross-sectional view of the cochlea. The three chambers are called the scala vestibuli, scala media, and scala tympani. The latter two chambers are connected at the top of the cochlear spiral. This connection allows for pressure waves to travel along the scala media to the tip of the cochlea and back through the scala tympani to the round

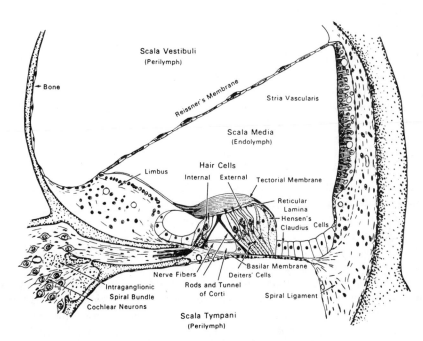

**Figure 12–2.** Cross-section of the cochlea: basilar membrane and hair cells. *(From Moore [1995],* Perceptive Consequences of Cochlear Damage *[Oxford University Press].)*

window. The round window provides a termination to the pressure wave in the cochlea. As the oval window moves in, the round window moves out.

The cochlea contains two membranes. The first, Reissner's membrane, is thin and flexible. It plays a role in the chemistry of the inner ear but, since it readily transmits pressure fluctuations between the scala vestibuli and the scala media, it essentially has no influence on the motion of fluid waves through the cochlea and the two chambers it separates can be considered as one. The second, the basilar membrane, separates the scala media from the scala tympani except where they join at the very top of the cochlear spiral.

The basilar membrane is supported by the sides of the cochlea, but it is not tightly stretched. When sound is introduced into the cochlea via the oval window it flexes the basilar membrane and sets up a traveling wave along its length. The membrane is narrow and stiff at the oval window and becomes wider and more flexible along its length. A motion of the oval window produces a fluid wave that gradually grows in amplitude to a resonant peak at a certain point along the basilar membrane and then quickly fades out. The point of maximum amplitude occurs at the point along the basilar membrane where its width and flexibility is conducive to resonate at the frequency of the incoming sound.

The basilar membrane supports a structure called the organ of Corti. This structure contains the mechanisms for converting the mechanical or hydraulic energy in a fluid wave resonance into electrical signals which can be recognized and interpreted by the brain.

Figure 12–2 shows the main components of the organ of Corti, including the hair cells that play a principal role in the conversion of hydraulic energy contained in fluid waves into electrical stimuli. The cochlea is thought to contain 4,000 inner hair cells (IHCs) and 12,000 outer hair cells (OHCs) arranged with one IHC and three OHCs spaced every ten microns apart along the length of the basilar membrane (Berlin, 1996). The tectorial membrane lies on top of the organ of Corti separated by a thin fluid layer of approximately four to six microns. When a fluid wave reaches a resonant peak at a particular point of the basilar membrane, enough energy is released to move the basilar membrane relative to the tectorial membrane. This causes motion in the hair cells. Hair cells are mechanoelectrical transducers. The mechanical displacement of the hair cell causes electrical current pulses to flow through the hair cell. These electrical pulses are sent along the auditory nerve, usually referred to as the VIII nerve, to be interpreted by the auditory center in the brain.

The vibrations created in the basilar membrane are structured in such a way that sounds are broken down—purely mechanically—into different frequencies. The resulting high and low frequencies resonate in different places on the membrane and stimulate different hair cells. Roughly speaking, the cochlea acts like a spatial filter bank. Each point on the basilar membrane is tuned to a different frequency, providing an audible frequency range in a healthy ear from 20 Hz to 16 kHz. Given that the cochlea is approximately 35 mm long, the spatial gradient along the cochlea is 0.2 octaves/mm.

It is important to distinguish between the functionality of the two types of hair cells, each of which plays a very different, but important, role. The so-called inner hair cells (IHCs), act purely as sensors whose job it is to conduct acoustic information to the brain in the form of electrical impulses. The outer hair cells (OHCs) play an "active" role in the analysis of sound by the inner ear. The OHCs primarily receive electrical impulses from the brain. By altering their length, OHCs actively influence the oscillations in the basilar membrane by boosting or dampening them. The active influence on the inner-ear mechanism by OHCs is an extremely complex, nonlinear process, whose individual stages and mechanisms have yet to be fully explained. Nevertheless, this mechanism is one of the reasons why both extremely loud and extremely soft sounds can be perceived with a high degree of differentiation between the levels and frequencies contained in the signal. The ear, or to be more precise, the inner ear, is not merely a passive receiver but an active amplifier. If it is damaged, the functionality of both the passive receiver and the active amplifier are likely to be compromised. In other words, the first stage in the sound-processing and signal analysis process is faulty. This naturally has a marked influence on human auditory capabilities, not only on the "audibility" of sounds, but also on their "intelligibility."

In the case of an inner-ear hearing impairment, both IHCs and OHCs are damaged (panels A, B, and C in Figure 12–3). Here, the sensors in the inner ear that pick up sounds—as well as the OHCs that permit a very precise analysis of the physical properties of a sound—are damaged. In a case of inner-ear hearing loss, then, the sound receiver and transducer are not only less sensitive, which would have meant "restoring audibility also restores intelligibility," but the entire inner ear's signal-processing system is seriously altered because the OHCs have suffered severe damage. Hence, the active amplifier in the inner ear no longer functions properly to make quiet sound audible.

## AUDITORY PERCEPTION—PSYCHOACOUSTICS

To look at the issue from a different angle than the purely physiological, briefly consider the psychoacoustic aspects of the problem. How does our hearing apparatus process sound and what are the effects of inner-ear damage on perception? As described previously, the construction of the inner ear is such that it is able to carry out extremely detailed analyses of the frequencies contained in a sound signal in purely mechanical terms. In other words, the inner ear is capable of analyzing precisely how many high and low frequencies are contained in an acoustic signal.

To put this in very simple terms, it is almost like having a piano keyboard in the inner ear (Figure 12–4). If a complex sound, such as speech, for example, enters the ear from outside, each of the tones finds its own key on the keyboard and strikes it. This type of frequency analysis is very precise and depends on the outer hair cells functioning correctly. The mechanism gives us the ability to differentiate between speech, music, and many other types of signals. Take two words as similar as "love" and "live." The tone differs only slightly in frequency, but it is this small difference which enables us to tell the two words apart. Precise analysis of the frequency content of sound is essential if we are to distinguish between different voices, or among male, female, and children's voices. It is also what enables us to recognize musical instruments and the different tones in a sound.

Most of the sounds we hear in our everyday lives are dynamic, that is, the signal level can fluctuate widely from very loud to soft within a single sentence. Changes in level and softer sequences in a speech signal mark the intervals between words and sentences. Sounds that have the same frequencies, but at different levels, generate different tones—an effect that helps us tell one musical instrument from another. Of course, one of the requirements for perceiving the changes in the levels of a sound is an auditory system that is able to follow these fluctuations. Another important aspect of the processing mechanism is the contribution made by the

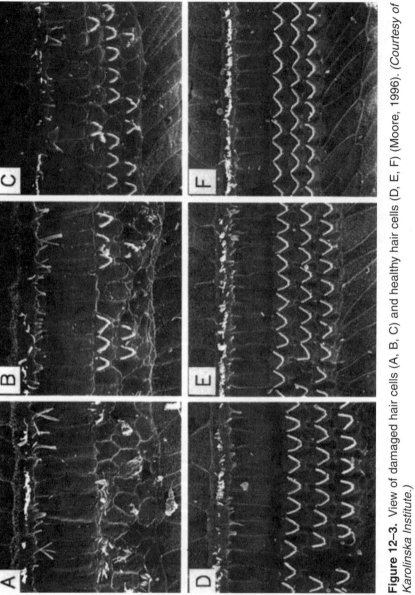

**Figure 12–3.** View of damaged hair cells (A, B, C) and healthy hair cells (D, E, F) (Moore, 1996). *(Courtesy of Karolinska Institute.)*

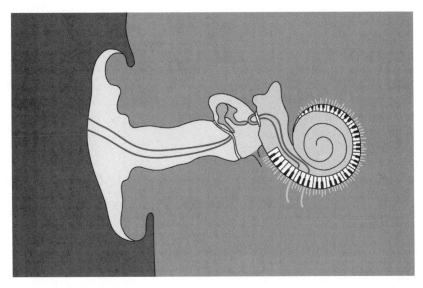

**Figure 12–4.** Representation of the inner ear as a piano keyboard. *(Courtesy of Phonak AG.)*

outer hair cells, which enable the inner ear to deal with an astonishingly wide range of sounds. In physical terms, sounds that occur at the auditory threshold, sounds that we are just barely able to hear, are a million times quieter in a healthy ear than sounds that occur at the other end of the auditory range. In physical terms, this represents a sound range of 120 decibels (see Figure 12–5). Furthermore, within this vast dynamic range, our auditory system is able to detect extremely fine differences of about 1 dB between two signals.

## PSYCHOACOUSTICS IN THE HEARING IMPAIRED

In the event of hearing loss in the inner ear, both of these processes—analysis of sound frequency and the ability to recognize different sound levels—are seriously impaired, making it very difficult for the affected person to hear or understand. The reason for this is usually that the hair cells, particularly the outer hair cells, have been damaged. As a result of the loss of outer hair cells, the function vital to normal hearing—active amplification in the inner ear—is lost. Using two examples of auditory perception, frequency analysis and loudness perception, we shall now consider the consequences of this type of damage on our perception of acoustic signals.

In the previous section, the inner ear's ability to analyze signals was compared to a piano keyboard. In the case of a hearing impairment in the inner ear, we no longer have so many keys, and three or four keys may have fused together into a single, wider one, which strikes several strings at once (see Figure 12–6). When this happens, speech characteristics which we distinguish by their different frequencies—"o" is low, "i" is high—can no longer be separated. We can see this for ourselves with words like "live" and "love" or "tip" and "top." Virtually the only difference between these words is the frequency content of the vowels. If our frequency analyzer no longer functions properly, we have immense difficulty telling words like

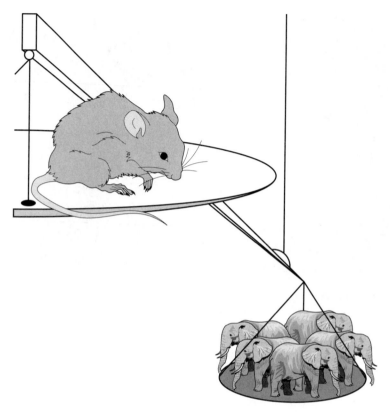

**Figure 12–5.** A dynamic range of 120 dB represents the ratio between the weight of a mouse and that of five elephants.

these apart. Individual frequency components no longer "play" different strings, but are bunched together on the same ones. Alternatively, groups of keys or strings may be completely missing leading to dead regions in the cochlea. A second important aspect of this is the way in which we perceive the physical levels of a signal and the time factor. Here, too, individuals suffering from hearing loss perceive sound in a radically different way. They may no longer be able to hear soft sounds, but hear louder ones as well as people with normal hearing. This limitation in perceptible volume or sound level range is called "recruitment." A person with normal hearing can hear and process sounds between 10 dB (very soft) and 100 dB (very loud) extremely well. In a person with impaired hearing, this range is much smaller and, depending on the degree of hearing loss, may only go from 50 dB (very soft) to 100 dB (very loud). As a result, this person's perception of loudness changes much more rapidly than in the case of an individual with normal hearing. Much smaller changes in the sound level result in a corresponding change in the way loudness is perceived. To understand this, it is only necessary to think of how a person with normal hearing is startled when he hears a sudden, very loud noise.

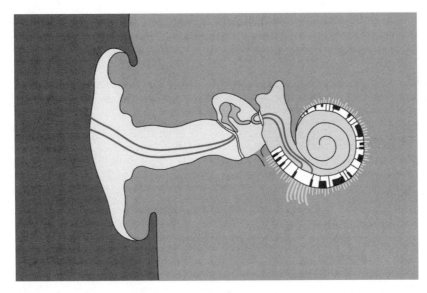

**Figure 12–6.** Representation of the impaired inner ear as a piano keyboard with missing keys. *(Courtesy of Phonak AG.)*

Another consequence with a huge bearing on intelligibility is the fact that fluctuations in the volume of an acoustic signal, like language or music, are perceived by the hearing impaired in very different ways; these differences in level contain very important information about the meaning of the sound. Very quiet components in a speech signal—soft vowels, soft consonants—are inaudible and the pauses signalling breaks between words are difficult to recognize. High sound levels, on the other hand, are almost too loud, which means that acoustic signals are very distorted. Overall perception no longer hovers within the range that persons with normal hearing would describe as "moderate" or "pleasant" but in a range between "quiet" and almost "loud."

## EFFECT OF HEARING LOSS ON OUR ABILITY TO COMMUNICATE

In the previous section we looked at two forms of perception—frequency and loudness—in an attempt to explain that an impairment in the inner ear does not merely involve a softer signal but also a change in the way in which sound is perceived. Of course, both forms of damage to the inner ear's ability to analyze sound have a whole range of further effects on the auditory perception and the communicative ability of hard-of-hearing individuals (Moore, 1995; Moore, 1996). These effects occur particularly in acoustically demanding surroundings such as noisy restaurants, places with a great deal of echo and reverberation (concert halls, churches), or on the telephone, to name but a few. Communication in noise calls for an effective form of signal processing and is, therefore, one of the most daunting problems facing the hearing impaired. One way of measuring how clearly a signal, such as the voice of the person we are talking to, stands out against background interference like noise in a busy restaurant or factory is the signal-to-noise ratio (SNR). This ratio shows how much stronger the desired signal is than the surrounding noise.

The healthy ear makes effective use of various mechanisms to separate the signal we wish to hear from unwanted noise. With normal hearing, communication is still possible when the signal-to-noise ratio is very bad, even in situations when the interference is physically louder than the desired signal (a negative signal-to-noise ratio situation). A whole range of mechanisms combine to make the auditory system efficient. These include binaural hearing (i.e., the comparison of signals by both ears), analysis of the sound frequency, pitch perception, and, possibly, tone perception.

The auditory system also provides us with a wide range of other information about our fellow human beings and our environment. The pitch and tone of a person's voice, for example, not only tell us whether a man, woman, or child is speaking but also much about the physical and mental state of that person and whether a sentence is a statement or a question. They also tell us whether speech is intended as a signal to warn us about something in the immediate surroundings, such as a person approaching us in a room or a car coming up from behind. People with impaired hearing are naturally often easily shocked because they tend not to hear signals increasing gradually in volume, but, as a result of the recruitment effect described earlier, hear them suddenly and very loudly.

It is important to understand that loudness is a perceived sensation. The ear picks up a signal and the brain interprets how loud the perceived signal is. On the other hand, the intensity of the perceived sound is a physical aspect of sound that can be quantified with the aid of an instrument like a sound level meter. Sound intensities can vary over such a wide range that the accepted convention of expressing sound intensity is to express it not as an absolute value, but as a ratio in decibels. The following section explains this unit of measure.

# DECIBELS AND HEARING

## THE DECIBEL

The term *decibel* (abbreviated dB) always means the same thing, but decibels may be calculated in several ways.

The decibel is not an absolute unit of measure in the same sense that a meter or a kilogram is. Meters and kilograms are defined quantities of distance and mass. (You can go to the National Bureau of Standards and look at a meter and a kilogram if you need to.) By contrast, a decibel is a relative quantity. A decibel is a relationship between two values of power.

Decibels are designed for talking about numbers of different magnitude, such as 23 horsepower (hp) versus 4,700,000,000,000 hp. The numbers are so vastly different, that the hardest task is getting the number of zeros right. Scientific notation helps, but a comparison between $2.3 \times 10^1$ hp and $4.7 \times 10^{12}$ hp is still awkward. A useful solution to this problem is to calculate the ratio between the two numbers and convert that ratio into a logarithm to the base ten as follows:

$$\log_{10}\frac{4,700,000,000,000}{23} = 11.3$$

The result is 11.3 and the unit for this number is a Bel. In practice it is more convenient to measure power ratios in a smaller unit, namely one-tenth of a Bel. This quantity is known as a decibel, or a dB. The outcome of this comparison is that 4.7 trillion hp is 113 dB greater than 23 hp.

Decibels are therefore defined by the formula:

$$\textit{Power Difference in dB} = 10 \log_{10} \frac{powerA}{powerB}$$

The usefulness of all this becomes apparent when one considers how the human ear perceives loudness. It is well-known that the ear is very sensitive. The softest audible sound has a power of about 0.000000000001 watt/m². At the other end of the scale, the threshold of discomfort is measured to be around 1 watt/m². The range between audibility and discomfort is calculated to be 120 dB according to the formula:

$$\textit{Power Difference} = 10 \log_{10} \frac{1}{0.000000000001} = \frac{1}{10^{-12}} = 10 \log_{10} 10^{12} = 120 \; dB$$

Not only does the dB allow convenient comparisons of large numbers, the comparison is perceptually meaningful because perception of relative loudness is somewhat logarithmic. If a sound has ten times the power of a reference (i.e., greater by 10 dB), it is perceived as twice as loud. If the power of a sound is doubled (an increase of 3 dB), the difference is just noticeable.

The calculations for these dB relationships go like this:

For a 10:1 relationship in power, the log of ten is one, and ten times one is ten.

For a 2:1 relationship in power, the log of two is 0.3, and ten times 0.3 is three.

If the ratio goes the other way, with the measured value less than the reference, we get a negative dB value, because the log of 1/10 is −1.

## CONVERTING VOLTAGE OR PRESSURE RATIOS TO DECIBELS

Remember that the dB is used to describe a power ratio. Power (P) is not often conveniently measured, especially in electronic devices. It is convenient to measure voltage (V), current (I), and resistance (R), and to use the formula $P = VI = V^2/R$ to calculate the power. When a ratio of powers is calculated, the result is a ratio of the squares of the voltages, since the $R$ cancels. The log of a squared quantity is two times the log of the quantity, so squaring a value doubles its logarithm. In terms of voltage, the dB formula becomes:

$$\textit{Power Difference in dB} = 20 \log_{10} \frac{voltage \; A}{voltage \; B}$$

Sound power varies as the square of pressure, so this formula is also appropriate for the calculation of SPL (sound pressure level) differences:

$$\textit{Power difference in dB} = 20 \log_{10} \frac{pressure \; A}{pressure \; B}$$

## REFERENCE LEVELS

The concept of relative power can be confusing. The question "relative to what?" has no single answer. The standard level (0 dB) is chosen to be some convenient value for the application. For acoustics, 0 dB often means the threshold of hearing. This of course varies from person to person, but for the purpose of sound pressure level measurements, the threshold of hearing is defined as 0.00002 newton/meter$^2$ or 20 micropascals ($\mu$Pa). A pascal is approximately equal to one hundred thousandth of normal atmospheric pressure. Acousticians deal with positive values and call their measurements dB SPL (dB sound pressure level).

Electrical engineers use several references for 0 dB. It is common to add a letter to the dB symbol to indicate the intended reference level. Some examples of different reference levels are given below.

0 dBj = 1 millivolt

0 dBk = 1 kilowatt

0 dBm = 1 milliwatt at 600 ohms

0 dBv = 1 volt

There are many more. The power calculations must also take the frequency content of the signals into account. It is not correct to compare a broadband noise signal to a sine wave without some correction factor. The simple rule is to always compare similar signals.

## dBVU

The standard reference which is often used in electronic music is 0 dBVU. dBVUs are calculated just like dB with some extra restrictions on bandwidth and the amount of damping used in the measuring apparatus. The VU (or volume unit) system is a hangover from early radio usage when 0 VU meant 100% of the legal modulation for the particular radio station. The level meters were all marked with percentage numbers as well as dBVU, and the numbers above zero were in red. When tape recorders were invented, the same meters were used, and 0 dBVU came to mean the recommended operating point for the tape in use. The tape manufacturer supplied calibration tapes, and the machines were adjusted to give a 0 dBVU reading on the meter when those tapes were played.

While 0 VU is the accepted maximum allowable signal on analog tape recorders, most tape decks will cope with +6 or even +15 for brief times (but such levels might damage the VU meters if sustained) and other devices will cope with up to +25. Any operating area above 0 VU is called the headroom. However, 0 VU is the maximum allowable signal on digital tape recorders. Exceeding that level will usually cause gross distortion in such devices. The level of the ever-present system noise limits the minimum useful signal. This floor may be as high as −40 VU on a cassette deck or as low as −100 VU on a digital recorder.

## DECIBELS AND HUMAN HEARING

A healthy human ear can hear everything from your fingertip brushing lightly over your skin to a loud jet engine. In terms of power, the sound of the jet engine is about 1,000,000,000,000

**Table 12–1.** Examples of common sounds and their dB ratings.

| Near total silence | 0 dB SPL | A lawnmower | 90 dB SPL |
|---|---|---|---|
| A whisper | 15 dB SPL | A car horn | 110 dB SPL |
| Normal conversation | 60 dB SPL | A rock concert or a jet engine | 120 dB SPL |
| Shouted conversation | 90 dB SPL | A gunshot or firecracker | 140 dB SPL |

times more powerful than the smallest audible sound. On the decibel scale, the smallest audible sound (near total silence) is 0 dB. A sound ten times more powerful is 10 dB. A sound 100 times more powerful than near total silence is 20 dB. A sound 1,000 times more powerful than near total silence is 30 dB. The jet engine is 120 dB higher than the hearing threshold. The ear requires its incredible sensitivity range because it needs to hear a broad range of sounds. Table 12–1 lists some common sounds and their decibel ratings.

The full range of the human ear is incredibly large, but it is also a complicated function of frequency and the sound pressure level. In 1933 Fletcher and Munson provided the first complete picture of the complicated details of the human auditory system in the form of equal-loudness contours. These have been refined since that time by many researchers including Robinson and Dadson (1956) and, in 1961, the International Organization for Standardization (ISO) published Recommendation R226 which described normal equal-loudness contours for pure tones and normal hearing under free field listening conditions. These equal-loudness contours are shown in Figure 12–7 in a graph with a horizontal frequency axis and a vertical dB SPL axis. The graph shows a number of curved lines, each marked with a number indicating the perceived loudness level. The lowest solid line is marked with a loudness level of 10 phon. A phon is a unit for subjective loudness sensation. A loudness level of 10 phon is as loud as a 1-kHz tone presented at 10 dB SPL. Similarly, 50 phon is as loud as a 1-kHz tone presented at 50 dB SPL. From about 500 Hz to roughly 1,500 Hz, the line is flat and a tone presented at 10 dB SPL in this frequency range is perceived with a loudness of 10 phon. The 10-phon line begins to dip at just before 2 kHz which means that the ear is most sensitive between 2 and 5 kHz. From this it is evident that the ear is most sensitive in the 2,000- to 5,000-Hz range and progressively less sensitive at lower and higher frequencies. The average measured threshold of hearing is the dashed curve in Figure 12–7, which is 4 dB SPL at 1 kHz. The standard threshold of hearing is nominally taken to be 0 dB SPL.

A simple physical explanation for the increased sensitivity in the 2,000- to 5,000-Hz range is that the ear canal has a natural resonance in this frequency range which serves to amplify these frequencies. This is beneficial because many of the cues for speech intelligibility are found in this frequency range. While our ears are capable of hearing the lower frequencies, our bodies feel them more than we actually hear them. This is the reason why many people who are nearly or completely deaf can still enjoy music—they can feel the low-frequency vibrations in their bodies.

As the overall loudness level increases, the equal-loudness contours flatten out at low frequencies because at higher SPLs the ear is more sensitive to these lower frequencies. Also, as the SPL increases, the ear is less and less sensitive to the frequencies above 6,000 Hz. This is why soft music seems to sound less rich or full than louder music. The louder the music is, the more the ear perceives the lower frequencies, and the fuller and richer it sounds. Many stereo systems have a loudness switch to boost the low and some of the high frequencies of the sound at normal listening levels between 50 and 70 phon.

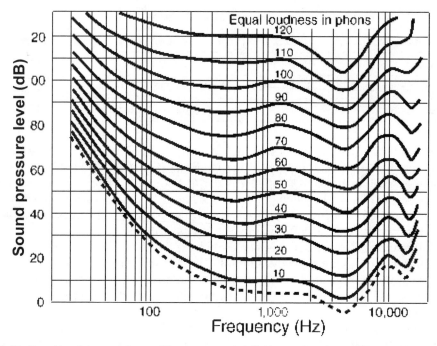

**Figure 12–7.** Equal loudness contours. *(The terms and definitions taken from ISO 226:2003 Acoustics— Normal equal-loudness-level contours, Figure A.1, are reproduced with the permission of the International Organization for Standardization, ISO. This standard can be obtained from any ISO member and from the Web site of the ISO Central Secretariat at the following address: www.iso.org. Copyright remains with ISO.)*

## dBA AND OTHER WEIGHTING FUNCTIONS

The dBA is a sound pressure level measured on a weighted frequency scale. The dBA was developed for sound pressure level meters. SPL meter microphones react to all frequencies equally but the electronics in an SPL meter filter the microphone signal in a number of ways. Measurements are weighted with "flat response," or weighted by the A, B, and C curves shown in Figure 12–8.

A weighting closely mirrors the ear's sensitivity at low SPL levels (40 phon). This means that the sensitivity of the measurement device changes to mirror the ear's sensitivity at the threshold of hearing. B weighting mirrors the loudness contour at a medium SPL level (70 phon), and C weighting mirrors the loudness contour at a high SPL level (100 phon). Thus, it is best to make measurements with an A-weighting setting to determine how the ear responds to the sound. At the same time, it is interesting to look at the C-weighted response because this measurement includes the low frequencies that may be present but which are inaudible to the ear. During heavy rock music or a Fourth-of-July fireworks celebration, the difference between A-weighted and C-weighted measurements can be 10 dB or more. A specialized D weighting has also been developed for aircraft noise measurements.

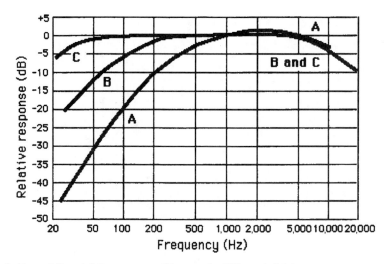

**Figure 12–8.** A, B, and C weighting curves. *(Courtesy of Phonak AG.)*

A weighting is the most widely used since the B and C weightings do not correlate well with subjective tests. One reason for this is because the equal-loudness contours derived from pure tone measurements. Most common sounds are not pure tones, but very complex signals made up of many different tones.

## SAFE SOUND EXPOSURE

Any sound above 85 dB SPL can cause hearing loss if the exposure time is long enough. An ambient noise level of 85 dB SPL requires speaking with a raised voice to be heard by somebody else. Continued unprotected exposure to sound at 90 dB SPL for periods longer than eight hours can cause damage to the ear. Any exposure to sounds in excess of 140 dB SPL can cause immediate inner-ear damage (and causes actual pain).

The International Standards Organization (ISO) and the U.S. Occupational Safety and Health Administration (OSHA) make recommendations for exposure limits in industrial settings. Exposure limits are recommended for people in industrial settings. Most industrial countries in the world have standards on unprotected occupational noise exposure to steady-state sound. The majority specify an eight-hour exposure limit at 90-dBA sound pressure levels and a halving rate of 5 dB. This means that at 95 dBA the exposure is limited to four hours, at 100 dBA, exposure is limited to two hours, with an overriding limit set at 115 dBA. These requirements are summarized in Table 12–2.

Some countries do have more stringent regulations. In particular, Sweden specifies the eight-hour exposure level at 85 dBA with a 3-dB halving rate, while the United Kingdom, Denmark, and Australia use the 90-dBA limit with a 3-dB halving rate. The 3-dB halving rate is recommended by the International Standards Organization (ISO) and differs from the 5-dB

**Table 12–2.** Permissible noise exposure (OSHA).

| Duration per Day (hours) | Sound Level (dBA) |
|:---:|:---:|
| 8 | 90 |
| 4 | 95 |
| 2 | 100 |
| 1 | 105 |
| ½ | 110 |
| ¼ or less | 115 |
| Maximum impact noise | 140 |

halving rate because it does not allow for the recovery of hearing during quiet periods. Some countries also limit exposure to impulsive sounds to 100 impulses of 140-dB peak per day.

It is interesting to note that the threshold of hearing is some 5,000,000,000 times less than, or approximately 194 dB below, normal atmospheric pressure. The threshold of pain (140 dB SPL) is 500 times smaller than, or 54 dB below, a pressure fluctuation with amplitude of one atmosphere of pressure. Stated another way, the dynamic range of the human ear extends from $2 \times 10^{-10}$ to 0.002 atmospheres.

## SUMMARY

1. Sounds are heard when their sound pressure level is above the hearing threshold and they are audible.
2. Understanding signifies the meaning of an audible sound is perceived.
3. The outer ear collects sound and the ear canal channels sound to the eardrum. The outer ear and the ear canal provide a small amount of frequency-selective amplification.
4. The middle ear mechanically transforms the force that air vibrations exert on the eardrum to a larger force the stapes exerts on the oval window to produce traveling waves in the fluid of the cochlea. The assembly of the malleus, incus, and stapes match the low mechanical (stiffness) of the eardrum to the higher mechanical impedance (stiffness) of the inner ear (cochlea).
5. Different frequencies resonate at different places along the cochlea where the mechanical resonances stimulate the hair cells on the organ of Corti on the basilar membrane. The hair cells produce electrical signals that are transmitted to the brain on the auditory nerve.
6. One row of inner hair cells and three rows of outer hair cells extend the length of the cochlea from the oval window to the top of the cochlear spiral.
7. When hair cells are damaged, loudness sensation and frequency selectivity of the ear are impaired.

8. The decibel is a relationship between two values of power.
9. Acoustic power is proportional to the square of acoustic pressure.
10. dB SPL is calculated by multiplying the base-ten logarithm of the ratio of a given sound pressure and sound pressure at the hearing threshold by twenty.
11. The hearing threshold of a healthy ear is 0 dBDSPL.
12. The dynamic range of the ear is approximately 120 dB.

## REVIEW QUESTIONS

1. What is the difference between hearing and understanding?
2. Describe the main parts of the ear.
3. What are the functions of the outer ear, the middle ear, and the inner ear?
4. What is the shape and size of the cochlea?
5. Which part of the cochlea plays an essential part in the transduction process?
6. Describe the function of the hair cells. Distinguish between inner hair cells and outer hair cells.
7. Define a decibel. Why is the decibel a useful unit of measure?
8. Describe equal-loudness contours.
9. Describe the different types of frequency weightings and what they represent.
10. Describe the basic rules for noise exposure.

# CHAPTER 13

# Interference in a Digital World

## INTRODUCTION

Human ears hear frequencies from 20 to 16,000 Hz, but hearing instrument design has historically been concerned primarily with the lower half of this audibility range. This is because the miniature loudspeakers, or receivers, that are available to hearing instrument designers generally do not produce significant outputs above 8,000 Hz. Until recently, frequencies outside the human audibility range were of little concern because interference from devices operating at such high frequencies was a rare occurrence. When problems did exist, they were most often caused when the hearing instrument reacted to ultrasound frequencies in the 30- to 60-kHz range. These frequencies are used in commercial security and energy management systems. However, this problem was relatively easily managed. Low-pass filters prevented such signals from affecting the operation of the hearing instrument amplifier. During the 1990s, the rapid growth in digital cell phone use introduced a new and significant source of radio interference for hearing instruments. This chapter discusses the causes of cell phone interference with hearing instruments.

## A BRIEF HISTORY OF RF AND THE RF SPECTRUM

AM and FM radio, VHF and UHF television, Citizens Band (CB) radio, cell phones, garage door openers, antitheft devices, and even baby monitors depend on radio frequency (RF) waves to function. In contrast with the human audio bandwidth of approximately 20,000 Hz, the radio spectrum extends well into the GHz range. The whole electromagnetic spectrum extends from very low frequencies, through the AM and FM radio ranges, the TV frequency bands, cellular phone range, and eventually to the infrared and visible light range, as shown in Figure 13–1.

Common frequency band allocations for radio and television, and selected wireless technologies are summarized in Table 13–1.

Why is the AM radio band allocated between 550 kHz and 1.7 MHz, while FM radios operate between 88 and 108 MHz? The reason is that AM radio preceded FM radio by many

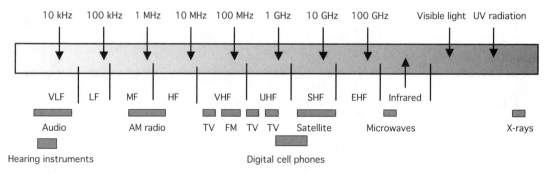

**Figure 13–1.** The RF spectrum. *(Courtesy of Unitron Hearing.)*

**Table 13–1.** Frequency band allocations for selected wireless applications.

| Application | Allocated frequency band |
|---|---|
| AM radio | 535 kHz–1.7 MHz |
| Short wave radio | 5.9 MHz–26.1 MHz |
| Citizens Band (CB) radio | 26.96 MHz–27.41 MHz |
| Television (Channels 2–6) | 54 MHz–88 MHz |
| FM radio | 88 Hz–108 MHz |
| Television (Channels 7–13) | 174 MHz–220 MHz |
| Garage door openers, alarm systems, etc. | ~40 MHz |
| Standard cordless telephones | 40–50 MHz |
| Baby monitors | 49 MHz |
| Radio-controlled airplanes | ~79 MHz |
| Radio-controlled cars | ~l75 MHz |
| Wildlife tracking collars | 215 MHz–220 MHz |
| MIR space station | 148 MHz–437 MHz |
| Cell phones–low band | 824 MHz–849 MHz |
| Cell phones–high band | 1.4 GHz–2 GHz |
| 900-MHz cordless phone | ~900 MHz |
| Air traffic control radar | 960 MHz–1.215 GHz |
| Global positioning system | 1.227 GHz–1.575 GHz |
| Deep space communications | 2.290 GHz–2.300 GHz |
| Bluetooth | 2.45 GHz |

years. The first AM radio broadcasts occurred during the 1920s. Government agencies were soon established to regulate the allocation of parts of the RF spectrum for specific devices and services. In the United States for example, Congress established the predecessor to the Federal Communications Commission (FCC) in 1927. During the 1920s, radio and electronic capabilities were relatively limited, hence the relatively low frequencies for AM radio. FM radio was invented to make it possible to broadcast high fidelity (and static-free) music. In the United States, the first FM radio station was built in 1939, but FM did not become popular until the 1960s. Radio technology advances had made higher frequencies for FM possible.

Television stations were essentially nonexistent when the FCC allocated commercial broadcast bands for TV in 1946, but by 1949, 1 million people owned TV sets and by 1951 there were 10 million TV sets in America. The allocations for bandwidth evolved over time as technologies developed and the need for non-interfering communication and entertainment channels became evident.

Every application has its own reference or product standards and unique frequency allocation. The FCC mandates these in the United States. Recently, the European Union has issued a number of electromagnetic compatibility (EMC) directives for Europe. In the United States, the Food and Drug Administration concerns itself with EMC for medical equipment and devices.

EMC is attracting increased attention because wireless devices are proliferating at an accelerating rate. Digital cellular telephones cause interference in hearing aids, and other electronic equipment. Because of this potential danger, the operation of almost all electronic devices is prohibited on airplanes during take off and landing because of concerns about potential interference with aviation control and communications systems.

Radio waves are electromagnetic waves propagated into air by a transmitting antenna and received at a remote location by a receiving antenna. A transmitting antenna usually radiates energy uniformly in all directions and at a distance of several wavelengths away the antenna begins to look like a point source. The receiving antenna senses the energy of interest because it is looking for signals at a predetermined frequency, but picks up only a very small fraction of the transmitted energy. In fact, the energy available to the receiving antenna is reduced by the inverse of the square of the distance between the transmitting and receiving antennas. This is due to the principle of conservation of energy which states that the total energy radiated from the antenna is spread over a sphere which grows in size with increasing distance from the transmitting antenna. If the antenna transmits one watt of energy (i.e., 1/100 the energy consumed by a 100-watt light bulb), then at a distance of ten meters the receiving antenna must be able to detect signals smaller than 0.01 watt. This is usually not a problem for systems such as baby monitors, garage door openers, and cordless phones since their ranges of operation are usually confined to a house, driveway, or backyard.

# FREQUENCIES FOR WIRELESS HEARING INSTRUMENT ACCESSORIES

Radio emissions are of interest to hearing aids because radio technology is now beginning to enable wireless hearing aid accessories. Auditory trainers have been used in educational settings for some time now but even these useful devices have suffered from the vagaries of bandwidth allocations. The North American allocation is different from the allocations in Europe and other countries. Some typical allocations are given in Table 13–2. It is noted that many countries have for many years used frequencies between 30 to 45 MHz as well as between 72 and 76 MHz. More recently, since 1996, many countries have applied for bandwidth allocations in the 170- to 223-MHz range for wireless microphones and auditory trainers.

It is evident that the rather large number of available frequencies for wireless accessories makes it extremely difficult for health care workers as well as educators to deal with these devices. Equipment manufacturers obviously incur additional expense to comply with many different requirements and standards in one country as well as between countries.

Aside from auditory trainers specialized for use in classrooms, recent developments have focused on individual use of wireless accessories outside the learning environment. In most instances, such use is limited to a single user in a space and there is little potential for interference from other transmitters, like in the home or in the car. It is possible, therefore, to design such an accessory without the need for multiple carrier frequencies which normally require the user to exchange crystals in the transmitter and receiver. Such a small, single-frequency receiver can be attached to, or integrated into, an audio input shoe. These devices work with an RF transmitting microphone operating at RF carrier frequencies summarized in Table 13–2. Furthermore, it is now possible to design and produce a synthesizing receiver that recognizes the carrier frequency in use in a particular space and automatically adjusts the receiver's carrier frequency to receive and demodulate the transmitted signal.

## INTERFERENCE BETWEEN EQUIPMENT AND APPARATUS

While auditory trainers and personal wireless accessories work over relatively small distances, cell phones operate with much greater distances between transmitters and receivers. Furthermore, they are integrated into larger systems that can operate around the world. These very sophisticated systems make use of worldwide networks of base stations, high-speed cable, fiber optics, and satellite communications systems. An individual cell phone signal is received by a base station, the originating and destination phone numbers are decoded from the signal, the signal is amplified and retransmitted as required.

Given the vast number of wireless devices and services that rely on frequencies all over the radio wave spectrum, it is not unusual to experience electromagnetic interference on a fairly regular basis. Every effort is made in the design of such equipment to ensure electromagnetic compatibility (EMC). In a nutshell, EMC is concerned with two issues. First, equipment should not interfere with other legitimate communications services. For example, computers have been known to generate emissions at frequencies of authorized broadcasts that jam radios or cause cross-hatching interference on television sets. Second, equipment should be designed to operate reliably in its intended environment. For example, equipment must be designed to achieve sufficiently high levels of immunity to any electrical and electromagnetic disturbance.

In spite of these considerations, digital cell phones are a source of interference for a number of electrical and electronic devices. Some cell phones in use near a computer can produce static in the computer's loudspeakers every time the cell phone and the base station exchange information. A car's tape player can emit static every time a cell phone is used in a car. A baby

**Table 13–2.** International frequency allocations for wireless hearing instrument accessories.

| Country | Allocated bands | # of bands & bandwidth | Comments |
|---|---|---|---|
| Belgium | 181.4–184.2 MHz | | |
| Canada | 72–76 MHz | 10 200-kHz bands or 40 50-kHz bands | |
| Denmark | 34.9–37.9 MHz<br>173.81–173.96 MHz | 16 200 kHz bands<br>5 bands | Max. power = 1 mW<br>25-kHz channel separation |
| England | 173.5–175.02 MHz | 20 bands | |
| France | 32.8–36.4 MHz &<br>39.2 MHz<br>32.8–36.4 MHz &<br>175.4–178.5 MHz<br>183.5–186.5 MHz | > 200 kHz | Radiated power < 1 W, fixed antenna<br><br>Radiated power < 10 mW, fixed or mobile antenna |
| Finland | 43.425–43.575 MHz | 7 200-kHz bands | |
| Germany | 36–39 MHz<br>173.990 MHz<br>180–225 MHz | 21 bands | |
| Iceland | 173–175 MHz | | |
| Ireland | 169.275–169.525 MHz | | |
| Liechtenstein | 174.12–181.90 MHz | | |
| Luxembourg | 173.35–173.65 MHz | | |
| Netherlands | 26 MHz, 30 MHz, 37 MHz<br>207.85–208.10 MHz<br>230 MHz<br>434–436 MHz | | |
| Norway | 40.9–43.5 MHz | 16 200-kHz bands | |
| South Africa | 72–76 MHz | 10 200-kHz bands<br>40 50-kHz bands | |
| Sweden | 40.9–43.5 MHz<br>173.81–173.96 MHz | 16 200-kHz bands<br>5 bands | Max. power = 1 mW<br>25-kHz channel separation |
| USA | 72–76 MHz<br>216–218 MHz | 10 200-kHz bands<br>40 50-kHz bands | |

monitor can also pick up signals from a cell phone and there have been reported cases of baby monitors interfering with air traffic radios or FM radios picking up CB traffic. Technically, none of these things should be happening.

However, all transmitters have some tendency to transmit at a lower power on harmonic side bands, and this is how FM radios can pick up a CB transmission. In the case of the cell phone affecting the computer speakers, the wire to each speaker is acting like an antenna and it picks up side band signals in the audible range.

Many hospitals have installed wireless networks for medical equipment. For example, heart monitors are equipped with antennas that transmit vital information to a monitor in the nursing station via the network. If a cell phone is used and it creates interference, it can disrupt these transmissions. That is true even if the cell phone is simply turned on. The cell phone and the base station communicate with each other at regular intervals and the phone periodically sends a burst of data to and receives data from, the base station.

# COMPATIBILITY OF CELL PHONES AND HEARING INSTRUMENTS

During the early 1990s a new cellular telephone system—GSM (Global System for Mobile communication)—attracted the attention of both hearing instrument manufacturers and associations for the hearing impaired. The rapid spread of this wireless mobile service in Europe and its introduction to North American consumers highlighted a serious interference problem for hearing instruments in areas of cell phone use. Interference with other electronic equipment was also observed, but this discussion will focus primarily on the hearing instrument issue.

## CELL PHONE TECHNOLOGIES

Three technologies used by cell phone networks to transmit information:

- ▼ Frequency division multiple access (FDMA)
- ▼ Time division multiple access (TDMA)
- ▼ Code division multiple access (CDMA)

The first word identifies the access method. The second word, division, means that it splits calls based on the access method. The last two words of each name means that more than one user can have access to the service. This is accomplished in different ways:

- ▼ FDMA puts each call on a separate frequency
- ▼ TDMA assigns each call a certain portion of time on a designated carrier frequency
- ▼ CDMA gives a unique code to each call and spreads it over a range of available frequencies

FDMA assigns uniform pieces of bandwidth to distinct voice channels. One piece of bandwidth is selected to carry the transmitted signal while a second piece carries the received portion of a telephone conversation. FDMA is used mainly for analog transmission, and while it is certainly capable of carrying digital information, it is not considered to be an efficient method for digital transmission.

TDMA is the access method used by the Electronics Industry Alliance and the Telecommunications Industry Association for Interim Standard 54 (IS-54, operating in the 800-MHz band) and Interim Standard 136 (IS-136, operating in the 1,900-MHz band). In TDMA, a narrow band 30 kHz wide and 20 ms long is split into three time slots, each 6.7 ms long. This can be done because speech is digitized and compressed. The compressed digital signal takes less time to be transmitted than the original uncompressed digital signal. Since the transmission is completed in 6.7 ms, three phones can share that particular frequency band, each phone transmitting a compressed segment of speech in one of the three 6.7-ms time slots and receiving a compressed segment of speech in a similar time slot in a different frequency channel (as shown in Figure 13–2). This North American TDMA therefore has a duty cycle of 1:3. The compressed speech segments are then decompressed in the telephone to produce a real-time signal that occupies the whole 20-ms time frame.

GSM is the international standard in Europe, Australia, and much of Asia and Africa. GSM operates in the 900-MHz and 1,800-MHz bands in Europe and Asia and in the 1,900-MHz band in the United States. GSM uses TDMA technology but in a somewhat different and incompatible way from IS-136. It uses a 217-Hz repetition rate and 0.58-ms time slots to provide a 1:8 duty cycle (see Figure 13–3). That is, eight different cell phones are each assigned a 0.58-ms time slot in each 4.6-ms (1/217-Hz) frame in two different frequency bands.

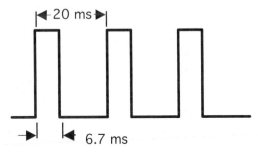

**Figure 13–2.** U.S. TDMA waveform: 50 Hz, 1/3 duty cycle. *(Courtesy of Unitron Hearing.)*

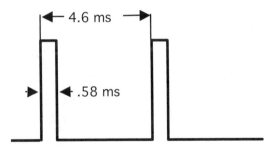

**Figure 13–3.** GSM/TDMA waveform: 217 Hz, 1/8 duty cycle. *(Courtesy of Unitron Hearing.)*

CDMA takes a different approach to TDMA. After digitizing the speech signal, CDMA spreads the data out over the entire available bandwidth. Multiple calls are overlaid on each other in the channel, but each call is assigned a unique sequence code. CDMA is a form of spread spectrum, which simply means that data are sent in small packets using any one of a number of the discrete frequencies available for use at any time in the specified range. CDMA technology is the basis of Interim Standard 95 (IS-95) and operates in both the 800-MHz and 1,900-MHz frequency bands.

## SIMPLE RADIO FREQUENCY ANTENNAS

Before proceeding to a discussion of cell phone interference in hearing aids, it is instructive to review very basic concepts for transmitting and receiving radio frequency signals using simple antenna concepts.

Figure 13–4 shows four antenna types for transmitting and receiving radio frequency signals. The dipole antennas shown in Figures 13–4(a) and (b) are fabricated from two lengths of wire, while the antennas in Figures 13–4(c) and (d) are wire loop antennas. Each type can be used to transmit and receive radio signals.

When an electric voltage is applied between the two wires in the dipole antenna of Figure 13–4(a), electric and magnetic fields are radiated from the antenna. Close to the wires, in the "near field" (closer than approximately 1/6 of the wavelength) the E (electric) field domi-

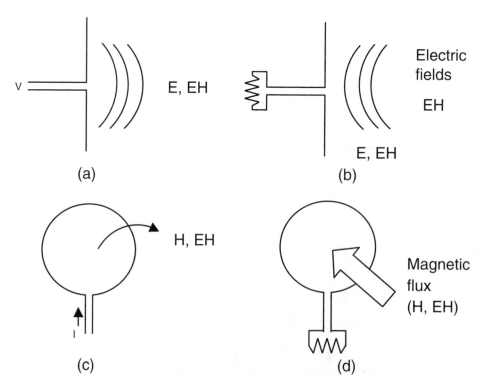

**Figure 13–4.** Different types of transmit and receive antennas.

nates, although there is some H (magnetic) field. In the far field, the magnetic and electric fields propagate together as an electromagnetic signal.

The dipole transmitting antenna of Figure 13–4a) can also act as a receiving antenna. This situation is in Figure 13–4b) where a resistive load replaces the voltage source. The dipole responds to electric fields in its vicinity by developing a voltage across the load. The sensitivity of the antenna is proportional to its size (length) and the amount of charge or current flow in the dipole. This proportionality exists at frequencies where the structure is small compared to the wavelength of the radio waves it receives. (Note that the wavelength of a radio wave at 1 GHz is 30 cm, or 11.75 inches.)

The alternative to the open-circuited electric field antenna is the current loop shown in Figure 13–4c). If a dc current flows, only a magnetic (H) field is generated. With an ac current, near fields are predominantly magnetic, with a small electric component, but the far field is a combination of the two, namely an electromagnetic field. Whether the source is a dipole or a loop antenna is irrelevant in the far field since electromagnetic radiation dominates the field at far-field distances.

The receiving complement to the magnetic transmitting antenna is the loop with a load shown in Figure 13–4d). Variation in the magnetic flux through the plane of the loop will cause a current to flow that in turn develops a voltage on the resistive load. The magnitude of the voltage developed across the load depends on the amount of magnetic flux passing through the loop, which is proportional to the loop area.

## THE CELL PHONE INTERFERENCE MECHANISM

In practice, the wires and circuit tracks in a hearing instrument act as antennas and pick up the RF field generated by the cell phone as it transmits information to the base station. Wire lengths terminated by a high-impedance load act like dipole antennas, while wire loops in the hearing instrument amplifier can act like loop antennas and respond to the electromagnetic fields produced by the cell phone.

Since hearing instrument amplifiers are designed to process and amplify audio band signals, they are essentially immune to continuous (unmodulated) RF signals, generally referred to as the RF carrier. The frequency of these signals is outside the passband of the hearing aid filters and can cause no harm.

Cell phones cause interference because they do not emit a continuous RF signal. Instead, cell phones operate by transmitting information in bursts as shown in Figures 13–2 and 13–3. The repetition rate of these bursts, or the modulation frequency of the RF carrier frequency, is in a portion of the audio band the hearing instrument amplifier is designed to amplify. When such a modulated RF signal is received in the hearing aid, the pulse envelope is demodulated from the carrier (800 or 1,800 MHz) at the first transistor junction or cold solder joint or any other component in the amplifier that can perform a rectifying function. Since the envelope is a square wave function, with fundamental and harmonic frequencies in the hearing aid's passband, the hearing aid amplifier readily amplifies this signal and reproduces the signal as a fundamental and its harmonics which the hearing aid user perceives as a loud and annoying buzz.

The pulse rate for the US TDMA and GSM cell phones are 50 and 217 Hz respectively. US TDMA interference should be less severe than GSM, by virtue of its lower pulse rate and by virtue of the fact that US TDMA operates at lower power levels than GSM. Although the 50-Hz fundamental frequency may receive less gain from the hearing aid amplifier than the 217-Hz fundamental, the higher harmonics of both signals receive essentially equal amounts of amplification, and in both cases the buzz is clearly audible.

A number of factors affect the loudness of the interference in the hearing instrument user's ear. The maximum operating power of the system has an effect. GSM is rated at a maximum transmit power of two watts at 800 MHz and one watt at 1,800 MHz while U.S. cell phone service operates at maximum power levels of 0.6 watts. The distance between the cell phone antenna and the hearing instrument plays a significant part. The further away the hearing instrument is from the antenna the less severe is the interference. The hearing instrument can be exposed to electric fields between 2 and 3 V/m at a typical bystander distance of 2 m from a cell phone. At a user distance of 10 cm from the antenna, the hearing instrument is exposed to more than 50 or 75 V/m, depending on the frequency band and the power rating of the cell phone (see Figure 13–5).

## ELECTROMAGNETIC COMPATIBILITY STANDARDS

Methods for measuring cell phone interference in hearing instruments have been developed in two standards: IEC 60118-13 (2004): "Hearing Aids—Electromagnetic Compatibility (EMC)" and ANSI C63-19 (2001): "Methods of Measurement of Compatibility between Wireless Devices and Hearing Aids."

Both standards employ an input related interference level (IRIL) to express the strength of the interfering signal. To make the IRIL value independent of the gain setting in the hearing aid, it is necessary to subtract the hearing instrument's gain value from the measured output level in dB. This is similar to the method for deriving the equivalent input noise level for a hearing instrument (see Chapter 9). IEC 60118-13 establishes immunity requirements for both a bystander condition and a cell phone use condition. When a hearing instrument is used at a

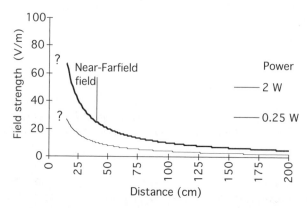

**Figure 13–5.** Reduction in field strength with distance from the cell phone at 0 cm. Field strength at 0 cm is difficult to determine and the value is indicated by "?." *(Courtesy of Phonak AG.)*

two-meter distance from a person using a cell phone, the hearing instrument user is considered to be a bystander. Bystander interference is measured at electric fields strengths of 3 V/m in the 800- to 960-MHz frequency range and 2 V/m in the 1.4- to 2.0-GHz range. When a hearing instrument is used with a cell phone, the two devices are separated by a 10-mm distance. The field strengths for measuring user interference are therefore much higher: 75 V/m for the 800- to 960-MHz range and 50 V/m for the 1.4- to 2.0-MHz range. A hearing instrument is bystander and user compatible if IRIL is less than or equal to 55 dB when tested with the field strengths described above. Almost all modern hearing instruments are bystander compatible and many are now user compatible.

ANSI C63.19 (2001) specifies measurement methods for determining cell phone emission ratings and hearing instruments immunity ratings. Telephone emissions are rated from U1 (highest emission level) to U4 (lowest emission level) while hearing instrument immunity is rated from U1 (lowest immunity level) to U4 (highest immunity level) as shown in Table 13–3.

The best performance will be achieved when the cell phone has the lowest possible emission (U4) and the hearing instrument has the highest possible immunity (U4). Clearly, this is not always the case. Table 13–4 provides typical hearing instrument/cell phone system performance classifications.

ANSI C63.19 (2001) is now undergoing a revision. The next edition of this standard will include the IEC 60118-13 measurement methods as a normative method. (Note that a pass rating according to IEC 60/18 = 13 is equivalent to a U2, or better, immunity rating according to ANSI C63.19.) It will also include modified terminology by replacing the U rating label with an M rating label when the rating is obtained with the hearing instrument operating in the microphone mode.

**Table 13–3.** Summary of rating scales for cell phone emissions and hearing instrument immunity.

|  | U1 | U2 | U3 | U4 |
|---|---|---|---|---|
| Telephone emission rating | High ← | | → | Low |
| Hearing instrument immunity rating | Low ← | | → | High |

**Table 13–4.** Estimated performance of hearing instruments with cell phones as a function of their combined immunity and emissions ratings.

| System Classification | | |
|---|---|---|
| System Classification | Articulation Index | U Category Sum |
|  | AI | Hearing aid U category + cell phone U category |
| Useable | 0.3 | 4 |
| Normal use | 0.5 | 5 |
| Excellent performance | 0.7 | 6 or greater |

## REGULATORY RULINGS

In the United States, the FCC issued a ruling in 2003 requiring cell phone manufacturers and service providers to make available, within two years of the ruling, two cell phone models that comply with the "U3" emission rating according to ANSI C63.19 (2001). These handsets, when used together with hearing instruments that exhibit at least a "U2" immunity rating, are expected to provide acceptable performance with an Articulation Index = 0.5, as shown in Table 13–4.

## IMPROVEMENTS IN HEARING INSTRUMENT IMMUNITY

Hard-of-hearing persons can use their hearing instruments with an increasing number of cellular phones, but not all. The immunity of hearing instruments to cell phone interference has been significantly improved since 1995. The first successful contributions were made when component manufacturers reduced RF sensitivities at the microphone input, the point in the hearing instrument where it could do the most damage. These improvements became part of an overall effort throughout the hearing instrument design process to bypass RF signals wherever possible in the mechanical and electrical layout of the hearing instrument. The conversion of hearing instruments from primarily analog-to-digital technology has improved average RF immunity of recent and current instruments by more than 30 dB over a period of five years (see Figure 13–6).

Investigations at the University of Zurich, Switzerland, show that radiation to the head from various GSM phones in normal use positions differ by factors of up to 4.75. These variations are due to various design factors and antenna orientation during phone use. If excessive interference prevents phone at ear level, an inductive neck loop developed by Nokia can be considered. In this case, the phone is worn at the belt, to move it beyond the nearfield range (see Figure 13–7). The loop has a built-in lapel-style microphone which replaces the microphone in the handset. The receiver signal is fed inductively via the neck loop to the hearing aid T-coil. The RF assistive device (see Figure 7–10) described in Chapter 7 is compatible with Bluetooth enabled cell phones. This device eliminates interference during cell phone use.

## SENSITIVITY OF OTHER DEVICES TO GSM INTERFERENCE

Hearing instruments are not the only electronic devices to experience interference from TDMA signals. A 1993 ETSI Technical Report "GSM EMC Considerations" listed the tolerance of a number of electronic devices to GSM/TDMA interference. The extrapolated mean/median peak TDMA field intensities at which various types of equipment would suffer visible or audible, but not annoying, interference are listed in Table 13–5.

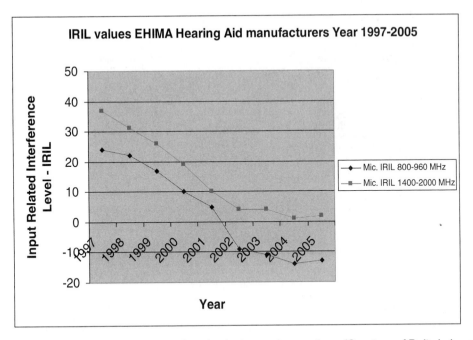

**Figure 13–6.** Immunity improvements in hearing instruments over time. *(Courtesy of Delta Laboratories, Odense, Denmark, and EHIMA, Wemmel, Belgium.)*

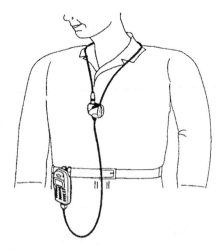

**Figure 13–7.** Neck loop for use with digital cell phone.

**Table 13–5.** TDMA intensities at which visible or audible interference occurs in various types of electronic equipment.

| Type of Equipment | Field Intensity V/m |
|---|---|
| Hearing aids | 4.1 |
| Television receivers | 4.0 |
| Video cassette recorders | > 13.9 |
| Satellite television receivers | 9.5 |
| Tuners/amplifiers | > 8.3 |
| Cassette decks | > 2.9 |
| CD players | > 13.9 |
| Portable radios & cassette players, etc. | 5.6 |
| Telephones | > 7.6 |
| Computers | > 8.5 |
| Computers (home/games) | > 13.5 |
| General electrical/electronic equipment | > 7.5 |

## SUMMARY

1. Continuous radio frequency (RF) transmissions pose no difficulty for hearing instruments.
2. Pulsed RF creates interference when the pulse rate is in the hearing instrument's passband.
3. Cell phone transmission methods use pulsed RF.
4. Cell phones cause audible interference in hearing instruments.
5. Hearing instruments have over the last five years achieved, on average, a 30-dB improvement in immunity or resistance to cell phone interference. Digital hearing instruments are generally more immune to cell phone interference than analog instruments.
6. Standards specify methods to measure hearing aid immunity and cell phone emissions.
7. Assistive devices can reduce cell phone interference in a hearing instrument by allowing the cell phone to be used at a greater distance from the hearing instrument.

## REVIEW QUESTIONS

1. What does EMC stand for?
2. Name the three main transmission methods used by cell phones.
3. Why do cell phone transmissions interfere with hearing instruments?

# CHAPTER 14

# Data Transmission

## INTRODUCTION

The personal computer (PC) is an integral part of the dispensing process and this tool offers new opportunities for fitting and assessing digital hearing systems. Hearing instrument fitting has traditionally been conducted in a well-controlled acoustic space like a sound room or a hearing health care professional's office. These locations eliminate natural environmental sounds during hearing aid adjustment and they generally do not facilitate testing the performance of the hearing instrument in a real-world environment, where it is ultimately used. It is, therefore, not surprising that additional office sessions are often required to fine-tune the instrument to best accommodate the user's lifestyle.

It may be inconvenient to send the patient into the street to determine how well the instrument performs in a normal noisy situation, but it is entirely reasonable to expect a dispensing clinic to have the capability to evaluate the performance of a newly prescribed hearing instrument in a wide variety of different real-world situations. Many different sound scenes can be recorded, digitized, and stored in the computer in an appropriate format. These audio files can be presented to the hearing aid user over loudspeakers or directly into the hearing aid.

Uncompressed good-quality audio files are large. They require a large amount of hard drive space and transmission bandwidth if they are to be used in an uncompressed manner. The file compression methods and the various communication protocols discussed in this chapter will find an increasing number of applications during the hearing instrument fitting and adjustment process. Downloading audio files, representative of the patient's lifestyle, directly to the hearing instrument is likely to become an integral part of verifying and validating the effectiveness of the prescription.

Data transmission has become an important element of digital hearing instrument technology. Analog signals are converted to numbers, processed with mathematical operations, and converted back to the analog signal domain to achieve an amplified, filtered, and clean signal that optimally overcomes a particular hearing impairment. Throughout this sequence of events, the hearing aid operates on data. During programming, data are transmitted from the programming terminal, usually a personal computer, to the hearing aid. When a remote control is used, data are sent to the hearing instrument to change the volume or to select a different program.

Information that is arranged in a standardized format that the various parts of the data communication system can interpret and respond to is referred to as data. The smallest unit of information is a bit, and these bits are usually grouped in a larger unit called a byte. The following paragraphs describe these basic concepts.

# BITS AND BYTES

Computers work with bits and bytes. These terms refer to how big a document is; it may be a file size, the amount of unused space on a hard drive, etc. It is common to hear advertisements about a computer with a thirty-two-bit Pentium processor with 128 megabytes of RAM and thirty-two gigabytes of hard disk space. What do these numbers mean and how are they derived?

# DECIMAL NUMBERS

First, it is useful to review some numbers and a numbering system that is intuitive and easily understand because it is such an integral part of daily life. This system is the decimal system and it is made up of digits. In the decimal system, a digit is a single place that can hold a numerical value between zero and nine. Digits are combined together in groups to form larger numbers. For example, the decimal number 7,691 is made up of four digits. It is understood that in the number 7,691, the one fills the ones place, the nine fills the tens place, the six fills the 100s place, and the seven fills the 1,000s place. To be very explicit, the number can be expressed in the following way:

$$(7 \times 1,000) + (6 \times 100) + (9 \times 10) + (1 \times 1) = 7,000 + 600 + 90 + 1 = 7,691$$

Another way to express it would be to use powers of ten. For convenience, we can represent the "places" in the decimal system by "ten raised to the power of n" so that $1,000 = 10^3$, $100 = 10^2$, $10 = 10^1$, and $1 = 10^0$. Now we have another way to express the number 7,691 as:

$$(7 \times 10^3) + (6 \times 10^2) + (9 \times 10^1) + (1 \times 10^0) = 7,000 + 600 + 90 + 1 = 7,691$$

It is evident that in a decimal system number, each digit in the number is a placeholder for the next higher power of ten, starting with the first digit with ten raised to the power of zero.

The next fact about number systems is that there is nothing that forces the use of ten different values for a digit. The base-ten number system was likely developed because mankind had ten fingers. If mankind had six fingers instead, a base-six number system would have been logical. There are good reasons to use different bases in different situations.

# BITS

Computers are based on electronic technology that, in its most fundamental implementation, uses two states. Computers are made up of millions of transistors that are combined to essentially operate as switches. A switch has two states; either open or closed. Transistors are used to construct microprocessors, memories, and other logic functions and operate like a switch (either on or off) in a binary (two state) mode.

Computers, therefore, use a base-two or a binary number system instead of a decimal system. One could wire up and build computers that operate in base-ten, but they would be much more expensive than a base-two or binary computer.

Whereas decimal digits can have ten possible values ranging from zero to nine, binary digits have only two possible values: zero and one. The word *bit* is the abbreviation for "binary digit."

Therefore, a binary number is composed of only zeros and ones, like this: 1011. The value of such a binary number is determined in the same way as was done for the decimal number 7,691, but using a base of two, instead of a base of ten:

$$1011 \text{ (binary)} = (1 \times 2^3) + (0 \times 2^2) + (1 \times 2^1) + (1 \times 2^0)$$
$$= (1 \times 8) + (0 \times 4) + (1 \times 2) + (1 \times 1) = 11 \text{ (decimal)}$$

In the binary number system, each bit holds the value of increasing powers of two. Starting at zero and counting to twenty in decimal and binary looks like this:

| Decimal | | Binary |
|---|---|---|
| 0 | = | 0 |
| 1 | = | 1 |
| 2 | = | 10 |
| 3 | = | 11 |
| 4 | = | 100 |
| 5 | = | 101 |
| 6 | = | 110 |
| 7 | = | 111 |
| 8 | = | 1000 |
| 9 | = | 1001 |
| 10 | = | 1010 |
| 11 | = | 1011 |
| 12 | = | 1100 |
| 13 | = | 1101 |
| 14 | = | 1110 |
| 15 | = | 1111 |
| 16 | = | 10000 |
| 17 | = | 10001 |
| 18 | = | 10010 |
| 19 | = | 10011 |
| 20 | = | 10100 |

In this sequence, zero and one are the same for the decimal and the binary systems. At the number two, one is added to one so the bit becomes zero and the next bit becomes a one. In the transition from fifteen to sixteen, this effect rolls over through four bits turning 1111 into 10000.

## BYTES

Bits are rarely used alone in computers. They are almost always bundled together into eight-bit groups, and these groups are called bytes. The eight-bit byte was adopted because it was sufficient for the earliest standard codes, like the ASCII code.

With eight bits in a byte, it is possible to represent 256 values ranging from 0 to 255. In other words, when an analog value is represented by a byte or eight bits, its value can be represented by 256 steps. A ten-volt signal can be converted into a binary value in 10 V/256 = 39.1-mV steps.

$$
\begin{array}{rcl}
0 & = & 00000000 \\
1 & = & 00000001 \\
2 & = & 00000010 \\
.... & & ..... \\
254 & = & 11111110 \\
255 & = & 11111111
\end{array}
$$

CDs use sixteen bits or two bytes per sample. That gives each sample a range from 0 to 65,535, like this:

$$
\begin{array}{rcl}
0 & = & 0000000000000000 \\
1 & = & 0000000000000001 \\
2 & = & 0000000000000010 \\
... & & ..... \\
65,534 & = & 1111111111111110 \\
65,535 & = & 1111111111111111
\end{array}
$$

A CD player can therefore represent a ten-volt signal in 0.1525-mV steps.

Prefixes like kilo, mega-, and giga, as in kilobyte, megabyte, and gigabyte (also shortened to K, M, and G, as in Kbytes, Mbytes, and Gbytes) are commonly used to express data rates, memory size, or hard drive capacity. The following table shows the multipliers:

| Name | Abbr. | Size |
|------|-------|------|
| Kilo | K | $2^{10} = 1{,}024$ |
| Mega | M | $2^{20} = 1{,}048{,}576$ |
| Giga | G | $2^{30} = 1{,}073{,}741{,}824$ |
| Tera | T | $2^{40} = 1{,}099{,}511{,}627{,}776$ |
| Peta | P | $2^{50} = 1{,}125{,}899{,}906{,}842{,}624$ |

It is evident from the chart that kilo is about a thousand, mega is about a million, giga is about a billion, and so on. When a computer has a two-gig hard drive, it means that the hard drive stores two gigabytes, or approximately 2 billion bytes, or exactly 2,147,483,364,648 bytes. That appears to be a vast quantity of data. To put this into perspective, this amounts to just the contents of three compact disks (CDs), each of which can hold up to 650 megabytes. Terabyte databases are now fairly common and there are probably a few Petabyte databases in use.

## BINARY MATHEMATICS

Binary math works just like decimal math except that the value of each bit can be only zero or one. First add 452 and 751:

$$
\begin{array}{r}
452 \\
+ \quad 751 \\
\hline
1{,}203
\end{array}
$$

To add these two numbers together, start at the right : $2 + 1 = 3$.

Next, $5 + 5 = 10$; save the zero and carry the 1 over to the next place.

Next, $4 + 7 + 1$ (because of the carry) $= 12$; save the 2 and carry the 1.

Finally, $0 + 0 + 1$ (again because of the carry) $= 1$; the answer is 1,203.

Binary addition works exactly the same way:

$$
\begin{array}{r}
010 \\
+ \quad 111 \\
\hline
1001
\end{array}
$$

Again, starting at the right, $0 + 1 = 1$. No carry here.

Next, $1 + 1 = 10$ for the second digit; save the 0 and carry the 1.

For the third digit, $0 + 1 + 1$ (for the carry) $= 10$; save the 0 and carry the 1.

Finally, $0 + 0 + 1$ (for the carry) $= 1$. So the answer is 1001 which is equal to 9 in decimal. Translating everything over to the decimal system shows this is correct: $2 + 7 = 9$.

## ASCII (AMERICAN STANDARD CODE FOR INFORMATION INTERCHANGE)

Bytes are frequently used to denote individual characters in a text document. In the ASCII character set, each binary value between 0 and 127 is given a specific character. The standard 127 ASCII character set is given on the next page in Table 14–1. Most computers extend the ASCII character set to use the full range of 256 characters available in a byte. The upper 128 characters handle special things like accented characters from common foreign languages.

Table 14–1. ASCII code.

| | ASCII | Binary | | ASCII | Binary | | ASCII | Binary |
|---|---|---|---|---|---|---|---|---|
| 0 | NUL (null) | 00000000 | 43 | + | 00101011 | 86 | V | 01010110 |
| 1 | SOH (start heading) | 00000001 | 44 | , | 00101100 | 87 | W | 01010111 |
| 2 | STX (start of text) | 00000010 | 45 | - | 00101101 | 88 | X | 01011000 |
| 3 | ETX (end of text) | 00000011 | 46 | . | 00101110 | 89 | Y | 01011001 |
| 4 | EOT (end of transmit) | 00000100 | 47 | / | 00101111 | 90 | Z | 01011010 |
| 5 | ENQ (enquiry) | 00000101 | 48 | 0 | 00110000 | 91 | [ | 01011011 |
| 6 | ACK (acknowledge) | 00000110 | 49 | 1 | 00110001 | 92 | \ | 01011100 |
| 7 | BEL (bell, beep) | 00000111 | 50 | 2 | 00110010 | 93 | ] | 01011101 |
| 8 | BS (backspace) | 00001000 | 51 | 3 | 00110011 | 94 | < | 01011110 |
| 9 | TAB (horizontal tab) | 00001001 | 52 | 4 | 00110100 | 95 | — | 01011111 |
| 10 | LF (line feed) | 00001010 | 53 | 5 | 00110101 | 96 | ` | 01100000 |
| 11 | VT (vertical tab, home) | 00001011 | 54 | 6 | 00110110 | 97 | a | 01100001 |
| 12 | FF (form feed) | 00001100 | 55 | 7 | 00110111 | 98 | b | 01100010 |
| 13 | CR (carriage return) | 00001101 | 56 | 8 | 00111000 | 99 | c | 01100011 |
| 14 | SO (shift out) | 00001110 | 57 | 9 | 00111001 | 100 | d | 01100100 |
| 15 | SI (shift in) | 00001111 | 58 | : | 00111010 | 101 | e | 01100101 |
| 16 | DLE (data line escape) | 00010000 | 59 | ; | 00111011 | 102 | f | 01100110 |
| 17 | DC1 (device control 1) | 00010001 | 60 | ∨ | 00111100 | 103 | g | 01100111 |
| 18 | DC2 (device control 2) | 00010010 | 61 | = | 00111101 | 104 | h | 01101000 |
| 19 | DC3 (device control 3) | 00010011 | 62 | ∧ | 00111110 | 105 | i | 01101001 |
| 20 | DC4 (device control 4) | 00010100 | 63 | ? | 00111111 | 106 | j | 01101010 |
| 21 | NAK (negative acknowledge) | 00010101 | 64 | @ | 01000000 | 107 | k | 01101011 |

*(Continued)*

**Table 14–1.** ASCII code (continued).

| | ASCII | Binary | | ASCII | Binary | | ASCII | Binary |
|---|---|---|---|---|---|---|---|---|
| 22 | SYN (synch. idle) | 00010110 | 65 | A | 01000001 | 108 | l | 01101100 |
| 23 | ETB (end transmit block) | 00010111 | 66 | B | 01000010 | 109 | m | 01101101 |
| 24 | CAN (cancel) | 00011000 | 67 | C | 01000011 | 110 | n | 01101110 |
| 25 | EM (end of medium) | 00011001 | 68 | D | 01000100 | 111 | o | 01101111 |
| 26 | SUB (substitute) | 00011010 | 69 | E | 01000101 | 112 | p | 01110000 |
| 27 | ESC (escape) | 00011011 | 70 | F | 01000110 | 113 | q | 01110001 |
| 28 | FS (file separator) | 00011100 | 71 | G | 01000111 | 114 | r | 01110010 |
| 29 | GS (group separator) | 00011101 | 72 | H | 01001000 | 115 | s | 01110011 |
| 30 | RS (record separator) | 00011110 | 73 | I | 01001001 | 116 | t | 01110100 |
| 31 | US (unit separator) | 00011111 | 74 | J | 01001010 | 117 | u | 01110101 |
| 32 | Space | 00100000 | 75 | K | 01001011 | 118 | v | 01110110 |
| 33 | ! | 00100001 | 76 | L | 01001100 | 119 | w | 01110111 |
| 34 | " | 00100010 | 77 | M | 01001101 | 120 | x | 01111000 |
| 35 | # | 00100011 | 78 | N | 01001110 | 121 | y | 01111001 |
| 36 | $ | 00100100 | 79 | O | 01001111 | 122 | z | 01111010 |
| 37 | % | 00100101 | 80 | P | 01010000 | 123 | { | 01111011 |
| 38 | & | 00100110 | 81 | Q | 01010001 | 124 | | | 01111100 |
| 39 | ' | 00100111 | 82 | R | 01010010 | 125 | } | 01111101 |
| 40 | ( | 00101000 | 83 | S | 01010011 | 126 | ~ | 01111110 |
| 41 | ) | 00101001 | 84 | T | 01010100 | 127 | DEL | 01111111 (delete) |
| 42 | * | 00101010 | 85 | U | 01010101 | | | |

# MODEMS

The word *modem* is a contraction of the words *modulator-demodulator*. A modem is typically used to send digital data over a telephone line. The sending modem modulates the data into a signal that is compatible with the phone line and the receiving modem demodulates the signal back into digital data. Wireless modems convert digital data into radio signals and back.

Modems were developed in the 1960s to connect computers over the phone lines. People got along with 300 bit-per-second (bps) data rates for quite some time. The reason this speed was tolerable was because 300 bps represents about thirty characters per second, which is much faster than a person could type or read. But when people began to transfer large programs and files, the 300-bps data rate became intolerable. Modem speeds rapidly became faster.

| | | |
|---:|:---:|:---|
| 300 bps | — | 1960s through to approximately 1983 |
| 1,200 bps | — | gained popularity in 1984 and 1985 |
| 2,400 bps | | |
| 9,600 bps | — | first appeared in late 1990 and early 1991 |
| 19.2 Kbps | | |
| 28.8 Kbps | | |
| 33.6 Kbps | | |
| 56 Kbps | — | became the standard in 1998 |
| ADSL–up to 8 Mbps | — | gained popularity in 1999 |

## 300-BPS MODEMS

The 300-bps modem is extremely easy to understand. These devices use frequency shift keying (FSK) to transmit digital information over a telephone line. In frequency shift keying, a different tone (frequency) is used for different bits. When a first modem (the original modem) dials a second modem, it transmits a 1,070-Hz tone for a zero and a 1,270-Hz tone for a one. The second modem (the answer modem) transmits a 2,025-Hz tone for a zero and a 2,225-Hz tone for a one. Because originate and answer modems transmit different tones, they can use the line simultaneously. This is known as full-duplex operation. Modems that can transmit in only one direction at a time are known as half-duplex modems, but these are seldom used now.

When two terminals are connected with 300-bps modems, and one user types the letter *a*, the terminal generates the ASCII code 01100001 for the letter "a," and the UART (universal synchronous receiver/transmitter) in the transmitting modem sends this code one bit at a time through the terminal's RS-232 port (also known as a serial port) to the answer modem. The answer modem is connected to the RS-232 port, so it receives the bits one at a time and decodes them to reproduce the letter *a*.

## FASTER MODEMS

Modem speed was limited with the FSK technique. Newer encoding techniques, such as phase-shift keying (PSK) and quadrature amplitude modulation (QAM), allowed data rates up to 56 kbps to be transmitted over the 3,400-Hz bandwidth available in a normal voice-grade telephone line. These high-speed modems incorporated the concept of gradual degradation which meant they could test the phone line and fall back to lower data rates if the line could not support the higher data rates.

The next step in the evolution of the modem was asymmetric digital subscriber line (ADSL) modems. These modems are asymmetric because they send data faster in one direction than they do in the other. An ADSL modem takes advantage of the fact that any normal home, apartment or office has a dedicated copper wire running between it and the telephone company's nearest central office. Digital subscriber line (DSL) modems have a capacity near 1 million bits per second (Mbps) between the home and the telephone company (upstream) and 8 Mbps between the telephone company and the home (downstream) under ideal conditions. The same line can transmit both a phone conversation and the digital data.

Today, modems connect to an Internet service provider (ISP), and the ISP connects the subscriber into the Internet. The Internet enables connections to any machine in the world. The computer, the ISP, and the Internet, no longer send individual characters. Instead, the modem uses TCP/IP (transmission control protocol/Internet protocol) to send packets of data between the computer and any desired destination on the Internet.

## DATA COMPRESSION

There are two ways to transmit more data in a given time. One is to increase the speed or data rate over the data link with faster modems and high-capacity connections as discussed in the preceding sections, and the other way is to reduce the amount of data that needs to be transmitted. This is accomplished with data compression techniques. The following sections describe how data compression is accomplished, ending with a description of a familiar compression technique, MP3, that has found application in the music industry, and which may also be applied to allow streaming audio data to hearing aids for the purpose of hearing aid fitting validation, in particular, auditory scene analysis.

A disadvantage of MP3 is that the compression calculations require a long time. A signal which is first compressed and then decompressed has a delay of more than 100 ms from the original signal, and MP3 cannot be used in a real-time compression system.

Many programs and files are downloaded from the Internet as zip files. These files contain a reduced number of bits so they can be transmitted faster and take up less space on a disk. Once such a file is downloaded, the computer unzips the file and expands it back to its original size. If everything works correctly, the expanded file is identical to the original file before it was compressed.

Most types of computer files contain redundant information. The same information occurs over and over again. File-compression programs simply eliminate the redundancy. A file-compression program lists a piece of information once, assigns it a code, and refers back to it whenever it appears in the original program.

Most compression programs use a variation of the LZ adaptive dictionary-based algorithm to shrink files. "LZ" refers to Lempel and Ziv, the algorithm's creators, and "dictionary" refers to the method of cataloging pieces of data. The system for arranging dictionaries varies, but it could be as simple as a numbered list. Repeated words are put into a numbered index. Then, the number is used instead of writing out the whole word. Compression programs also look for patterns, and in order to reduce the file size as much as possible, it carefully selects which patterns to include in the dictionary.

In this way, a reduction of 50% or more is typical for a good-sized text file. Most programming languages are also very redundant because they use a relatively small collection of commands, which frequently go together in a set pattern. Files that include a lot of unique information, such as MP3 files, cannot be compressed much with this system because patterns are usually not repeated (more on this in the next section).

## THE MP3 FORMAT

MPEG is the acronym for Moving Picture Experts Group. This group has developed compression systems used for video data. For example, DVD movies, HDTV broadcasts, and DSS satellite systems use MPEG compression to fit video and movie data into smaller spaces. The MPEG compression system includes a subsystem to compress sound, called MPEG Audio Layer-3, or MP3 in the abbreviated form.

The MP3 format is used to store music on CDs. A CD stores an audio as digital information. The data on a CD uses an uncompressed, high-resolution format. When a CD is created, music is sampled 44,100 times per second. The samples are two bytes (sixteen bits) long. Separate samples are taken for the left and right channels in a stereo system.

A CD stores a large number of bits for each second of music: 44,100 samples/second × 16 bits/sample × 2 channels = 1,411,200 bits per second; 1.4 million bits per second equals 176,000 bytes per second. The average three minute long song on a CD consumes about 32 million bytes of space. A 56K modem requires close to two hours to download one song.

An MP3 compresses a 32-MB song on a CD to about 3 MB. This downloads in minutes rather than hours, and hundreds of songs can be efficiently stored on a computer's hard drive.

The compression algorithm uses a technique called *perceptual noise shaping*. It is "perceptual" partly because the MP3 format uses characteristics of the human ear to design the compression algorithm. It uses the fact that the human ear cannot hear certain sounds and the fact that the human ear hears some sounds much better than others. If two sounds are playing simultaneously, the louder one is heard but the softer one is not (masking). Using facts like these, certain parts of an audio passage can be eliminated without significantly hurting overall quality for the listener. Compressing the rest of the material with well-known compression techniques produces a data reduction of approximately ten times. The MP3 version of the song does not sound exactly the same as the original CD song because some of it has been removed, but it is very close.

## DATA COMMUNICATION PROTOCOLS

When any two devices communicate with each other, they agree on several points before the conversation begins. The first point of agreement is physical: will they talk over wires, or through some form of wireless signals? If the answer is wires, how many are required—one, two, eight, twenty-five? Once the physical attributes are decided, several more questions arise. Information can be sent one bit at a time in a scheme called *serial communication,* or in groups of bits (usually eight or sixteen at a time) in a scheme called *parallel communication.* A desktop computer uses both serial and parallel communications to transmit data to different devices. Modems and keyboards communicate over serial links, while printers tend to use parallel links.

All the parties in an electronic discussion need to know what the bits mean and whether the message they receive is the same message that was sent. In most cases, this means developing a language of commands and responses known as a protocol. Some types of products have a standard protocol used by virtually all manufacturers of those products so that the commands for one product will have the same effect on another. Modems fall into this category. Other product types each speak their own language, which means that commands intended for one specific product have no meaning, or an incorrect meaning if received by another. Printers are like this and use multiple standards like PCL and PostScript.

Companies that manufacture computers, entertainment systems, and other electronic devices have realized that the incredible array of cables and connectors involved in their products make it difficult for even expert technicians to correctly set up a complete system on the first try. Communication protocols like RS-232, USB, Bluetooth, and others, are intended to solve these interconnection problems.

## RS-232

In the 1960s, a standards committee known today as the Electronic Industries Association developed a common interface standard, RS-232, for serial data communications over analog telephone voice lines. The standard specifies signal voltages, signal timing, signal function, a protocol for exchange, and mechanical connectors.

## USB

USB stands for Universal Serial Bus, which is a single standardized way to connect up to 127 devices to a computer using cables and connection points called *hubs.* Hubs can be powered or unpowered. The power comes from the computer. Up to 500 milliamps at five volts can be drawn to power low-power devices like a mouse or a digital camera. Self-powered devices like scanners and printers are connected using an unpowered hub. The powered hub has its own transformer and supplies power to the device so the device does not overload the computer's supply. Individual cables can be as long as five meters. Each device can consume up to 6 Mbps of bandwidth, which is fast enough for the vast majority of peripheral devices that most people want to connect to their machines.

The original version, USB 1.1, provides for data rates of 12 Mbps. Version USB 2.0 allows data rates from 120 to 240 Mbps. Most computers and peripherals made today use USB.

## BLUETOOTH

Bluetooth is a standard developed by a group of more than 1,000 electronic manufacturers, the Bluetooth Special Interest Group. Bluetooth allows any sort of electronic equipment—from computers to cell phones to keyboards to headphones—to make its own connections, without wires, cables, or any direct action from a user.

Bluetooth is an RF interconnect scheme which, unlike infrared, does not require line-of-sight between two devices. It operates at 2.45 GHz, which is part of the ISM band allocated to industrial, scientific, and medical devices. Other devices in this band are baby monitors, garage door openers, and the newest generation of cordless phones.

To avoid interfering with other systems, Bluetooth operates with very weak signal levels, typically 1 mW, which limits its range to approximately ten meters. By comparison, cell phones operate in the 0.6- to 3-watt range. Up to seventy-nine individual bands, each 1 MHz wide, are available. The likelihood of any two transmitters being on the same channel is minimized by transmitting data in discrete 625-μs time slots and hopping through the available channel frequencies 1,600 times a second. Each device forms a small personal-area network (PAN) and uses a range of addresses assigned to the device by the manufacturer. A PAN may interconnect a number of devices within a room or operate over a smaller distance, such as the distance between the cell phone on a belt clip and the headset on the user's head.

A major advantage of the Bluetooth protocol is that it is wireless, relatively low cost, and the system setup is automatic. While North America and Europe have adopted the same frequencies and channels, seventy-nine 1-MHz channels between 2.402 and 2.48 GHz, Japan has adopted twenty three channels between 2.472 and 2.497 GHz. One major disadvantage includes interference in large installations where more than six PANs operate simultaneously, and as more devices are added to a PAN, the latency between devices increases. At this time, Bluetooth cannot be integrated into a hearing instrument because the technology requires more power than a hearing instrument battery can supply.

## WI-FI (WIRELESS FIDELITY)

Wi-Fi, like Hi-Fi for high fidelity in audio equipment, essentially means that the manufacturer's product is compliant with a variation of the IEEE specification known as 802.11b. This specification drops the frequency hopping spread spectrum (FHSS) part of the standard and focuses instead on the direct sequence spread spectrum (DSSS) method of communicating because of the higher data rate it can obtain. This is possible because in DSSS each byte of data is split into several parts and sent concurrently at different frequencies. DSSS operates in the 2.4-GHz range and uses frequency-shift keying (FSK) technology.

Some advantages of Wi-Fi are:

▼ It is fast (11 Mbps)
▼ It is reliable
▼ It has a long range (1,000 feet or 305 meters in open spaces and 250 to 400 feet or 78 to 122 meters in closed areas)
▼ It is easily integrated into existing wired-Ethernet networks
▼ It is compatible with original 802.11 DSSS devices

Some disadvantages are:

▼ It is expensive
▼ It can be difficult to set up
▼ Speed can fluctuate if signal strength fluctuates or interference disrupts data

**Table 14–2.** IEE 802.11 Wi-Fi standards.

| Standard | Band (GHz) | Data Rate (Mbps) | Channels | #Range (m) |
|---|---|---|---|---|
| IEEE 802.11 a | 5.2 | 54 | 18 | 50 |
| IEEE 802.11 b | 2.4 | 11 | 3 | 100 |
| IEEE 802.11 g | 2.4 | 54 | 3 | 100 |

Wi-Fi standards are still evolving and by the end of 2003, three major standards were in use. These are being deployed as "hot spots" to provide wireless interconnects to the World Wide Web. The most commonly used scheme, IEEE 802.11 b, and others are listed in Table 14–2.

## SUMMARY

1. Data is information arranged in a standardized format that the various parts of a communications system can interpret and respond to.
2. Data consists of a string of bit (zero and one) groupings that follow a standard protocol like the ASCII protocol.
3. Modems are used to transmit data over telephone lines and dedicated transmission channels at data rates of up to 8 Mbps.
4. More data can be transmitted in a given time by increasing transmission rates or by compressing the amount of data that needs to be sent.
5. File compression algorithms eliminate redundant information.
6. An MP3 is used to compress audio files by a factor of up to ten.
7. An MP3 uses techniques based on perceptual coding. If a sound is masked by a louder sound, it is rejected and not encoded.
8. Standard data transfer protocols are used in hearing instrument systems.
9. Bluetooth is used in some hearing instrument accessories, but its use in hearing instruments is not yet possible due to high power requirements.

## REVIEW QUESTIONS

1. How many bits make up a byte?
2. Computers use what type of numbering system?
3. The initial data rate of modems was 300 bps. What is the data rate of current modems?
4. List two ways that are used to transmit more data in a given time.

5. File compression works on the principles of:
   A. Removing long words      A ☐
   B. Recognizing and coding patterns      B ☐
   C. Recognizing and coding words that are used many times      C ☐
   D. Removing redundancies      D ☐
6. Compression methods can reduce the size of text files by:
   A. 10%      A ☐
   B. 90%      B ☐
   C. 50%      C ☐
   D. 0%      D ☐
7. What does MP3 stand for?
8. By how much is an MP3 music file reduced from its original size?
9. What psychoacoustic effect does the MP3 compression method exploit?
10. RS-232 is a interface standard for:
    A. Serial data transfer      A ☐
    B. Parallel data transfer      B ☐
11. How many devices can a USB connect to a computer?
    A. 25      A ☐
    B. 50      B ☐
    C. 1,000      C ☐
    D. 127      D ☐
12. Why can Bluetooth not be used in hearing instruments?
13. The Wi-Fi 802.11 b protocol has the following properties:
    A. Eighteen channels      A ☐
    B. A data rate of 11 Mbps      B ☐
    C. Operates in the 2.4-GHz band      C ☐
    D. Has a range of 100 meters      D ☐

# CHAPTER 15

# Implanted Devices

## INTRODUCTION

Hearing instrument development continues to exploit the ear's acoustic pathway but much work is also devoted to bypassing the ear canal and eardrum to stimulate instead areas of the middle or inner ear. A number of devices pursue this line of development:

- ▼ bone conduction hearing instruments,
- ▼ bone anchored hearing aids (BAHA),
- ▼ middle-ear implants,
- ▼ cochlear implants (CI), and
- ▼ auditory brainstem implants.

Although acoustic hearing instruments are by far the most numerous hearing correction devices in use today, nonacoustic devices meet specific needs and address types of impairment that would otherwise not be corrected with acoustic amplification alone.

The bone conduction instrument and the BAHA overcome outer- and middle-ear conditions that prevent the use of a hearing aid by delivering bone-conducted vibrations directly to the cochlea. The middle-ear implant overcomes similar problems by stimulating bones in the middle ear and delivering vibrations to the stapes and the basilar membrane. The cochlear implant, however, corrects for inner-ear problems which may have left an individual profoundly impaired or deaf, bypassing the outer, middle, and inner ear completely and directly stimulating the auditory nerve in the cochlea.

All these devices are distinguished from acoustic path hearing instruments in that they require some degree of surgical intervention. The only exception is the basic bone conduction instrument. This device is a modified power BTE in which the acoustic output receiver is replaced by a bone vibrator transducer. This bone vibrator is electrically connected to the hearing instrument amplifier and is attached to one end of a head band so that the bone vibrator can be positioned and held against the temporal bone usually behind the outer ear. The bone anchored hearing instrument is a more recent development and it does require a surgical procedure.

Some components of implanted and semi-implanted devices are not visible outside the ear, but invariably, these devices require an acoustic input from a microphone and a device for processing the acoustic signal processor into a form that is appropriate to drive the implanted transducer. The microphone and the signal processor are worn externally on the head, usually behind the ear. The implanted portion of these devices usually contains a receiver. This term is used in conventional hearing instrument terminology to mean at the electroacoustic transducer, or the miniature loudspeaker. In the case of implanted devices, signals are transmitted by the outside portion of the device to the implanted portion using some form of wireless transmission. The receiver is the implanted part of this transmission mechanism.

A thorough discussion of implanted devices is well beyond the scope of this book, and this chapter provides only a brief overview introductory discussion.

# BONE CONDUCTION HEARING INSTRUMENTS

Diagnoses of chronic otitis media, malformed ears, and conductive or mixed hearing loss are common in clinical otology. When amplification is needed to rehabilitate patients with these conditions, and the use of air conduction hearing instruments is precluded, they may be candidates for bone conduction instruments. The principal otologic indications for such devices are:

▼ chronic otitis media, at times accompanied by external otitis.
▼ middle- or external-ear congenital malformation that cannot be surgically corrected.
▼ otosclerosis or tympanosclerosis in certain cases.

The conventional bone conduction hearing instrument described does not require surgery. Patient discomfort and poor sound quality are common complaints expressed by patients wearing such a bone conduction hearing instrument. Patient discomfort can occur because the bone conductor must be applied with steady pressure to the mastoid region of the temporal bone. This pressure causes, to various degrees, pain, headache, irritation of the skin, and eczema. The quality of the transmitted sound has relatively poor sound quality and low fidelity due to an effect referred to as soft tissue attenuation. Occasional variations in the quality of the transmitted sound occur because the bone conductor is not applied at exactly the same place each time.

## THE BAHA SYSTEM

The principle of the BAHA system (see Figure 15–1) is to provide a direct bone conduction signal. It consists basically of two parts: an external part, referred to as the sound processor, and an implanted part, comprising the titanium bone implant and the skin-penetrating titanium abutment.

The use of titanium implants for treatment of patients who have no teeth started in Goteborg, Sweden, in 1965. Pioneering work was done on osseointegration and showed that titanium implants can remain stable. Titanium implants for the attachment of bone anchored hearing aids have been in clinical use in Sweden since 1977 (Hakansson, 1990).

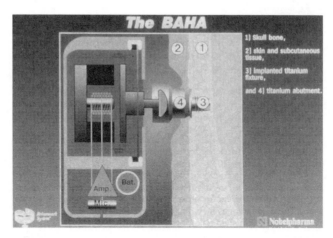

**Figure 15–1.** The bone anchored hearing aid (BAHA). *(Courtesy of Phonak AG.)*

The titanium fixture is surgically implanted into the bone behind the ear. The titanium fixture and the bone bond together by a process called *osseointegration*, after which the skin-penetrating titanium abutment is attached to the implant. Both surgeries can be performed under local anesthetic. After a healing process of three months, the titanium abutment is firmly integrated with the bone and the BAHA can be used and removed as often as the patient likes. The hearing health care professional can then fit the BAHA as a conventional hearing instrument.

The surgical procedures are reversible. If for some reason the patient does not want to keep the skin-penetrating coupling, it is easy to remove without any future complications.

Compared with conventional hearing instruments or conventional bone conductors for hearing-impaired patients with chronically draining ears, malformed ear, or otosclerosis, the BAHA has several advantages. These advantages include: improved quality of sound, improved comfort, and diminished risk of ear infections.

## MIDDLE-EAR IMPLANTS

Unlike a hearing instrument that picks up a sound signal, amplifies it, and transmits it to the eardrum, the middle-ear implant (see Figure 15–2) converts the sound signal into micromechanical vibration and transmits it directly onto the ossicular chain. The three tiny bones of the ossicular chain are built like a chain through the middle ear, and transmit the sound that was produced by the hearing instrument to the oval window, the entrance to the inner ear.

The middle-ear implant consists of an outer and inner part. The outer part consists of the microphone, the battery, and the electronics that convert sound pressure into an electromagnetic signal (wireless at about 150 kHz). This signal is transmitted to the inner part. The most recent middle-ear implants are implanted in the back of the ear canal under the skin. This means the microphone is situated at an acoustically optimal place and is protected fully

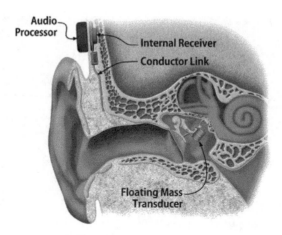

**Figure 15–2.** Middle-ear implant from Symphonix. *(Courtesy of Vibrant MED-EL.)*

against outer influences. The electronics are also implanted into bone so that the hearing instrument is not visible. It is, in fact, a completely implanted instrument. The accumulator (also implanted), which is responsible for the electricity supply for the middle-ear implant, can be charged up inductively (i.e., without touching).

The inner part consists of a receiver, cable, and vibrator that convert sound into micromechanical vibration and put the ossicular chain into movement. The vibrator is one of the essential parts of the middle-ear implant. It has to be very small and light so that it does not influence the normal functioning of the ossicular chain. The middle-ear implant can be fixed on the skull with a magnet. An appropriate magnet is also found in the inner part of the middle-ear implant.

Many problems that arise with conventional hearing instruments do not occur with middle-ear implants because the middle-ear implant is not situated in the ear canal. Problems like feedback, occlusion, and obstruction with earwax are avoided.

The acoustical qualities are usually very good, especially in the high-frequency range. Currently, the use of middle-ear implants is restricted to patients with mild-to-moderate hearing loss. The primary disadvantage is obviously the high cost and potential complications that arise from a two-hour surgery.

## COCHLEAR IMPLANTS (CI)

For many years people believed that it was impossible to restore hearing to the deaf. About forty years ago researchers first began to experiment with stimulating the auditory nerve in an attempt to restore auditory sensation. Progress was slow, but this work eventually led to the development of a cochlear implant (CI), a prosthetic device that is implanted in the inner ear to restore partial hearing to profoundly deaf people.

A cochlear implant is very different from a hearing instrument. Instead of amplifying sound, cochlear implants compensate for damaged or non-working hair cells in the inner ear by stimulating the auditory nerve directly. If the auditory nerve is functional, the CI can restore auditory sensation and in many cases it can restore speech understanding.

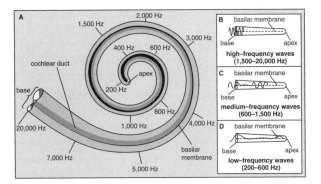

**Figure 15–3.** Places of maximum sensitivity to different frequencies along the basilar membrane in the cochlea.

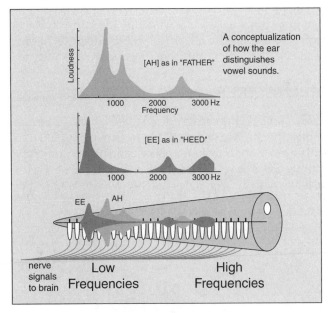

**Figure 15–4.** Formant structure of two vowel sounds and approximately where on the cochlea they would stimulate hair cell and nerve activity. *(From HyperPhysics by Rod Nave, Georgia State University.)*

It was discussed in Chapter 12 that frequencies are detected at specific places along the basilar membrane. Figure 15–3 shows this distribution of frequency selectivity. Sounds are not simply tones. Our vocal tract produces sounds that are characterized by unique spectral shapes. In vowels, the dominant characteristics are the formant frequencies at which intensity peaks occur in the response. The frequencies of the first three formants contain sufficient information for the recognition of vowels as well as other voice sounds. Formant movement is also important for the perception of unvoiced sounds (i.e., consonants). Figure 15–4 shows the formant structure of two different vowel sounds and where on the cochlea they would stimulate hair cell or nerve activity.

## CANDIDACY

Persons who receive little or no benefit from conventional hearing aids are considered to be candidates for a cochlear implant. Not all people with hearing impairment are candidates for cochlear implantation. Certain audiological criteria need to be met. First, the hearing loss has to be profound and bilateral and the candidate has to obtain sentence recognition scores of 30% correct or less under best aided conditions. Children with profound sensorineural loss in both ears are also candidates for cochlear implants.

Approximately 70,000 people worldwide have received cochlear implants. In the United States alone, about 13,000 adults and nearly 10,000 children have undergone implant procedures. Growth rate is estimated at 20% annually. Learning to interpret the sounds created by a cochlear implant takes time and practice and speech therapists and audiologists are invariably involved in this learning process.

The implantation of a CI is final and irreversible. Inserting an electrode into the cochlea results in the destruction of any residual hearing, and the decision to proceed with this procedure should be well considered with input from professionals as well as family members.

## COCHLEAR IMPLANT TYPES

Similar to the middle-ear implant, the cochlear implant (CI) consists of two parts. Sound signals are received from the microphone, usually in a BTE type of housing, and transmitted to the speech processor via a cable. The processor transforms speech and other sounds and delivers them to the receiver via a transmitting coil. The second part of the system is the receiver/stimulator (see Figure 15–5) that is implanted, with the electrodes (twenty-two electrodes at most).

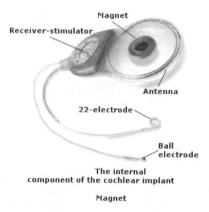

**Figure 15–5.** Implanted components of a CI system.

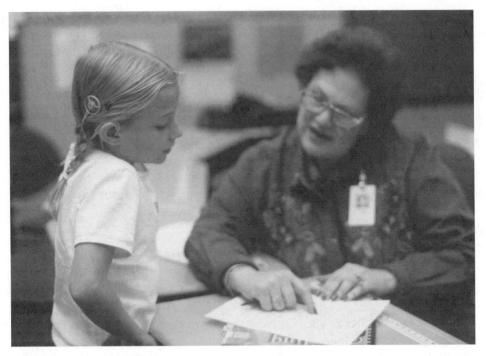

**Figure 15–6.** CI system components on the head. *(Courtesy of the Central Institute for the Deaf.)*

The transmitting coil has to be placed exactly above the receiver coil since not only speech signals but the whole power supply for the implanted system have to be transferred without wires (see Figure 15–6).

## HOW THE CI WORKS FROM "1" TO "7"

1. Sounds are picked up by the microphone.
2. The cable sends the sound from the microphone to the speech processor.
3. The speech processor filters, analyzes, and digitizes sound into coded signals.
4. These coded signals are sent from the speech processor to the transmitting coil via the cables.
5. The transmitting coil sends the signals across the skin to the implanted receiver/stimulator via an FM radio or a magnetic signal.
6. The receiver/stimulator delivers the correct amount of electrical stimulation to the appropriate electrodes.
7. The electrodes along the array stimulate the remaining auditory nerve fibers in the cochlea.

The receiver/stimulator decodes the information and, according to the instructions, delivers signals to the electrodes. The electrodes are placed in the cochlea and the electrical energy stimulates the surviving auditory nerve fibers in the inner ear. The actual output of the implant is the electrode. The electrode is very flexible so it can be inserted easily into the cochlea.

The initial cochlear implants in the 1970s consisted of a single electrode which provided electrical stimulation at a single place in the cochlea. These were simple in design and the spectral information a patient could receive was restricted to frequencies below 1 kHz. The House/3M and the Vienna/3M are two examples of single-channel implants. Although people could differentiate to some degree between vowels, there was insufficient information to discriminate consonants and very few patients could obtain speech understanding with these single-channel devices.

Multichannel implants appeared in the 1980s and two different signal-processing strategies were developed for these instruments. The first, a waveform-processing strategy, attempted some type of analog or pulsed waveform stimulation of the auditory nerve while the second, a feature extraction strategy, presented formants and other spectral features (Loizou, 1998).

## PROCESSING STRATEGIES

A compressed analog (CA) approach is used in the Ineraid device (manufactured by Symbion Inc.) and the UCSF/Storz device (which is now discontinued). The CA approach first uses AGC to compress the incoming signal, and then filters it into four adjacent bands centered on 500, 1,000, 2,000, and 3,400 Hz. The filtered waveforms are again passed through an AGC stage and then sent to four electrodes each separated by 4 mm from the other, each in the cochlea.

This approach enables many patients to obtain varying degrees of speech understanding (median scores of 45% correct for word identification in CID sentences) because this multichannel system provided considerably increased frequency resolution than the single-channel device.

In a second approach, continuous interleaved sampling (CIS), the signal is passed through a six-channel bandpass filter. The envelopes of the filtered waveforms are rectified, low-pass filtered, and finally compressed to modulate biphasic pulses. Compression is used to fit the pulses to the patient's electrically evoked dynamic range of hearing. These pulse trains are presented to six electrodes at a constant rate.

The CIS approach is currently used in three commercially available implant devices: the Clarion device, the Med-El device, and the Nucleus CI24M device (see Figures 15–7 to 15–9).

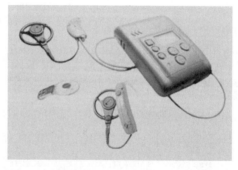

**Figure 15–7.** A Nucleus cochlear implant system. *(Pictures courtesy of Cochlear Americas.)*

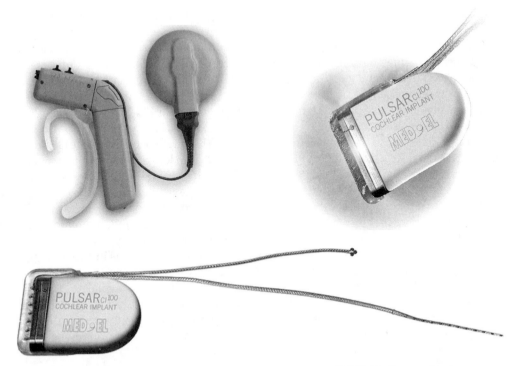

**Figure 15–8.** Two Med-El cochlear implant systems. *(Courtesy of MED-EL Corporation.)*

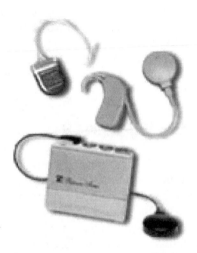

**Figure 15–9.** A Clarion cochlear implant system. *(Courtesy of Advanced Bionics Corporation.)*

The Nucleus multielectrode implant was developed at the University of Melbourne in Australia and is manufactured by Nucleus Ltd. It was first introduced in the early 1980s and has seen a number of improvements since that time. Initially it used a feature extraction approach which was fundamentally different from the CA and the CIS approaches. The Nucleus processor contained specialized algorithms to extract spectral features, such as formants, and more recently uses a filterbank approach to extract spectral maxima. This strategy is currently used in the commercially available Nucleus Spectra 22, manufactured by Cochlear Pty Ltd in Australia. This implant device uses a 22-electrode array in the cochlea. The electrodes consist of twenty-two platinum rings connected to twenty-two insulated wires. The length of the complete electrode that can be inserted into the cochlea is typically between 15 to 20 mm long; the diameter about 0.5 mm.

State-of-the-art implant devices are now produced by a number of manufacturers. The Clarion cochlear implant system from Advanced Bionics was developed at the University of California in San Francisco. It can be programmed for either CA or CIS processing. In one study, thirty-two of the first forty-six patients fitted with the Clarion implant obtained moderate to excellent open-set speech recognition scores (30–100% correct on CID sentence tests) twelve months after implantation. This device has undergone continuous improvements such as smaller speech processor, improved bandpass filters with 30 dB/octave roll-offs, and enhanced preprocessing.

The Med-El processor is widely used in Europe and is manufactured by the Med-El Corporation in Austria. It features very soft electrode technology which allows very deep, up to 30 mm, insertion into the cochlea thereby being able to stimulate a larger number of perceivable channels. The processor implements a CIS strategy.

## COCHLEAR IMPLANTS IN CHILDREN

Language can be acquired only if it can be heard. Speech skills develop through an iterative process of refining speech utterances under the influence of auditory feedback. For deaf children, cochlear implants can provide the necessary feedback. Research has shown that the intelligibility of speech produced by children with cochlear implants as well as the speech perception abilities of children with cochlear implants improves over time. Both pre-lingually and post-lingually deafened children obtain benefits from cochlear implants. The implications of successful implants are far greater in a young child than in an adult and age is therefore extremely crucial for the child's language and cognitive development for speech production and perception.

## AUDITORY BRAINSTEM IMPLANTS

The auditory brainstem implant (ABI) is performed on patients who have severed auditory nerves as a result of surgery to remove tumors on or around the auditory nerve. This type of implant is designed to penetrate into the auditory portion of the brainstem, stimulate the cochlear nucleus, and send signals to the brain. The ABI is the only device that can restore limited hearing for people with no remaining auditory nerve. ABIs have been implanted in 350 people worldwide. In the United States, the Food and Drug Administration (FDA) approved the ABI as a medical device in 2000.

## SUMMARY

1. Cosmetic appearance is a powerful motivator for continuous improvement in miniaturization. It is clear that hearing instruments have undergone massive transformations in size from body-worn instruments all the way to being located completely in the ear canal.
2. Technical innovations have played a major role in hearing instrument miniaturization and will also play major roles in the continuous miniaturization of semi- and fully implanted devices.
3. Figure 15–8 clearly shows that progression is under way. The processor portion of a CI is already reduced from a body- or pocket-worn device to a BTE-style unit.
4. Dedicated, low-power, and efficient integrated circuits have had a significant impact on hearing instruments and they will also have an impact on semi-implanted and CI processors.
5. Properly protected electret microphones can already be implanted under the skin in the ear canal. Further size reduction could be achieved with silicon microphones that are now finding application in communications devices.
6. Silicon microphones, or arrays of silicon microphones, could be integrated into the signal processor IC reducing size as well as eliminating some of the interconnect requirements. Smaller size coupled with lower power requirements and the application of efficient wireless battery charging techniques, will make these devices candidates for full implantation.

## REVIEW QUESTIONS

1. List four hearing device developments that do not exploit the acoustic pathway of the ear.
2. Name two disadvantages of the traditional bone conduction hearing instrument.
3. What is osseointegration?
4. List three problems that often occur with conventional air conduction hearing instruments that middle-ear implants overcome.
5. What is the principal difference between a middle-ear implant and a cochlear implant?

# CHAPTER 16

# Glossary of Digital Signal Processing and Psychoacoustics

## DIGITAL SIGNAL PROCESSING

### ADAPTIVE FILTER

An adaptive filter can change its filter characteristics. It can be used to eliminate unwanted background noise or to eliminate feedback. Unlike conventional filters, its frequency response is not fixed. Usually it is a digital filter with variable filter coefficients. A control loop compares the output signal from the filter to a desired signal. The difference between these two signals that can be seen as an error is minimized by the algorithm of the adaptive filter. One type of algorithm of adaptive filters is called *LMS* (least mean squares), which minimizes the sum of squared errors. As shown in Figure 16–1, two input signals are needed to build an adaptive filter. For a feedback canceller, for example, the input signal is compared to a delayed version of itself. The desired signal is the same signal as the input and the input will be delayed. Periodic components of the signal (feedback) can be detected and eliminated. The output (two different signals) will contain the wanted signal with attenuated feedback components.

### ALGORITHMS

An algorithm is a sequence of instructions and calculations. Digital or digitally programmable instruments require mathematical relationships of the most varied character to determine or calculate the amplification properties in relation to a certain hearing loss: the algorithms. Algorithms are also used to specify to the processor in the digital hearing instrument how it should change or switch over its properties in certain situations. Algorithms are the heart of digital signal processing as they contain the mathematical description of empirical or theoretical founded models for compensation hearing loss.

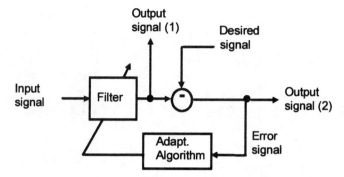

**Figure 16–1.** Schematic diagram of an adaptive filter. This is a very general concept. For specific applications, the desired signal has to be chosen appropriately and the output signal may be collected at different points on the control loop. *(Courtesy of Phonak AG.)*

## ALIASING

Signal components at frequencies above half of the *sampling frequency* are mirrored to lower frequencies and may become audible. This leads to nonlinear distortions. Cf. *Sampling theorem.*

## ANALOG SIGNAL

Its characteristic is continuity in time and amplitude. At any particular moment of time you can measure the signal and it would have some value. The resolution in time is infinite. The amplitude of the signal as well may have any value and is not restricted to a set of finite values.

## ANALOG-TO-DIGITAL CONVERTER (ADC)

An ADC converts analog continous signals (i.e., electrical voltage), which can have arbitrary value, to digital form, which can be processed by a computer. The digital form consists of integer numbers within a range that is determined by the *data word width* (e.g., sixteen-bit ADC). During analog-to-digital conversion, a quantization of amplitudes and sampling at uniform discrete time points of the signal is performed. Information about the amplitude between sample points is lost. A special type of ADC with low-power consumption is the *sigma-delta converter*; this type is preferably used in hearing aids.

## ANTIALIAS FILTER

An antialias filter is an analog low-pass filter in the beginning of the processing chain. It is required to fulfill the *sampling theorem.* Hence, the cutoff frequency must be half of the *sampling rate.*

## BINARY NUMBERS

In a computer all information is represented in the state of semiconductor switches. The memory of a computer consists of millions of these switches. There are two states for the memory: on and off or high/low. These two states can be seen as zeros and ones, with every number that is stored in the memory in principle a sequence of zeros and ones. Binary numbers use the same mathematical operations as decimal numbers.

## BIT (BINARY DIGIT)

Representation of numbers in digital technique. The information is stored in memory that has two discrete states (on/off, 0/1), as *binary numbers*. Every decimal number is represented as a sequence of binary digits. The table below shows all numbers that can be represented with three bits. There are $2 \cdot 2 \cdot 2 = 2^3 = 8$ different values. A sixteen-bit number allows for $2^{16} = 64,536$ different values.

| decimal | 0 | 1 | 2 | 3 | 4 | 5 | 6 | 7 |
|---------|-----|-----|-----|-----|-----|-----|-----|-----|
| binary | 000 | 001 | 010 | 011 | 100 | 101 | 110 | 111 |

## CHAIN OF DIGITAL SIGNAL PROCESSING

1. The hearing aid microphone turns sound into an analog electric signal. 2. Frequencies above the audible range are removed by an *anti-aliasing filter*. 3. The filtered analog signal goes to the A/D converter, which changes it to a numerical digital signal at a very fast rate. An FFT filterbank 4. transforms the signal to *frequency domain* and then the digital representation is processed by a DSP. 5. The DSP chip can be hard-wired or freely software programmable to perform any number of numerical operations (e.g., filtering, noise reduction, feedback cancellation, or loudness compensation), depending on the algorithms that are used. The complexity of the operations is limited only by the available computational power, since the processing must be in real-time (without perceivable delay). 6. The digital signal is reverted to a time signal using inverse FFT and *overlap-add* synthesis. Hereafter, the processed signal goes to a D/A converter 7. that changes it back to analog. It is low-pass filtered 8. and can be reproduced via a loudspeaker or receiver. For hearing aid applications the last part of the processing chain may look different, since a direct digital output drive (DDD) may be used to share the benefits from a Class D amplifier. A block diagram of the processing steps is shown in Figure 16–2.

## CHANNELS/FREQUENCY BANDS

The frequency resolution of signal processing in the frequency domain depends on the number of points of the FFT and the sampling rate. For example, at 20 kHz a 256-point FFT has a

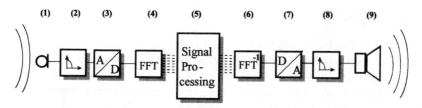

**Figure 16–2.** Block diagram of a digital signal-processing circuit. The blocks are described in the text. *(Courtesy of Phonak AG.)*

frequency resolution of $20,000/256 \sim 78$ Hz. The output of the 256-point FFT can be interpreted as a filterbank with a filter bandwidth of 78 Hz for each output channel.

## CHIP TECHNOLOGY

The chip technology describes dimensions of structures on the silicon (e.g., $0.5\ \mu$, $0.35\ \mu$; $\mu$ designates a micron which is one millionth of a meter.). With decreasing size of the structures, the overall size, operation voltage, and power consumption decreases, and the speed of operation and overall performance increases.

## CLASS D AMPLIFIER

The signal information is coded in the modulation of the pulse width. The amplitude of the pulse does not carry any information, and it can be as high as the battery voltage. Class D end amplifiers have a lower current consumption than other end amplifiers and this is especially important for low-voltage systems such as hearing aids.

## COMPLEMENTARY METAL OXIDE SEMICONDUCTOR (CMOS)

A semiconductor fabrication technology designed for very low-power consumption.

## DATA WORD WIDTH

The data word width expresses how many pieces of binary information (bits) are used for representing a sampled value. The data word width has a direct influence on the accuracy (resolution) of the digital representation of signals. Cf. *Quantization error*.

The following rule of thumb applies: a one-bit increase of the data word width improves the dynamic response by 6 dB. The dynamic range is expressed in dB and is derived from the quotient of the biggest and the smallest number that can be represented.

| Data word width | 8 bit | 12 bit | 16 bit | 20 bit | 22 bit |
|---|---|---|---|---|---|
| Max. dynamic range | 48 dB | 72 dB | 96 dB | 120 dB | 132 dB |

In a digital system with complex mathematical operations, it may be necessary to perform internal calculations with higher accuracy when fixed-point calculations are performed. The problem with fixed-point arithmetic is that all numbers are represented with the number of digits. If two big numbers of the same range are subtracted, the difference is of a much smaller magnitude. Further, calculations with this small number have a smaller precision because the number of significant digits is reduced. In numerical calculations with floating-point numbers, these problems do not occur. Floating-point DSPs are much more complex and expensive to design than fixed-point DSPs.

## DIGITAL DIRECT DRIVE (DDD)

In a digital direct drive output stage no explicit D/A converter is needed. It is a combination of a Class D amplifier (pulse-width modulation output stage), which is driven by a sigma-delta converter ($\Sigma$-$\Delta$ converter), as in the input stage. The $\Sigma$-$\Delta$ converter produces a high-speed, one-bit stream. This bit stream can be demodulated into audible sounds by the induction coil of the hearing aid receiver. A low-pass filter at the analog output, like the antialias filter at the input stage, is not needed, since the receiver itself has low-pass characteristics.

## DIGITAL FEEDBACK SUPPRESSION (DFS)

Digital feedback suppression is a feedback cancelling system that eliminates acoustical feedback due to sound transmission through the leak between the ear canal and earmold, and/or the vents in the earmold. The idea is to adapt a filter in the signal path so that the sound from the receiver that is transmitted to the microphone just compensates for the ringing feedback signal. It is performed by an *adaptive filter.*

## DIGITAL SIGNAL

A digital signal is, in principle, a sequence of numbers. It may be stored as a table of values and is an appropriate form for numerical processing. Each number represents a sample of the analog signal. The samples are taken at a constant rate, the sampling rate.

## DIGITAL SIGNAL PROCESSOR (DSP)

A digital signal processor is a processor that is optimized for numerical calculations, especially the "multiply and add" operation required to perform an FFT or to filter digital signals. The DSP differs from a multipurpose processor like the CPU of a personal computer in that it is optimized for rapid and efficient numerical calculations. There are two different types of DSPs. A general-purpose (open platform) DSP can be freely programmed with different algorithms and can therefore be used for a wide variety of arithmetic tasks. These processors are bigger in size and power consumption than the hardwired DSPs, but may be the solution for future hearing instrument applications. The hardwired (closed platform) DSP is optimized for a specific application (e.g., one hearing aid algorithm). The algorithm running on the machine cannot be changed, but there may be hundreds of parameters that can be altered by the dispenser/clinician or user. The first digital hearing aids were all of the hardwired type. Many second-generation digital hearing instruments are of the first type (open platform). Here, the hardware is a freely programmable DSP and different algorithms can be installed in this hardware platform.

| Benefits from DSP technology | Limitations of DSP technology |
| --- | --- |
| • Higher system dynamic range | • Loss of data is critical |
| • Increased signal-to-noise ratio (SNR) | • Overdrive leads to severe distortions (similar to PC) |
| • Insensitivity against variations of temperature or working voltage | • Power consumption is rather high |
| • No distortions | • Significantly higher development costs |
| • Extreme variability in signal-processing strategies and flexibility | • Increased cost |
| • Low noise circuits | • Size limitations? |
| • Improved noise reduction algorithms | • Training |
| • Improved internal noise reduction | • Number of fitting parameters |
| • Enhanced frequency shaping | • Speech processing for optimal intelligibility still has to be found |
| • Advanced compression circuits | |
| • Improved intelligibility in quiet? | |
| • Improved intelligibility in noise? | |

## DIGITAL-TO-ANALOG CONVERTER (DAC)

A DAC converts a digital sequence of numbers to a continous analog electric signal that can be amplified and be reproduced via a receiver or loudspeaker. The DDD is a special type of DAC optimized for hearing aid applications.

## DIGITALLY PROGRAMMABLE VS. FULLY DIGITAL HEARING AID

A digitally programmable hearing aid has a number of different hearing programs that can be programmed via a PC with a special interface (e.g., Hi-PRO) or a stand-alone programming device. The audio signal path, however, is an analog signal path. The audio signal is manipulated by analog filters or compression circuits, but is not converted to a digital signal. In a fully digital hearing aid the audio signal is converted to a digital signal via an ADC, is processed numerically with more or less complex algorithms, and is then reconverted to analog with a DAC. The calculations on the signal can be performed in the *time domain* (e.g., filtering with digital filters) or in the *frequency domain*.

## DIRECTIONAL MICROPHONES

A conventional directional microphone has two openings through which sound enters the microphone case compared to one opening for the omnidirectional microphone. The sound from the second opening is delayed acoustically and is fed to the backside of the transducer diaphragm. The difference in pressure and phase for sound arriving from different directions produce a fixed directivity pattern. Combining the signal from two omnidirectional microphones separated by a specific distance and with one microphone delayed by an additional delay (e.g., AudioZoom), produces a directivity superior to that of a single directional microphone. When the directional characteristic is changed by adapting the delay to the direction of the incoming noise in order to achieve a maximum suppression of the noise, the microphone is called an *adaptive directional microphone* (adaptive beamformer). The directivity pattern can be changed from a cardioid (max. suppression of signals from 180°) to a figure-eight characteristics, meaning that sound incident from ±90° is mostly attenuated.

## DUAL COMPRESSION

Dual compression has two characteristics in its time response. Corresponding to the behavior of the signal triggering the control action, dual compression reacts with different attack and release responses. For large, short-duration amplitude changes, the attack and release times are short. For small, long-duration amplitude changes, the attack and release times are long. For large, long-duration amplitude changes, the attack time is short and the release time is long. In this way a very quiet control behavior is achieved in spite of the rapid reaction to high-level peaks.

## DYNAMIC RANGE

The dynamic range is the difference (in dB) between the smallest occurring signal level in the instrument (noise) and the largest possible level that has not yet led to significant distortion. In a digital system it mainly depends on the data word width and is related to quantization error. For example, an optimal sixteen-bit ADC/DAC system has a dynamic range of 96 dB.

## ELECTROMAGNETIC COMPATIBILITY (EMC)

Electromagnetic compatibility describes the behavior and interference of electronic devices. The use of digital technology introduces growing problems with interference. As digital signals are of pulsive types, they produce broadband high-frequency electromagnetic radiation (radio frequencies). The widespread use of many electronic devices (computers, cellular telephones, etc.) leads to a new form of pollution: electromagnetic pollution. Digital cellular phones (GSM) are known to produce some interference in hearing aids because of their highly pulsive modulation scheme. The modulation frequency is in the audible range and can lead to audible interferences in the hearing aid. Any nonlinearity in the hearing aid circuit will demodulate these signals. Amplification of signal components in the audible range can then be heard as a buzz.

There are three different types of interactions concerning hearing aids and cellular phones:

1. Bystander interference occurs when a user of a GSM phone stands near a hearing aid user.
2. User interference occurs when a wearer of a hearing aid uses a cellular phone.
3. Hearing aid compatibility of the cellular phone means that the phone does not interfere with the hearing aid.

The most difficult situation is the user interference case because the interference increases with decreasing distances between the devices. Two measures can be taken: (1) increase the distance between the hearing instrument and telephone (e.g., handheld microphone) and (2) increase the immunity of the hearing aid to unwanted electromagnetic signals, called "hardening" of the HI. This can be done by electromagnetic shielding (metallic coating), by the use of bypass capacitors that will short circuit very high-frequency signals, or through an optimized design of wiring and circuit layout.

## FAST FOURIER TRANSFORM (FFT)

Fast Fourier transform is an efficient algorithm to transform a digital signal in time domain to frequency domain. The inverse operation is performed by an Inverse Fast Fourier Transform (IFFT). Filtering, signal analysis, and manipulation are easier and need less numerical calculations in frequency domain than in time domain. In the analog world a spectrum analyzer does the same thing. The frequency resolution of an FFT depends on the number of points (samples) that are transformed and the sampling rate, $\Delta f = F_s * N$ ($\Delta f$: Frequency resolution of FFT, $F_s$: sampling rate, $N$: Number of samples).

## FOURIER ANALYSIS

The French mathematician and physicist Jean Baptiste Fourier of the eighteenth and nineteenth centuries developed a mathematical tool for describing complex wave phenomena by a decomposition to simple sinusoidal tones, which today is called Fourier analysis. Every complex waveform (e.g., sound pressure) can be interpreted as a superposition (sum) of sinusoidal functions with harmonic frequencies. Hence every complex sound is composed of a number of simple tones.

## GLOBAL SYSTEM FOR MOBILE (GSM)

Global system for mobile communication is a standard for digital mobile telephone communication.

## MILLION INSTRUCTIONS PER SECOND (MIPS)

Million instructions per second is a measure of computational power. One MIPS means that a processor can do 1,000,000 additions or multiplications per second.

## NYQUIST RATE

The Nyquist rate is the lowest rate at which an analog signal can be sampled without loss of information. Converting such a signal back to analog will produce a perfect-replica of the original analog signal. Loss of information introduces signal distortion. According to the sampling theorem, the Nyquist rate is twice the highest frequency occurring in the analog signal.

## OVERLAP-SAVE/OVERLAP-ADD METHOD

The overlap-add method is used to break long signals into segments for processing. Multiplying an input segment of N samples by a filter function segment consisting of M samples produces an output signal segment of N + M + 1 samples. Padding the input segments with sufficient zeros (M + 1) accounts for this expansion in segment length after processing. During reconstruction, the segments are overlapped by M + 1 samples, to ensure no content is lost from the segment, and they are then added. For audio signals, the length of these segments or frames translates to several milliseconds (e.g., 5 ms) in the time domain.

## OVERSAMPLING

Sampling of an analog signal at a much higher rate than required by the sampling theorem. The sampling rate is far above twice the highest signal frequency.

*Advantage:* only a simple antialiasing filter is needed (no very steep filter characteristics), and signal-to-noise ratio (SNR) is improved.

## PULSE CODE MODULATION (PCM)

Digital representation of an analog signal (e.g., an audio CD contains sixteen-bit PCM signals at a sampling rate of 44.1 kHz).

## QUANTIZATION ERROR

The process of quantization is performed during ADC. The amplitude of a continous analog signal is rounded or truncated to discrete numerical values. Suppose you have an analog input signal ranging from 0 to 255 volts. When this signal is quantizised with an eight-bit data word width, the analog voltage is rounded to integers ranging from 0 to $2^8 - 1 = 255$. Hence, both analog values 254.51 and 255.49 volts are mapped to the digital representation 255. The relative error is then $1/255 \cong 0.39\%$. Another way to look at it is the dynamic range from the smallest to the biggest value of the digital representation, which in this case is 48 dB.

## SAMPLING RATE

To convert an analog signal to digital the signal is sampled (measured) at discrete time points. The inverse of the time interval between two samples is the sampling rate. The sampling rate limits the bandwidth of signals that can be processed and reconstructed to analog without losing information or having artifacts (sampling theorem).

## SAMPLING THEOREM NYQUIST/SHANNON THEOREM

The conversion of arbitrary broadband analog signals to digital form needs a low-pass filtering (antialiasing filter) of the analog signal with a cutoff frequency at the half of the sampling frequency $f_s/2$. Otherwise high unaudible frequencies in the original spectrum appear mirrored at audible low frequencies (see Figure 16–3) so the original analog signal can not be reconstructed from the PCM signal. During reconstruction of the analog signal, the digital signal that has a very broad spectrum needs to be passed through an anti-image filter, which is similar to the low-pass filter in the input stage, to avoid unwanted signal artifacts. The sampling theorem is frequently called the Nyquist theorem or the Shannon theorem. The Nyquist rate is the sampling rate that is exactly twice the highest frequency occurring in the signal.

## SIGMA-DELTA CONVERTER (Σ-Δ CONVERTER)

A special type of A/D converter that is easily implemented in modern low-power CMOS chip technology. The conversion is performed in two steps. First, a digital discrete time signal is generated, which roughly resembles the analog signal to be digitized. It can be viewed as a bit stream of zeros and ones corresponding to a decrease or increase of signal amplitude. This signal has a high factor of oversampling. Second, the high-rate digital signal is processed to produce a digital signal that more closely resembles the analog signal and is more closely sampled to the Nyquist rate of the analog signal.

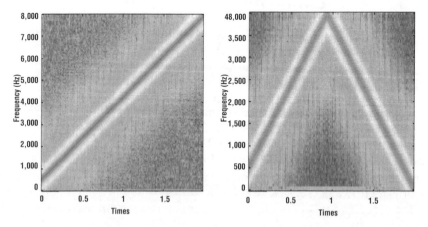

**Figure 16–3.** Spectrogram of a sweep signal to demonstrate the aliasing effect. In the left panel, a swept sine signal from 500 to 8,000 Hz is displayed. It is sampled at a rate of 16 kHz. According to the sampling theorem, only frequencies up to 16 kHz are displayed. You can see a straight line showing the increasing frequency of the signal in time. In the right panel, the same sweep signal is sampled at 8 kHz. Here, an alias error occurs: frequency components above 4 kHz, that is, half the sampling rate, are mirrored ("aliased") to lower frequencies. Finally, the 8-kHz tone is mirrored to the frequency of 0 Hz. *(Courtesy of Phonak AG.)*

The main advantages of $\Sigma$-$\Delta$ converters are the low-power consumption compared to ADC with other technologies and its low noise. It is appropriate that audio signals with a low bandwidth be compared to radio frequency applications, since here oversampling at 1 MHz is possible.

## TIME DOMAIN/FREQUENCY DOMAIN

In digital signal-processing numerical operations can either be performed as time sequence samples (time domain), or the sequence of sampled data can be transformed via a blockwise FFT to a sequence of short time spectra. This signal contains the same information as the time sequence, but the computational efforts for many calculations is much less for the spectral signal than for the time-domain signal.

This is similar to the processing of sounds in the inner ear. Different frequencies of an incoming sound wave are mapped to different locations of maximum excitation on the basilar membrane. This spatial mapping of different frequencies causes different frequencies to be processed separately in the brain. A picture for this is a harp with undamped strings that can vibrate freely. If an incoming sound has frequency components that match the resonant modes of a harp string, then these strings will start to resonate and will follow the incoming signal component. The harp can be seen as a "spectrum analyzer." Because the vibration of the strings is nearly undamped, they will ring long after the original stimulus has disappeared. From a technical point of view, they are very sharply tuned bandpass filters with a very high-frequency resolution but a bad time resolution. Once they start to resonate, the amplitude of vibration decays very slowly and hence the filter gets insensitve to rapidly fluctuating signals.

The human cochlea has filters that are not so sharply tuned. This means that even fast modulation, as they occur in speech signals, can be detected with high accuracy. In signal processing there is a general trade-off between the resolution in frequency and time. Very high-frequency resolution requires a long averaging time. If, on the other hand, the time structure of fast fluctuating signals is to be examined, the frequency resolution is poor. To illustrate, the spectrograms of the word "Tomas" are displayed in two versions in Figure 16–4. One shows a good resolution in frequency (harmonics of the tonal components), the other shows a good temporal resolution (vibration of the glottis can be seen and only the raw structure of formants).

## WINDOWS AND FRAMES

In most applications of digital signal processing it is necessary to work with short terms or frames of the signal, especially when nonstationary variable signals such as speech are to be analyzed. This can be done by putting a window function over the signal and multiplying the signal with this window. The window function used should have a low-pass spectrum and a good suppression of high frequencies. Otherwise the spectrum of the signal may be distorted. The simple rectangular window has poor side lobe suppression and therefore a poor spectral response. When an ideal rectangular window is implemented in a physical system, its filter response outside the passband contains low-level amplitude ripple decreasing with distance from the passband. These ripples are referred to as the side lobes of the filter response. The often-used Hamming window suppresses sidelobes outside the passband about 20 dB better than the rectangular window.

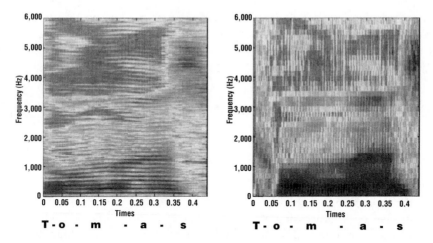

**Figure 16–4.** Spectrogram of the German word "Tomas" uttered by a male speaker in different temporal/spectral resolution. A spectrogram is a temporal spectral diagram of a signal. The horizontal axis is a time axis; the frequency is displayed on the vertical axis. The amplitude of the signal is coded by different colors or intensity. The intensity ranges for blue, green, yellow, red, and brown from low to high values. For the left-hand figure, the frequency resolution is 10 Hz. Here, the fundamental frequency and its harmonics are clearly visible for the voiced parts "o-m-a." The consonant "s" at the end can be seen as bandpass noise from 3 to 6 kHz. The very short plosive "T" at the beginning is not resolved because of the long time frame of averaging (here, a time frame is about 0.1 s long). The frame on the right shows the spectral resolution is only 172 Hz. Here, on the contrary, the impulses of glottal excitation can be seen clearly as vertical line structures (time frame 0.006 s), but the fine structure of fundamental frequency and the harmonic vibrations in the formant regions cannot be resolved. *(Courtesy of Phonak AG.)*

A longer window increases the spectral resolution when the signal is stationary at that time. However, a shorter window can better resolve the temporal structure of the signal. The process of windowing can be seen as averaging and analysis with a long time frame and cannot reveal the temporal fine structure of a signal.

# PSYCHOACOUSTICS

## BARK SCALE

The Bark scale is a physiological frequency scale. In the cochlea, the signals are processed in a kind of filter bank. The bandwidth and center frequency of these filters can be determined from psychoacoustic masking experiments. Twenty-four Barkbands cover the normal hearing frequency range up to 15 kHz. Below 500 Hz the bandwidth is 100 Hz, above 500 Hz the bandwidth is 20% of the center frequency. At high frequencies this is a logarithmic scale (see Figure 16–5).

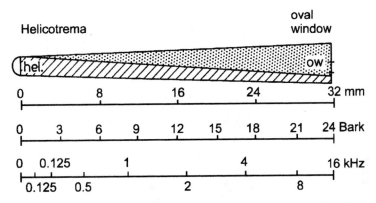

**Figure 16–5.** Comparison of the physiological scale that is given by the length of the unwound cochlea to the critical band scale (Bark scale) and the respective frequencies. The critical band scale is a linear scale but the frequency scale is not. *(Adapted from Zwicker & Fastl, 1990.)*

## CATEGORICAL SCALING OF LOUDNESS

Categorical scaling of loudness is a method for determination of individual loudness perception of different signals (mostly narrowband noise). The person is asked to classify the presented sounds into categories of "not heard" through "very quiet," "quiet," "medium loud," "loud," "very loud," and "too loud." From that measurement, an individual function of loudness growth can be determined.

## CRITICAL BANDWIDTH

A measure of the "effective bandwidth" of the auditory filters. It is often defined empirically by measuring some aspect of perception as a function of bandwidth of stimuli. A typical experiment to determine the critical bandwidth is the detection threshold of a sinusoidal tone in a narrowband noise as a function of bandwidth.

## DYNAMIC LOSS

Dynamic loss is referred to if the original difference between the hearing and discomfort threshold of a person with normal hearing is reduced by a sensorineural (recruitment) hearing loss in the hearing-impaired person.

## EXCITATION PATTERNS

The distribution of neural activity across the basilar membrane (BM) for different center frequencies is caused by excitation of hair cells on the BM. It describes the shape of auditory filters for different center frequencies and different levels of incoming sound. These curves can

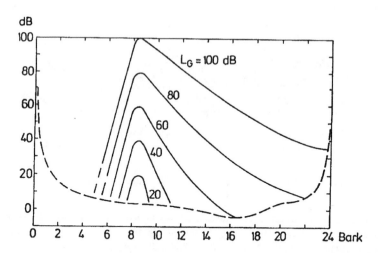

**Figure 16–6.** Excitation level as a function of critical band rate for different signal levels. It is calculated for a narrowband noise with a bandwidth of one critical band. The signal is centered at 1 kHz. The dashed line indicates the threshold in quiet. *(Adapted from Zwicker & Fastl, 1990.)*

be extracted from psychoacoustic masking experiments. As you can see in Figure 16–6, with higher levels of sound, the excitation pattern gets broader. The other thing that is obvious is the shallow slope of the filters at the high-frequency end. This effect is often called *upward spread of masking*, which means that a low-frequency tone can mask high-frequency signals much more effectively than the other way round.

## FILTER BANK

A filter bank is a number of contiguous bandpass filters that together cover a broad bandwidth. It is used to decompose a time signal in to its narrowband components. An analog filter bank gives the output of all frequency bands simultaneously. The individual filters must not have the same bandwidth for auditory signal processing. From the engineering point of view, the human cochlea may be seen as a filter bank (Bark scale).

## LOUDNESS

Loudness expresses the subjectively felt perception of sound intensity caused by a signal. For different persons, subjects of physically identical levels can cause very different perceptions of loudness. The loudness perception of persons with normal hearing can be calculated from the properties of the signal. For the purpose of hearing instrument fitting, the loudness is frequently measured by means of loudness scaling in special units, the so-called category units.

## LOUDNESS COMPENSATION

When hearing an acoustic event, the listener can normally assess very well the loudness of what he or she hears, and classify it into categories of "not heard" through "very quiet," "quiet," "medium loud," "loud," "very loud," and "too loud." With these categories both a person with normal hearing and a hearing-impaired person can assess what he or she hears. The assessment depends on the sound pressure level of the incoming signal and on the person's hearing ability. Hearing-impaired persons with recruitment demonstrate a steeper loudness curve.

The objective is to adjust the hearing instrument so that the hearing-impaired person makes the same assessment in all tone levels and at the same input levels as a person with normal hearing. Loudness compensation has then been achieved with the hearing instrument.

## LOUDNESS SUMMATION

If the bandwidth of a sound is increased progressively while maintaining a constant overall measured sound level, it is found that loudness remains constant from narrow bandwidths up to a value called the critical bandwidth. At larger bandwidths, the loudness increases as a function of bandwidth because of a process known as loudness summation. For example, the broadband sound of an orchestra playing a chord will be louder than the simple sound of a flute playing a single note even when the sounds have been adjusted to the same SPL. This is caused by the nonlinear signal processing in the cochlea. For hearing-impaired people the nonlinearity decreases, and as the system gets more linear, the effect of loudness summation decreases.

## MASKING

Masking is the amount or the process by which the threshold of audibility for one sound is raised by the presence of another masking sound. From masking experiments, the shape of auditory filters can be determined.

## PSYCHOACOUSTICS + SENSORINEURAL HEARING LOSS

If you compare the performance of hearing-impaired people to normal hearing in psychoacoustic experiments the following is found:

- ▼ Auditory filters (Bark filters) are broadened → loss of frequency selectivity
- ▼ Loudness growth is steeper (recruitment)
- ▼ Reduced loudness summation
- ▼ Higher SNR is required for the same level of understanding

## SIGNAL-TO-NOISE RATIO (SNR)

The signal-to-noise ratio is the quotient of total signal energy (the wanted signal, e.g., speech) to the total noise energy expressed in decibels. A good (high) SNR is needed for good speech intelligibility. For example, at an SNR = 0 dB (speech level = noise level) with speech and noise from the front, speech intelligibility is still no problem for a person with normal hearing; but for a person with a hearing impairment it becomes difficult. At an SNR = −10 dB even normal hearing subjects can hardly understand speech.

## SPEECH RECEPTION THRESHOLD (SRT)

The speech reception threshold is the lowest sound pressure level at which 50% of the spondaic test words (words with two syllables having equal stress) are repeated correctly.

## UPWARD MASKING (OR HEARING THRESHOLD FOR MASKING NOISE)

When the hearing threshold is measured in the presence of an interforming signal (e.g., narrowband noise), upward masking causes a threshold shift for tones of higher frequency than the narrow band noise.

Measuring a family of curves with different noise levels, it is apparent that with increasing noise levels the hearing threshold runs significantly flatter toward high frequencies than toward low frequencies. The higher-frequency useful signals are concealed/masked by the interference significantly more strongly than the low frequencies—thus the term *upward masking*.

# ANSWERS TO REVIEW QUESTIONS

## Chapter 1: Historical Overview

1. Mechanical and acoustic resonances
2. The transistor
3. The in-the-ear type (which includes the concha instrument and the canal instrument) and the completely-in-the-canal (CIC) instrument.
4. The CIC instrument
5. A

## Chapter 2: Hearing Instrument Components

1. a) See Figure 2–12
   b) The directional characteristic is related to distance between front and rear port, and time delay between front and rear port (acoustical or electrical delay).
2. The high-pass portion of the response of the directional microphone is moved by one octave to higher frequencies, therefore the sensitivity of the directional microphone will be reduced by 6 dB and therefore the noise of the directional microphone is increased by 6 dB. The directional characteristic will stay the same as long the internal delay of the front and the rear port is also reduced by a factor of two.
3. Advantages: better current consumption, reduced size because end amplifier is integrated in the receiver (today, no longer an advantage because end amplifiers are integrated on the digital chip); disadvantages: cost (cost of additional chip inside of a receiver), one more wire (cost, reliability), clock in the Class D amplifier can cause interference with the digital chip on board.
4. A, D
5. B
6. A, C
7. C
8. D
9. C, D

## Chapter 3: Digitally Programmable Hearing Instruments

1. D
2. Programmable hearing instrument, programming interface, personal computer and peripherals, programming software, cables for interconnection.
3. HI-PRO, NOAHlink, Microconnect

## Chapter 4: Signal Processing Strategies

1. AGCi: The user has control of the MPO (is able to reduce very loud sound); the user is not able to move the kneepoint, therefore, certain signals will attack and release all the time and the user is not able to control this.

   AGCo: The user has the possibility to move the kneepoint with the VC and get a higher linear range.

2.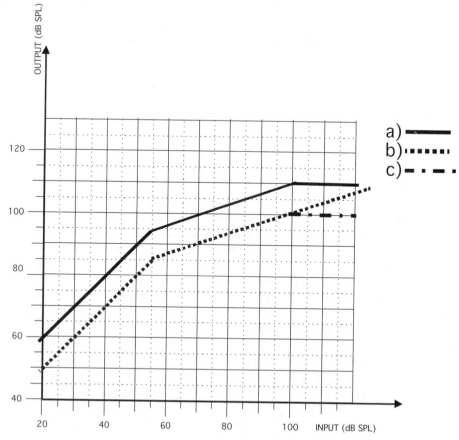

**3.** B, C
**4.** B
**5.** A, C, D
**6.**

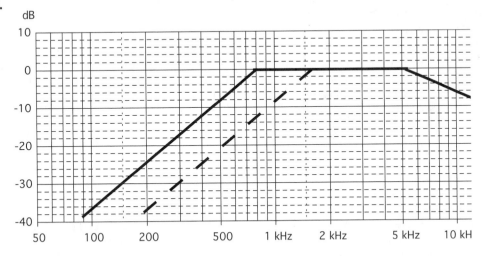

**7.** Diode compression: pros: low second order harmonic distortion, no attack and no re-lease times; cons: higher distortion than AGC, reduced fitting range

AGC: pros: low distortion; cons: attack and release time

Peak clipping: pros: no attack release time, highest output power (with additional distortion); con: distortion

Additional information: Regarding the pros and cons, AGC is recommended for mild-to-moderate hearing losses. Diode and peak clipping system have advantages for profound hearing losses where sound pressure level is more important than sound quality

## Chapter 5: Digital Hearing Instruments

**1.** B, C
**2.** D
**3.** B
**4.** The development of integrated circuits that operated at the voltage supplied by a hearing instrument battery, that consumed little current, and that were small.
**5.** The ASIC type has fixed functionality which requires a redesigned IC to change; the algorithm-based device can change functionality by installing a different algorithm.
**6.** Directional processing, noise reduction, feedback cancellation, auditory scene adaptation, and amplification and filtering.

## Chapter 6: Acoustic Path

1. a) The damping screens smooth out the frequency response, reducing the peak frequency response of BTE sound tubes, thereby reducing peak-to-valley value, improving sound quality, being less prone to feedback (also important for homologation in certain countries/standards).

   b) The closer the screen is to the hearing instrument receiver, the more consistent the damping is over the whole frequency response (overall damping). The further away from the receiver, the higher the damping of the tube resonance is at about 1 kHz. An etymotic frequency response is possible with a screen at the end of the hook.

2. B, D
3. C
4. D
5. C

## Chapter 7: Accessories

1. CROS: pros: signals also on the deaf side, more gain before feedback for severe and profound hearing losses, open fitting is possible because of the long distance between receiver and microphone; cons: needs a cable connection (if not wireless), requires learning or adaptation for directional hearing.

   BiCROS: pros: Signals from both side of the head will be amplified and can be heard even if one side is completely deaf; cons: BiCROS is not binaural, also requires a cable which can degrade and requires replacement.

2. Ultrasonic
   ▾ Receiver is already in the hearing instrument
   ▾ Remote requires line in sight, binaural control is not possible
   Infrared
   ▾ Well-known technology
   ▾ Requires line of sight, binaural control is not reliable
   Radio (FM)
   ▾ Good transmission properties, binaural is possible
   ▾ Sensitive to strong interferers (magnetic fields like PC monitors)
   Inductive
   ▾ Good transmission properties, binaural possible
   ▾ Sensitive to strong interferers (magnetic fields like PC monitors)

3. a) FM receiver, FM transmitter, hearing instrument with direct audio input
   b) FM+M, it is important that the level of the audio input (the FM) is adjusted to produce the same output level as the level of the hearing instrument microphone.

4. Zinc-Air: pros: large capacity, constant voltage during discharge; cons: quiescent current of about 5.0 μA as soon as the adhesive tab is removed; maximum current is limited by the amount of air that enters through the holes in the battery case.

5. D
6. A, B
7. B

## Chapter 8: Hearing Instrument Troubleshooting

1. Acoustic feedback (leakage from the earmold or vent), magnetic feedback (magnetic leakage between receiver and T-coil), mechanical feedback (receiver vibration picked up by the microphone), electrical feedback (too much electrical gain; the amplifier becomes unstable if the power-supply rejection ratio is not big enough and the instrument produces a "motorboating" sound).

2. a) Blocked earhook, failed receiver, blocked microphone, defective amplifier, depleted battery, corroded battery compartment
   b) T-coil is no longer in its proper position and may be within the magnetic field of the receiver causing magnetic feedback; receiver or microphone may not be properly seated in its suspension (hearing instrument may have been dropped on the floor) and is transmitting vibrations; receiver sound spout may have come loose and sound is leaking back to the microphone; earhook may be loose and leaking sound.

3. Check for obstructions in vent; check that the microphone opening is not obstructed; ensure the tip of the shell seals against the bony portion of the canal, ensure the instrument does not migrate out of the ear and if a canal lock would help prevent this.

4. Identify the area where discomfort occurs and modify the CIC shell to remove pressure at those points.

5. The hearing instrument or microphone is noisy, or there is a high level of ambient noise in the environment.

6. Reduce gain at frequencies where noise is predominant using tone controls; if the microphone is defective, replace the microphone; adjust the low-level expansion threshold or slope.

7. Send the instrument to the manufacturer for repair.

## Chapter 9: Hearing Instrument Measurements and Standards

1. The greater the influence of the head (the plot is no longer a circle), the higher the frequency.

2. The ear simulator curve should be about 5 dB higher up to 1 kHz, about 10 dB higher at 3 kHz and 15 dB higher at 6 kHz than the 2-cc curve.

3. The effect of the body, head, pinna, and ear canal will be measured; optimization of a hearing instrument (especially directional microphones located within the pinna) can be made. Insertion gain (In situ − REUG) can be measured.

4. The insertion gain = (aided in situ gain) − (unaided in situ gain) = REAG − REUG, see Figure 9–39.

5. A

6. A

7. B

8. A, B

## Chapter 10: Digital Mechanics

1. Poor fit and comfort.
2. The first and second in the ear canal, the tragus, helix, and concha are reproduced in the impression.
3. Laser scan the impression to produce a three-dimensional representation of the ear; create a virtual shell; place digitized models of hearing instrument components like amplifier, microphone, receiver battery, etc. in the virtual shell to determine if all components fit into the shell without interference; determine where the faceplate cut should be made; check the virtual model for fit in the virtual ear canal.
4. The hearing instrument can be designed electronically; predetermination is all components fit into the shell; evaluation of cosmetic appearance of finished product; decide if product can be built in the available space; this can be done before production is started.
5. Laser sintering using pigmented polyamide powder; stereolithography using colored acrylic resin.

## Chapter 11: Fitting, Verification, and Outcome

1. POGO, NAL-R, NAL-RP, NAL-NL1, DSL [i/o]
2. Moderate (HL is 49–60 dB); profound (HL is 80–110 dB)
3. NAL-RP is an extension of NAL-R to also cover severe-to-profound hearing losses.
4. In DSL [i/o] all data is converted to dB SPL with common reference values.
5. The RECD is used.
6. Loudness scaling determines hearing sensitivity for the whole auditory field between threshold and UCL, whereas threshold audiometry determines only the threshold of hearing.
7. Speech intelligibility in quiet and noise, sound quality judgments, loudness ratings, functional gain, probe microphone measurements.
8. APHAB, HHIE/HHIA, COSI

## Chapter 12: Audiology and Psychoacoustics

1. Hearing means you hear a sound. Understanding implies you perceive the meaning of that sound.
2. The outer ear consists of the pinna and ear canal; the middle ear consists of the ear drum and the ossicles: malleus, incus, stapes; the inner ear or the cochlea is a spiral-shaped, fluid-filled chamber separated into two by the basilar membrane which contains inner and outer hair cells.
3. The outer ear: (pinna, ear canal) pinna provides some frequency emphasis in the high frequencies and the ear canal provides some amplification and channels sound to the eardrum; the middle ear (ear drum and the ossicles: malleus, incus, stapes) act as an impedance converter to deliver sound energy to the oval window of the inner ear; the inner ear (cochlea) consists of fluid-filled chambers separated by the basilar membrane and hair cells transform vibrations into nerve impulses which are sent to the brain on the auditory nerve.

4. The cochlea has the shape of a spiral approximately 5 mm high, or about 35 mm long if it were to be stretched out.

5. The tympanic membrane contains the organ of Corti, which contains the hair cells.

6. The hair cells are arranged in one row of inner hair cells and three rows of outer hair cells. These rows stretch along the basilar membrane from the oval window to the tip of the cochlear spiral. Wave motion in the cochlea flexes the basilar membrane and stimulates the hair cells, causing them to generate electrical pulses that are sent along the auditory nerve to the brain. The inner hair cells send pulses to the brain when they are stimulated by mechanical motion. The outer hair cells receive information from the brain and alter their length to reduce the gap between the organ of Corti and the tectorial membrane. This occurs for quiet sounds and effectively increases the sensitivity of the inner hair cells for quiet sound.

7. A decibel is a measure of the ratio of two values of power. In acoustics it is used to calculate the magnitude of sound pressure level of a sound relative to the pressure at the hearing threshold. The decibel is used to compare large numbers.

8. Equal-loudness contours are points in the auditory space where a tone sounds as loud as a tone presented at 1 kHz. For example, when a 100-Hz tone presented at 85 dB SPL is judged equally loud to a 1,000-Hz tone presented at 80 dB SPL, the two tones lie on the same loudness contour.

9. A weighting mirrors the equal-loudness contour for quiet sounds (0 phon). B weighting mirrors the equal-loudness contour for moderate sounds (70 phon). C weighting mirrors the equal-loudness contour for loud sounds (100 phon).

10. Most countries set the level for unprotected noise exposure for eight hours at 90 dBA. For every increase of 5 dB, the exposure time is halved. So at 95 dBA, the maximum exposure is four hours, at 100 dBA it is two hours, etc. Unprotected exposure to more than 115 dBA should not occur.

## Chapter 13: Interference in a Digital world

1. Electromagnetic interference

2. Frequency division multiple access (FDMA), time division multiple access (TDMA), code division multiple access (CDMA)

3. Cell phone transmission occurs in short bursts with repetition frequency in the audio band. The hearing instrument detects and amplifies these frequencies which the user perceives as a buzz.

## Chapter 14: Data Transmission

1. 8

2. binary

3. up to 8 Mbps

4. a) increase the data rate
   b) decrease the amount of data by using data compression.

5. B, C, D

6. C

7. Motion Picture Experts Group (MPEG) Audio Layer-3.
8. A factor of ten
9. Perceptual noise shaping.
10. A
11. D
12. Bluetooth current requirements are too high for a hearing instrument battery.
13. B, C, D

## Chapter 15: Implanted Devices

1. Bone conduction instruments, middle-ear implants, cochlear implants, auditory brainstem implants.
2. Patient discomfort and poor sound quality.
3. Bonding of bone and implanted material.
4. Feedback, occlusion, obstruction with earwax
5. The middle-ear implant does not involve surgery to the cochlea while the cochlear implant does.

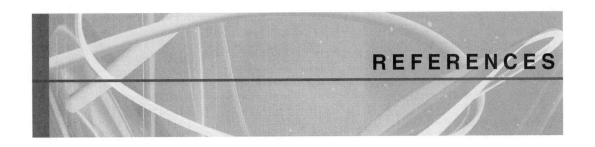

# REFERENCES

American Speech-Language-Hearing Association, Ad Hoc Committee on FM Systems. (1998, October). *Guidelines for fitting and monitoring FM systems* [Draft report]. Rockville, MD: ASHA.

ANSI (2003). *Specification of hearing aid characteristics: S3.22.* Acoustical Society of America, New York: Standards Secretariat.

ANSI (2004). *Method of measurement of performance characteristics under simulated real-ear working conditions: S3.35.* New York: Acoustical Society of America, Standards Secretariat.

Bächler, H., Knecht, W. G., Launer, S., & Uvacek, B. (1997). Audibility, intelligibility, sound quality and comfort. *High Performance Hearing Aid Solutions, 2,* 31–36.

Berger, K. W. (1984). *The hearing aid.* New York: National Hearing Aid Society.

Berger, K. W., Hagberg, E. N., & Rane, R. L. (1988). *Prescription of hearing aids: Rationale, procedure and results* (5th ed.). Kent, OH: Herald Publishing.

Berlin, C. I. (1996). *Hair cells and hearing aids.* San Diego: Singular Publishing.

Bregman, A. S. (1990). *Auditory scene analysis.* Cambridge, MA: MIT Press.

Brüel & Kjaer. (1981, April). *Handbuch, Ohrsimulator Typ 4157.* Berlin: Author.

Buechler, M. (2001). How good are automatic program selection features? *The Hearing Review, 8*(9).

Burkhard, M., & Sachs. (1975). Manikin for acoustic research. *Journal of the Acoustical Society of America, 58,* no. 1.

Byrne, D., & Dillon, H. (1986). The National Acoustics Laboratories' (NAL) new procedure for selecting the gain and frequency response of a hearing aid. *Ear and Hearing, 7,* 257–265.

Byrne, D., Parkinson, A., & Newall, P. (1991). Modified hearing aid selection process for severe/profound hearing losses. In G. Studebaker, F. Bess, & L. Beck (Eds.), *The Vanderbilt hearing aid report II.* Parkton, MD: York Press.

Cornelisse, L. E., Seewald, R. C., & Jamieson, D. G. (1995). The input/output (i/o) formula: A theoretical approach to the fitting of personal amplification devices. *Journal of the Acoustical Society of America, 97,* 1854–1864.

Courtois, J., Johansen, P., Larsen, B., Christensen, P., & Beilin, J. (1988). Open molds. In J. H. Jensen (Ed.), *Hearing aid fitting: Theoretical and practical views. 13th Danavox Symposium.* Copenhagen: Stougaard Jensen.

Cox, R. M., & Gilmore, C. (1990) Development of the profile of hearing aid performance (PHAP). *Journal of Speech and Hearing Research, 33,* 343–357.

Dallos, P., Popper, A. D., & Fay, R. R. The cochlea. *Springer Handbook of Auditory Research* (vol. 8). New York: Springer.

Dillon, H. (2001). *Hearing aids.* Turramurra, Australia: Boomerang Press.

Dillon, H., Birtles, G., & Lovegrove, R. (1999). Measuring the outcome of a national rehabilitation program: Normative data for the Client Oriented Scale of Improvement (COSI) and the Hearing Aid User's Questionnaire (HAUQ). *J. Amer. Acad. Audiol., 10*(2), 67–79.

Ditthardt, A. (1990, January). *Detailed application notes for the Knowles EP Integrated receiver.* Itasca, IL: Knowles Electronics, Inc.

Edwards, B. W., et al. (1998, September). Signal-processing algorithms for a new software-based digital hearing device. *The Hearing Journal, 51,* no. 9.

Fabry, D. A. Programmable and automatic noise reduction in existing hearing aids. In G. Studebaker, F. Bess, & L. Beck (Eds.), *The Vanderbilt hearing aid report* (pp. 65–78). Parkton, MD: York Press.

Fabry, D. A. (1998). Do we really need digital hearing aids? *The Hearing Journal, 51*(11), 30, 32–33.

Fabry, D. A., & Van Tassel, D. J. (1990). Evaluation of an articulation based model for predicting the effects of adaptive frequency response hearing aids. *Journal of Speech and Hearing Research, 33,* 676–689.

Fletcher, H., & Munson, W. A. (1933). Loudness, its definition, measurement and calculation. *JASA, 5,* 82–108.

Güttner, W. H. (1978). *Hörgerätetechnik.* Stuttgart, Germany: Thieme Verlag.

Hakansson, B. (1990). Ten years of experience with the Swedish bone-anchored hearing system. *Annals of Otolaryngology, 99*(10, pt 2, suppl. 151).

Hawkins, D., & Yacullo, W. (1984). Signal-to-noise ratio advantage of binaural hearing aids and directional microphones under different levels of reverberation. *Journal of Speech and Hearing Disorders, 49,* 278–286.

Hayes, D. (2004, September). The need for fine-tuning adaptive hearing aids. *Hearing Review,* 40–44.

Hays, L. V., (2002, April). Feedback cancellation improvements. US Patent 6,377,119, April 23, 2002.

IEC. Hearing aids: Hearing aids with induction pickup coil input. IEC Publ. No. 60118–1. Geneva, Switzerland: IEC.

IEC. Hearing aids: Measurement of electroacoustical characteristics. IEC Publ. No. 118–0. Geneva, Switzerland: IEC.

ISO (1961). Normal equal-loudness contours for pure tones and normal threshold for hearing under free field listening conditions. Recommendation R226.

Kates, J. M., & Mclanson, J. L. (2002, August). Feedback cancellation apparatus and methods utilizing adaptive reference filter mechanisms. US Patent 6,434,247, August 13, 2002.

Kiesling, J., Kollmeier, B., & Dillier, G. (1997). *Versorgung und Reabilitation mit Hörgeräten.* Stuttgart: Georg Thieme Verlag.

Killion, M. C., & Carlson, E. V. (1969, October). *A wideband miniature microphone.* Paper presented at the 37th Audio Engineering Society Convention, New York.

Killion, M. C., & Carlson, E. V. (1973, September). *A subminiature electret-condenser microphone of new design.* Paper presented at the 46th Audio Engineering Society Convention, New York.

Killion, M. C., Staab, W. J., & Preeves, D. A. (1990). Classifying automatic signal processors. *Hearing Instruments, 41,* 24–26.

Knowles Electronics. Datasheet: Miniature microphones and miniature receivers. Itasca, IL: Author.

Knowles Electronics. Directional hearing aid microphone application note. *Technical Bulletin, 21B.* Franklin Park, IL: Author.

Kochkin, S. (1994). Optimizing the emerging market for completely-in-the-canal instruments. *Hearing Journal, 47*(6).

Kochkin, S. (1995). Customer satisfaction and benefit with CIC hearing instruments. *Hearing Review, 2*(5).

Kuk, F. (2002, February). Understanding feedback and digital feedback cancellation strategies. *Hearing Review,* 36–41, 48–49.

Launer, S. (1995). *Loudness perception in listeners with sensorineural hearing impairment.* [in German]. Dissertation, Fachbereich Physik der Universität, Oldenburg, Germany.

Lazarus, H., Lazarus-Mainka, G., & Schubeius, M. (1985). *Sprachliche Kommunikation unter Larm.* Ludwigshaven, Germany: Friedrich Kiehl Verlag GmbH.

Loizou, P. C. (1998, September). Mimicking the human ear. *IEEE Signal Processing Magazine,* 101–130.

Madaffari, P. (1983). Directional matrix technical bulletin. Project 10554. In *Industrial Research Products, a Knowles company report.* Itasca, IL: Knowles Electronics.

McCandless, G. A., & Lyregaard, P. E. Prescription of gain/output (POGO) for hearing aids. *Hearing Instruments, 34,* 16–21.

Moore, B. C. J. (1995). Perceptual consequences of cochlear damage. Oxford Psychology Series No. 28. New York: Oxford University Press.

Moore, B. C. J. (1996). Perceptual consequences of cochlear hearing loss and their implications for the design of hearing aids. *Ear and Hearing, 17,* 133–160.

Moore, B. C. J. (2000). *Cochlear hearing loss.* London, England: Whurr Publishers.

Moss, C. F. (2001). Auditory scene analysis by echolocation in bats, *J. Acoust. Soc. Am., 110*(4), 2207–2226.

Mueller, H. G., Hawkins, D. B., & Northern, J. L. (1992). *Probe microphone measurements—Hearing aid selection and assessment.* San Diego, CA: Singular Publishing.

Mueller, H. G., & Killion, M. C. (1990, September). An easy method for calculating the articulation index. *The hearing Journal*, 14–17.

Murray, D. J., & Hanson, J. V. (1992). Application of digital signal processing to hearing aids: A critical survey. *Journal of the American Academy of Audiology*, 3(2), 145–152.

Newman, C. W., & Weinstein, B. E. (1988). The Hearing Handicap Inventory for the Elderly as a measure of hearing aid benefit. *Ear and Hearing, 9*, 81–85.

Niellsen, H. (1998). Defining "open platform" DSP, *The Hearing Review, 7*(1), 27, 59.

Pavlovic, C. V. (1987). Derivation of primary parameters and procedures for use in speech intelligibility predictions. *Journal of the Acoustical Society of America, 82*(2).

Popelka, G. R. (1998). Computer and hearing aids: A prediction of the future. *The Hearing Journal, 51*(11), 52, 57–62.

Powers, T. (1997). The use of digital features to combat background noise, *Supplement to the Hearing Review, 3*, 36–39.

Robinson, D. W., & Dadson, R. S. (1956). A re-determination of the equal-loudness relations for pure tones. *Br. J. Appl. Physics, 7*, 166–181.

Schum, D. J. (2004, July). Artifical intelligence: The new advanced technology in hearing aids. *Audiology Online*, http://www.audiologyonline.com/articles/arc_disp.asp?id=733.

Seewald, R. C. (1992). The desired sensation level method for fitting children: Version 3.0. *Hearing Journal, 45*(4), 38–41.

Smriga, D. (1999, January). Problem solving through "smart" digital technology. *The Hearing Review, 6*, no. 1, 58–60.

Soede, W. (1990). *Improvement of speech intelligibility in noise*. Dissertation, Delft University of Technology, The Netherlands.

Valente, M. (1994). *Strategies for selecting and verifying hearing aid fittings*. Thieme Medical Publishers Inc.,

Veit, I. (1978). *Technische Akustik, 2.* Auflage. Würzburg, Germany: Vogel Verlag.

Venema, T. H. (1998). *Compression for clinicians*. San Diego: Singular Publishing.

Voll, L. M., & Jones, C. (1998). CICs: Five years later, what have we learned? *Hearing Review, 8*(3).

Weidner, T. (2002, June 11). Method for feedback recognition in a hearing aid and a hearing aid operating according to the method. US Patent 6,404,895 B1.

Westermann, S., & Sandlin, R. E. (1997). Digital signal processing: Benefits and expectations. *Supplement to the Hearing Review, 2*, 56–59.

Zwicker, E. (1982). *Psychoakustik*. Berlin, Germany: Springer.

Zwicker, E., & Fastl, H. (1990). *Psychoacoustics: Facts and model*. Heidelburg, Germany: Springer Verlag.

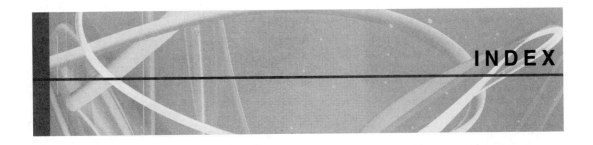

# INDEX